STUDY GUIDE
to accompany
Potter • Perry • Stockert • Hall

Basic Nursing

STUDY GUIDE
to accompany
Potter • Perry • Stockert • Hall

Basic Nursing

Seventh Edition

Patricia A. Castaldi, DNP, RN
Director
Practical Nursing Program
Union County College
Plainfield, New Jersey

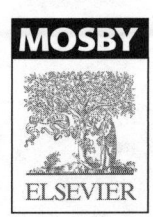

MOSBY
ELSEVIER

3251 Riverport Lane
St. Louis, Missouri 63043

STUDY GUIDE TO ACCOMPANY BASIC NURSING, Seventh Edition   ISBN: 978-0-323-06987-8

Copyright © 2011, 2007, 2003 by Mosby, Inc., an affiliate of Elsevier Inc.

All rights reserved. No part of this publication may be reproduced or transmitted in any form or by any means, electronic or mechanical, including photocopy, recording, or any information storage and retrieval system, without permission in writing from the publisher, except that, until further notice, instructors requiring their students to purchase STUDY GUIDE FOR BASIC NURSING, Seventh Edition, by Patricia A. Castaldi, may reproduce the contents or parts thereof for instructional purposes, provided each copy contains a proper copyright notice as follows:

Copyright © 2011, 2007, 2003 by Mosby, Inc., an affiliate of Elsevier Inc.

Notice

Knowledge and best practice in this field are constantly changing. As new research and experience broaden our understanding, changes in research methods, professional practices, or medical treatment may become necessary.

Practitioners and researchers must always rely on their own experience and knowledge in evaluating and using any information, methods, compounds, or experiments described herein. In using such information or methods they should be mindful of their own safety and the safety of others, including parties for whom they have a professional responsibility.

With respect to any drug or pharmaceutical products identified, readers are advised to check the most current information provided (i) on procedures featured or (ii) by the manufacturer of each product to be administered, to verify the recommended dose or formula, the method and duration of administration, and contraindications. It is the responsibility of practitioners, relying on their own experience and knowledge of their patients, to make diagnoses, to determine dosages and the best treatment for each individual patient, and to take all appropriate safety precautions.

To the fullest extent of the law, neither the Publisher nor the authors, contributors, or editors, assume any liability for any injury and/or damage to persons or property as a matter of products liability, negligence or otherwise, or from any use or operation of any methods, products, instructions, or ideas contained in the material herein.

The Publisher

International Standard Book Number: 978-0-323-06987-8

Editor: Tamara Myers
Senior Developmental Editor: Laura M. Selkirk
Publishing Services Manager: Anne Altepeter
Senior Project Manager: Beth Hayes

Printed in the United States of America

Last digit is the print number: 9 8 7 6 5 4

Working together to grow
libraries in developing countries

www.elsevier.com | www.bookaid.org | www.sabre.org

ELSEVIER   BOOK AID International   Sabre Foundation

To John and Dan for all of your love and support.
To the faculty, students, and all of my colleagues who have inspired me throughout the years.

Introduction and Preface

This guide is designed to correspond, chapter by chapter, to *Basic Nursing* (seventh edition). Each chapter in this guide contains study aids to assist in learning and applying the theoretical concepts from the text.

The comprehensive chapter review sections allow you the opportunity to evaluate your own level of comprehension after reading the text. Use of the study group questions with fellow students may help in your overall understanding of the nursing content, as well as provide a way to further evaluate your familiarity with that content. There are also more short-answer and multiple-response questions to promote your preparation for classroom examinations and the alternate-format items on the NCLEX® examination. You may find that there are questions that require you to apply information from other chapters or use other reference sources to answer them.

General study tips to use while reading, taking classroom notes, and preparing for and taking examinations are also included in this guide. Other students have found these ideas to be helpful in their nursing course experiences.

A skills performance checklist has been provided for each of the major skills and procedural guidelines presented in the text. These checklists may be used by faculty members to evaluate your ability to perform the techniques, as well as offer their comments and recommendations for improvement. The checklists represent generally accepted nursing principles and practice. You may need to adapt these skills to meet a patient's special needs or follow the particular policy of an institution.

Answers are available through your instructor for all of the questions and activities contained within this study guide.

Study Charts

While reading through the chapters in the text, you may create study charts to assist you to organize the material that is covered. The charts allow for a comparison of key concepts in the chapter. Suggestions for creating charts are provided in the chapters of this text. An example follows.

Routes of Injection

The learning activities presented in this study guide should assist in your review of the text material and your application of the nursing concepts to classroom and clinical experiences.

Route	Angle of Insertion/Needle Size/Maximum Amount of Medication
Intradermal	
Subcutaneous	
Intramuscular	

General Study Tips

While reading
- Read before the scheduled class: Highlight key points or outline content in the text that will be covered in the classroom.
- Look up definitions: Find the meanings of words you do not recognize while you are going through the text. It helps to have a medical dictionary and a regular dictionary handy!
- Make notes: Write down a list of topics that you do not understand while you are reading so that you may clarify them with the instructor.
- Compare notes: Use notes taken from the book and in class to create a complete picture of the content.
- Use study/comparison charts: Put facts and ideas in an organized form so that you can refer to them easily at a later point, such as when studying for an examination.
- Use references: Go back to texts and notes used in other courses (such as anatomy and physiology) to help in understanding new material.

In the classroom
- Make notes: Do not try to write everything down. Note the essential information from the class. Jot down questions that you may have as you go along so that you remember to ask them at some point. Before the end of the class, note any areas that you need to clarify with the instructor.
- Ask questions: Remember to take advantage of the expertise of the instructor. Do not go away from the class without trying to clear up areas of confusion!
- Audiotape: Make audiotapes of classroom discussions, only with instructor permission, if:
  1. There is time to listen to them at some point (such as in the car).
  2. There are positive results from this process, with better understanding of the material and improved examination grades.

On your own
- Use available resources: Take advantage of all of the resources at the school, such as the library, computer laboratory, and skill laboratory. Make time to practice nursing techniques, watch DVDs or videos, and complete computer learning programs.
- Join/create a study group: Get together with other students in your class to review material. Study groups offer an opportunity to share information, challenge one another, and provide mutual support.
- Use time management techniques: Use available time as efficiently as possible. For example, the time that is spent waiting for an appointment or riding on public transportation may be used to read over materials or complete assignments.

Before an examination
- Try to remain calm: Easy to recommend, but hard to do! Learn and use relaxation skills. Do not jump immediately into the examination. Relax and get focused first, then start the test.
- Be prepared: check with the instructor to be sure you have covered the content that will be on the examination. Bring the right materials: Pencils, pens, erasers, computer passwords, and so on. Leave enough time to get to the examination area so that there is no last-minute "rushing in."

During the examination
- Read the questions carefully: Determine what the question is asking. Stay focused on the actual question without reading into the situations. If allowed to mark on the examination paper, underline key words or cross out unnecessary information to assist in getting to the heart of the question.
- Do not keep changing your answers: Most of the time, the first answer selected is correct. Do not change an answer unless you have remembered the correct response.
- Stay focused: Take brief moments during the examination, if necessary, to stop and use relaxation techniques to compose yourself.

General suggestions for classroom-based and online courses
- Review the syllabus in advance to identify the course requirements and expectations.
- Make a calendar to keep track of dates for examinations, quizzes, and assignments.
- Schedule time to study or complete assignments.
- Connect with other students in the course electronically, by telephone, or in person.
- Take advantage of all of the available resources, such as online or on-campus tutorial programs.
- Keep in contact with the instructor! Do not forget to ask questions.
- Maintain professional behavior with your instructors and classmates.

Contents

UNIT I	CONCEPTS IN NURSING
1	Health and Wellness, 1
2	The Health Care Delivery System, 3
3	Community-Based Nursing Practice, 6
4	Legal Principles in Nursing, 8
5	Ethics, 11
6	Evidence-Based Practice, 13

UNIT II	PROCESSES IN NURSING CARE
7	Critical Thinking, 15
8	Nursing Process, 17
9	Informatics and Documentation, 21
10	Communication, 24
11	Patient Education, 28
12	Managing Patient Care, 31

UNIT III	ESSENTIALS FOR NURSING PRACTICE
13	Infection Prevention and Control, 33
14	Vital Signs, 44
15	Health Assessment and Physical Examination, 64
16	Administering Medications, 71
17	Fluid, Electrolyte, and Acid-Base Balances, 104

UNIT IV	PROMOTING PSYCHOSOCIAL HEALTH
18	Caring in Nursing Practice, 120
19	Cultural Diversity, 122
20	Spiritual Health, 125
21	Growth and Development, 127
22	Self-Concept and Sexuality, 130
23	Family Context in Nursing, 133
24	Stress and Coping, 135
25	Loss and Grief, 137

UNIT V	PROMOTING PHYSICAL HEALTH
26	Exercise and Activity, 139
27	Safety, 151
28	Hygiene, 157
29	Oxygenation, 177
30	Sleep, 191
31	Pain Management, 194
32	Nutrition, 199
33	Urinary Elimination, 209
34	Bowel Elimination, 218
35	Immobility, 235
36	Skin Integrity and Wound Care, 241
37	Sensory Alterations, 262
38	Surgical Patient, 265

Health and Wellness 1

CASE STUDY

1. A personal friend has been experiencing severe stomach and intestinal distress for a few months. She is 35 years old and is employed as an advertisement salesperson for a local newspaper. During the past year, she has been pressured to create more income for her department. When you ask her if she has sought medical treatment, she responds, "I don't have the time to go to the doctor." In addition to her job responsibilities, she is a single parent of a grade school child who enjoys several after-school activities.
   a. What physical and lifestyle factors are present in this situation?
   b. What initial responses/interventions may be helpful for this individual?

CHAPTER REVIEW

Match the description/definition in Column A with the correct term in Column B.

Column A

_____ 1. A person's definition and interpretation of symptoms and use of the health care system
_____ 2. A belief that patients have the authority to be active participants in determining their health and well-being
_____ 3. Longer than 6 months' duration
_____ 4. A subjective concept of physical appearance
_____ 5. Developmental stage, intellectual background, emotional and spiritual factors
_____ 6. Short term and severe
_____ 7. Addresses the relationship between a person's beliefs and behaviors

Column B

a. Health belief model
b. Internal variables
c. Body image
d. Holistic health
e. Illness behavior
f. Acute illness
g. Chronic illness

Complete the following:

8. Health is the absence of disease.
   True _____ False _____
9. Identify at least one health promotion concern for older adults.

10. Place Maslow's hierarchy of needs in order of priority from the lowest to the highest level.
    Love and belongingness _____
    Self-esteem _____
    Physiological needs _____
    Self-actualization _____
    Safety needs _____
11. Identify whether the following are internal or external variables that influence health beliefs and practices.
    a. Financial status

    b. Family health behaviors

    c. Cognitive abilities

    d. Cultural values

12. What is an example of a positive health behavior?

13. What is an example of a negative health behavior?

14. Identify all of the external variables that may influence a person's illness behaviors. Select all that apply.
    a. Visibility of symptoms _____
    b. Disruption of normal routine _____
    c. Accessibility of the health care system _____
    d. Acuity of the illness _____
    e. Cultural background _____
    f. Economics _____

Copyright © 2011, 2007, 2003 by Mosby, Inc., an affiliate of Elsevier Inc. All rights reserved.

CHAPTER 1 • Health and Wellness

Select the best answer for each of the following questions:

15. At the tertiary level of prevention, a nurse would prepare an educational program for a group requiring:
    1. Chemotherapy
    2. Cardiac rehabilitation
    3. Genetic screening
    4. Sex education
16. At the secondary level of prevention, what is the intervention that a nurse expects to assist with or provide instruction for?
    1. Immunization
    2. Referral to outpatient therapy for monitoring
    3. Performance of a biopsy
    4. Parent bathing a newborn
17. A nurse is working with a patient who is experiencing chronic joint pain. To assist the patient to manage or reduce the pain, the nurse decides to use a holistic health approach. With this in mind, the nurse specifically elects to include:
    1. Aroma therapy
    2. Wound care
    3. Hygienic care measures
    4. Analgesic medications
18. A nurse is completing an assessment for a patient who has gone to a medical clinic. Variables that influence the patient's health beliefs and practices are being determined. The nurse is aware that an internal variable for this patient is the:
    1. Way in which the patient celebrates family occasions
    2. Manner in which the patient deals with stress on the job and at home
    3. Frequency of the family's visit to the health care agency
    4. Amount of insurance coverage that is provided by the patient's employer
19. A nurse recognizes that primary prevention is a critical aspect in health care. The target group for a program on hand hygiene for this level of prevention is:
    1. Fourth grade children at the elementary school
    2. Patients in a cardiac rehabilitation program at the medical center
    3. Parents of a child with a congenital heart defect
    4. Patients with diabetes at the outpatient clinic
20. A nurse is leading a group of community members who are trying to quit smoking. In the precontemplation phase of health behavior change, the nurse anticipates that the group members will respond by:
    1. Discussing previous attempts at quitting
    2. Recognizing the benefits of not smoking
    3. Expressing irritation when the topic of quitting is introduced
    4. Requesting phone numbers of support people who have participated in the group
21. A young adult student has gone to the university's health center for a physical examination. The nurse conducting the initial interview is looking for possible lifestyle risk factors. The nurse is specifically alerted to the student's:
    1. Mild hypertension
    2. Mountain climbing hobby
    3. Family history of diabetes
    4. Part-time job at the auto factory
22. According to Maslow's hierarchy of needs, a patient's priority should be:
    1. Physical safety
    2. Psychological safety
    3. Self-esteem
    4. Adequate nutrition
23. To determine a patient's stage in the process of changing behaviors in reponse to being diagnosed with diabetes, a nurse can conclude that the patient is in the maintenance stage on basis of what response?
    1. "I don't believe I need injections because I feel okay."
    2. "I may need to adjust my diet a little."
    3. "I take my insulin daily as ordered."
    4. "I have been trying to learn the diet plan."
24. A nurse recognizes an environmental risk for illness upon learning that the patient:
    1. Works in a chemical plant
    2. Has a history of heart disease
    3. Admits to intermittent substance abuse
    4. Is older than 65 years of age

STUDY GROUP QUESTIONS

- What are the different health models and how can they be applied to different patient situations? What are the advantages and disadvantages of each model?
- What are the different internal and external variables that are present in health practices and illness behavior? Give specific examples of the different variables and possible nursing interventions.
- What behaviors may be observed in a patient during illness? What impact may the patient's illness have on the family and significant others?
- How do the levels of prevention relate to the nursing care of patients in different health care settings?

STUDY CHART

Create a study chart to compare the *Levels of Prevention* that identifies both patient and nursing activities associated with each level.

Answers available through your instructor.

The Health Care Delivery System 2

CASE STUDIES

1. A neighbor who has just accepted a new job with a different benefits package stops by to ask if you know anything about managed care. He then asks you what a PPO is and what it means to him. The neighbor also tells you that he received a "big book" full of hospital and doctor names that is really confusing.
   a. What information can you provide to this individual?
   b. How could you undertake assisting the neighbor to understand his PPO coverage?
2. An 80-year-old female patient has just been diagnosed with an inoperable cancerous growth in the brain. After being told of the poor prognosis, she opts to refuse chemotherapy.
   a. Where could this individual be referred for terminal care?

CHAPTER REVIEW

Match the description/definition in Column A with the correct term in Column B.

Column A

1. Nationwide health insurance program that provides benefits to individuals older than 65 years of age
2. Integration of best knowledge, clinical expertise, and patient values
3. Fixed amount of payment for services per enrollee
4. Short-term relief for persons providing care to ill, disabled
5. Income eligibility for coverage below the federal poverty level
6. Patient responses directly related to nursing care
7. Administrative control over primary health care services practice for a defined patient population
8. Worldwide in scope
9. Multidisciplinary treatment plan that patients need for a specific condition
10. A program to recognize health care organizations that achieve excellence in nursing practice

Column B

a. Medicaid
b. Capitation
c. Globalization
d. Managed care
e. Magnet status
f. Medicare
g. Respite care
h. Critical pathway
i. Nursing-sensitive outcomes
j. Evidence-based

Complete the following:

11. A(n) _____ is a system of family-centered care designed to allow patients to live with dignity while dealing with a terminal illness.

12. In an acute care setting, discharge planning begins:

13. Technology influences health care delivery by:

14. The main purpose of a utilization review is to:

15. Select the appropriate health care service level for each of the following:
    Primary care Secondary acute care
    Restorative care Preventive care
    Tertiary care Continuing care
    a. Well-baby care
    b. Intensive care treatment
    c. Cardiac rehabilitation program
    d. Visiting nurses
    e. Adult day care center
    f. Immunizations

Copyright © 2011, 2007, 2003 by Mosby, Inc., an affiliate of Elsevier Inc. All rights reserved.

g. Family planning clinic

h. Mental health counseling

i. Appendectomy surgery

j. Assisted-living facility

k. CT scans

l. Sports medicine

16. The role of the case manager is to:

    The focus of case management is on:

17. An example of a vulnerable population is:

18. Based on the dimensions of patient-centered care, select all of the following that patients want specifically with regard to *access* to health care.
    a. To schedule appointments at convenient times without difficulty _____
    b. To have a setting that focuses on the quality of life _____
    c. To receive accurate and timely information _____
    d. To have an environment that is clean and comfortable _____
    e. To see a specialist when a referral is made _____
    f. To interact with a competent and caring staff _____
    g. To find transportation when going to different health care settings _____
    h. To have family members involved in the plan of care _____

Select the best answer for each of the following questions:

19. The daughter of an older woman expresses her concern that while she is at work her mother, recently diagnosed with Alzheimer's disease, has been found wandering around the neighborhood in a disoriented state. This family may benefit from the services of a(n):
    1. Hospice
    2. Subacute care unit
    3. Adult day care center
    4. Residential community

20. While working in the community health agency, a nurse visits an older adult patient who is having difficulty performing activities of daily living (ADLs) in her own home. The patient recognizes that she needs some supervision with medications. In discussions with this patient, the nurse refers the patient to a(n):
    1. Subacute care unit
    2. Assisted-living facility
    3. Rehabilitation hospital
    4. Primary care institution

21. A patient is discharged from a medical unit and requires more constant nursing care at a level above a nursing center or extended care facility. The nurse recognizes that this patient will be referred to an:
    1. Subacute care unit
    2. Home health care agency
    3. Urgent care center
    4. Rural primary care facility

22. A nurse's next-door neighbor has recently experienced some health problems. The neighbor visits the nurse to ask about Medicaid coverage. The nurse informs the neighbor that this program is:
    1. Catastrophic long-term care coverage for older adults
    2. A fee-for-service plan that provides preventive health care
    3. A two-part federally funded health care program for older adults
    4. A federally funded and state-regulated program for individuals of all ages with low income

23. A graduate of a nursing program is interested in the occupational health field. The graduate nurse decides to pursue a position at:
    1. The local medical center
    2. A car manufacturing plant
    3. An urgent care center
    4. A physician's office

24. A patient is being discharged from the medical unit of the hospital. While working with the patient, the nurse identifies that intermittent supervision will be required. The patient will also need to rent durable medical equipment for use in the home. There is family support for the patient upon discharge. The nurse will refer this patient to:
    1. A subacute care unit
    2. An extended care facility
    3. A home health agency
    4. An urgent care center

25. The family of a patient has requested that the hospice agency become involved with the patient's care. The nurse recognizes that the services provided by hospice for this patient include:
    1. Extensive rehabilitative measures
    2. Daytime coverage for the working caregivers
    3. Residential care with an emphasis on a return to functioning
    4. Provision of symptom management and comfort measures for the terminally ill

26. Health care costs are generally reduced with:
    1. Treatment in an outpatient facility
    2. Use of new technology
    3. Prescription medications
    4. Identification of acuity levels for hospitalized patients

27. An individual has health insurance coverage that offers an extremely limited choice of providers, with

one health care organization to use and less access to specialists. The nurse recognizes that this individual is covered by a(n):
1. Managed care organization (MCO)
2. Preferred provider organization (PPO)
3. Exclusive provider organization (EPO)
4. Private insurance company

28. In a school health setting, the nurse expects to provide which service?
1. Communicable disease prevention
2. Physical assessment
3. Chronic pain management
4. Respite care

STUDY GROUP QUESTIONS

- What types of health care financing are available, who is eligible, and what services are covered?
- What does managed care mean to patients and health care providers?
- According to the health care services levels, what health care agencies and services are available, and what are the usual roles for nurses in each agency?
- What are some of the key competencies required of nurses today?

STUDY CHART

Create a study chart to compare the *Types of Health Care Delivery Agencies* that identifies the different health care services provided and the nursing roles and activities for each.

Answers available through your instructor.

3 Community-Based Nursing Practice

CASE STUDIES

1. A nurse lives in a community that has had a steady increase in the number of older adult residents. The nurse has been approached by some of these residents and asked a variety of health-related questions. The nurse decides to investigate the needs of older adults and the resources available to this population.
   a. For the older adult, what problems and needs should the nurse anticipate?
   b. What kind of programs or services may be available or could be offered in this community for the older adult residents?
2. A 54-year-old patient was discharged from the medical center after being diagnosed with diabetes mellitus. The patient will be taking oral medication and needs to maintain dietary restrictions. Patient teaching was started during the brief stay in the medical center, but the discharge planning nurse has contacted the community health agency to follow-up with the patient. You will be visiting this patient in his home today.
   a. What should you include in the assessment of the patient's home environment?
   b. What assessment data will you need to obtain from the patient?

CHAPTER REVIEW

Complete the following:

1. The focus of community-based care is to:

2. One challenge for community-based health care is:

3. The difference between public health and community health nursing is:

4. Identify a particular risk for individuals from the following vulnerable populations:
   a. Immigrant
   b. Poor and homeless
   c. Mentally ill
   d. Older adult

5. Identify the role of the nurse in community-based practice for each of the following examples:
   a. Coordinating the visits of physical and occupational therapists
   b. Demonstrating the use of an aerosol nebulizer

Select the best answer for each of the following questions:

6. A nurse is aware that the homeless population has a higher prevalence of:
   1. Diabetes mellitus
   2. Heart disease
   3. Mental illness
   4. Asthma

7. A nurse is working with a member of a vulnerable population within the community. What is the most appropriate intervention?
   1. Providing financial advice
   2. Setting priorities for the patient and family
   3. Focusing the assessment on only the needed information
   4. Considering the meaning of the patient's language and behavior

8. In completing an assessment of a community's social system, the nurse investigates the:
   1. Schools
   2. Economy
   3. Educational level of the population
   4. Distribution of the population by age

9. For an older adult with a cognitive impairment living in the community, a nurse should specifically plan to:
   1. Provide a well-lighted, glare-free environment
   2. Promote activities that reinforce reality
   3. Make arrangements for a hearing evaluation
   4. Encourage the use of self-help groups

CHAPTER 3 • Community-Based Nursing Practice

STUDY GROUP QUESTIONS

- What are the essential functions of public and community health?
- How does the community health nurse care for the community?
- What competencies are required of a community health nurse?
- What roles are assumed by the community health nurse?
- What are the special needs of vulnerable populations?
- How does the nurse approach and care for vulnerable populations?
- What is included in the assessment of the community?

Answers available through your instructor.

4 Legal Principles in Nursing

CASE STUDIES

1. In preparation for surgery, you are to have the patient sign the consent form for the procedure. During discussions about postoperative care, the patient does not appear to fully understand what will be done during the surgery.
   a. What are your responsibilities in this situation?
2. You are reviewing the doctor's orders for the medications to be given to the patient. One of the medication orders is very difficult to read. The nurse in charge tells you that she is sure it is Lasix 40 mg PO.
   a. What should you do in this circumstance?
   b. What legal implications may be involved if the order is incorrect?
3. A child arrives in the emergency department in critical condition. His parents are divorced.
   a. What issues concerning consent for treatment may be involved in this child's case?
4. You have been observing a nursing colleague on your unit, and she appears to be taking narcotics from the medication cart. There have been occasions where her behavior has been erratic.
   a. What, if any, are your legal responsibilities regarding this colleague's behavior?

CHAPTER REVIEW

Match the descriptions/definitions in Column A with the correct term in Column B.

Column A

_____ 1. Completed when anything unusual happens that could potentially cause harm to a patient, visitor, or employee
_____ 2. Any willful attempt or threat to harm another person
_____ 3. A civil wrong or injury for which remedy is in the form of money damages
_____ 4. A crime of a serious nature that usually carries a penalty of imprisonment
_____ 5. Limitation of liability for health care professionals offering assistance at the scene of an accident
_____ 6. Conduct that falls below the standard of care
_____ 7. Any intentional touching of another person's body without consent
_____ 8. A form of contemporary laws created by elected legislative bodies
_____ 9. Documents instructing physicians to withhold or withdraw life-sustaining procedures
_____ 10. A form of contemporary law created by judicial decision in court when cases are decided

Column B

a. Tort
b. Negligence
c. Living wills
d. Statutory law
e. Good Samaritan law
f. Assault
g. Common law
h. Battery
i. Incident report
j. Felony

Complete the following:

11. The best way for a nurse to avoid being liable for negligence is to:

12. Identify two areas in which standards of care are defined.

13. Informed consent requires that the patient:

14. A 9-year-old boy arrives at the hospital after a fall from a tree. He will need emergency surgery. The 25-year-old brother who has brought him to the hospital may give legal consent.
    True _____ False _____

15. Professional negligence is termed:

16. Select all of the following correct statements regarding the Good Samaritan Law (1998):
    a. Health care providers are not liable for care provided during an emergency, even if they are not trained in the care they offer. _____

b. In an emergency, nurses may treat minors without a parent's consent. _____
c. Health care providers must follow through on care that is provided in an emergency, transferring the victim to EMTs or other emergency personnel. _____
d. In the United States, nurses are not liable for failing to provide emergency care. _____

17. A verbal or telephone order from a physician usually needs to be signed within _____ hours.

18. The two standards for determination of death are:

19. A "Do not resuscitate" (DNR) order may be given verbally by a physician.
    True _____ False _____

20. The elements of malpractice are:
    a. _____
    b. _____
    c. _____
    d. _____

21. The coroner is notified if the patient's death is: _____

22. For informed consent, the nurse's role is to:

23. Advance directives act to:

24. Health care workers are required to report what incidents?

25. Provide an example of a preventable error.

Select the best answer for each of the following questions:

26. A clinical experience is planned for an acute care facility. The student nurse recognizes that his or her liability for patient care includes:
    1. No individual responsibility for actions while being supervised
    2. A shared responsibility with instructor, staff member(s), and health care agency
    3. Activities performed while working in another capacity, such as a nursing assistant
    4. Accountability for information and techniques that will be learned in the school

27. There has been a serious flu epidemic among the staff at a medical center. Upon arriving to work on the medical unit, a nurse discovers that all other nursing staff members have called in sick and there are no other nurses available in the facility. In this situation, the nurse should:
    1. Not accept the assignment and leave the unit
    2. Accept the assignment and identify the poor staffing in each patient's record
    3. Document the situation and provide a copy to nursing administration
    4. Inform the hospital administration that nursing responsibilities have been delegated to other personnel

28. While a nurse is preparing to administer medication, the patient states that he or she refuses the medication. The nurse knows that the medication is important for the patient and proceeds with the injection of the medication. This is considered:
    1. Invasion of privacy
    2. Negligence
    3. Assault
    4. Battery

29. The urgent care center in town is busy this evening. There are many walk-in patients of different ages waiting for treatment. The nurse recognizes that in a nonemergency situation the individual who may give consent for a treatment is:
    1. A 16-year-old student
    2. The grandparent of a minor
    3. A teenage parent
    4. The 14-year-old brother of a patient

30. A nurse observes the following actions and recognizes that an invasion of patient privacy has occurred when another nurse:
    1. Shares patient data with other agency personnel not involved in the patient's treatment
    2. Withholds the patient's diagnosis from the family members per the patient's request
    3. Provides details of a major scientific advancement to the public relations' department
    4. Reports an incidence of an infectious disease to the health department

31. A nurse enters the room of a patient and observes that an incident has occurred. The situation is appropriately documented as follows:
    1. "Patient fell out of bed. Physician notified and x-rays ordered."
    2. "Patient found on floor. Laceration to forehead."
    3. "Patient given incorrect medication, became dizzy, and slid to the floor."
    4. "Patient got out of bed without assistance and appeared to have fallen."

32. While working as a receptionist in a physician's office, a student nurse is offered the opportunity to provide an injection to one of the patients. This individual's liability is based upon the:
    1. Job description of a receptionist
    2. Educational level achieved in the nursing program

3. Physician's willingness to accept responsibility for this individual
4. Limits of the malpractice insurance held by the physician and this individual

33. A nurse has administered a medication to a patient with a documented allergy to that medication. A standard of care is applied when:
   1. There is a determination of an injury to the patient
   2. An amount of financial compensation is determined
   3. Criminal statutes from the federal government are investigated
   4. The nurse's action is compared to that of another nurse in a similar circumstance

34. Of the following actions, which one is considered to be assault?
   1. A nurse threatens to administer medication to a patient who refuses it.
   2. A surgeon operates on the wrong leg.
   3. A nurse fails to use aseptic technique.
   4. A nursing assistant restrains a confused patient.

35. The National Organ Transplant Act (1984) allows for or requires:
   1. Health care agency removal of organs with the family's consent
   2. Donor transplant without the patient's consent
   3. Physicians who certify death to participate in organ removal and transplant
   4. Health care providers to ask family members to consider organ and tissue donation

STUDY GROUP QUESTIONS

- What are the sources and types of laws?
- What are intentional and unintentional torts?
- How may intentional torts be applied to nursing situations?
- What criteria are necessary for negligence/malpractice to occur?
- How are the standards of care defined and applied?
- Which individuals may give consent for treatment?
- What is the role of a nurse in obtaining consent?
- What is the role of a nurse in situations related to death and dying, employment contracts, and organ and tissue donation?
- How can a nurse minimize his/her liability?
- What situations require reporting by a nurse?
- How is the profession and practice of nursing influenced by legal issues?
- What are some of the legal concerns for nurses working in specialty areas, such as obstetrics?

STUDY CHART

Create a study chart describing *How to Minimize Liability* that identifies the nursing actions that reduce possible liability for the following situations: short staffing, floating, patient occurrences, and reporting/recording.

Answers available through your instructor.

Ethics 5

CASE STUDIES

1. You are the home care nurse for a 42-year-old male patient who has severe multiple sclerosis. He tells you on several occasions that he is tired of living this way, of not being able to do anything for himself. He says that he has read about individuals who have been "helped to die," and he asks if you can assist him in finding out more about this procedure.
   a. Apply the steps for processing an ethical dilemma to this situation.
   b. What is the role of the nurse in this situation?
2. The son of one of your patients asks you if he can look at his mother's medical record. He insists that he needs to know what is happening so that he and his sister can plan for the mother's care.
   a. What should you do in this circumstance?

CHAPTER REVIEW

Match the description/definition in Column A with the correct term in Column B.

Column A
_____ 1. Supporting the patient's right to informed consent
_____ 2. Considering the patient's best interest
_____ 3. Avoiding deliberate harm
_____ 4. Keeping promises
_____ 5. Determining the order in which patients should be treated
_____ 6. Consideration of standards of conduct
_____ 7. Ethics within the field of health care
_____ 8. Judgment about behavior
_____ 9. Personal beliefs about the worth of an idea

Column B
a. Ethics
b. Fidelity
c. Justice
d. Morals
e. Bioethics
f. Autonomy
g. Beneficence
h. Nonmaleficence
i. Values or object

Complete the following:

10. According to the Health Insurance Portability and Accountability Act of 1996 (HIPAA), access to a patient's medical record by a family member requires:

11. Identify an end-of-life issue that has ethical implications for nurses.

12. Identify the ethical theory for each of the following descriptions:
    a. Proposes that actions are right or wrong based on the essence of right and wrong in the principles of fidelity, truthfulness, and justice
    b. Discusses how ethical decisions affect women
    c. Proposes that the value of something is based on its usefulness
    d. Discusses nursing, gender, and ethical dilemmas

13. For the following areas, provide a specific example of how ethical concerns may be involved:
    a. Cost containment

    b. Cultural sensitivity

Select the best answer for each of the following questions:

14. A professional code of ethics includes:
    1. Legal standards for practice
    2. Extensive details on moral principles
    3. Guidelines for approaching common ethical dilemmas
    4. A collective statement of group expectations for behavior

15. By administering medication to a patient on a unit in an extended care facility, a nurse is applying the ethical principle of:
    1. Justice
    2. Fidelity
    3. Autonomy
    4. Beneficence

16. A nurse has been working with a patient who had abdominal surgery. The patient is experiencing discomfort and has been calling for assistance often. The ethical principle of fidelity is demonstrated when the nurse:
    1. Changes the dressing
    2. Provides a warm lotion back rub
    3. Informs the patient of the actions of the medications administered
    4. Returns to assist the patient with breathing exercises at the agreed-upon times
17. A student nurse is assigned to work with parents who refuse to have essential medical treatment provided to their child. The medical center is pursuing a court order to force the family to accept the treatment plan that will assist the child. The nurse has strong feelings for the family's position, as well as the importance of the medical treatment. The first step for the nurse to take in attempting to resolve this ethical dilemma is to:
    1. Examine personal values
    2. Evaluate the outcomes
    3. Gather all of the facts
    4. Verbalize the problem
18. An example of advocacy in nursing practice is:
    1. Documenting care provided to a patient
    2. Giving medication to a patient
    3. Assessing the patient's comfort level after surgery
    4. Contacting the physician to discuss patient's response to the plan of care
19. The last phase in the processing of an ethical dilemma is to:
    1. Evaluate the action taken
    2. Consider treatment options
    3. Negotiate the options and outcomes
    4. Identify the problem

STUDY GROUP QUESTIONS

- What are ethics and what is the purpose of a code of ethics in a profession?
- What principles are promoted in a profession?
- How can a nurse be a patient advocate?
- What are the basic standards of ethics?
- What are values and how are they developed?
- How do values relate to ethics?
- How does a professional determine that an ethical dilemma exists?
- What are the steps for processing an ethical dilemma?
- What ethical dilemmas may arise in health care and nursing practice?

STUDY CHART

Create a study chart to identify and compare *Responsibility, Accountability, Confidentiality, Competence, Judgment, and Advocacy,* and provide examples of nursing behaviors for each.

Answers available through your instructor.

Evidence-Based Practice 6

CASE STUDIES

1. You are working in a home care agency. One of your assigned patients is having difficulty with managing his daily insulin intake. You discover that he is having difficulty in getting an accurate blood glucose reading with his monitor. Because of the problem, the patient is self-administering too much or too little insulin. You remember that some of the other home care patients are also having some trouble with this particular glucose monitor.
    a. Use the PICO format to develop a possible question.
    b. What type of trigger is present in this scenario?
2. As a nurse for a surgical unit in a local medical center, you will be involved in identifying some quality improvement (QI) projects for your unit.
    a. What possible areas may be important for you, your fellow staff members, and the patients on your unit?

CHAPTER REVIEW

Complete the following:

1. Evidence-based practice is:

2. Identify three valuable sources of nonresearch-based evidence.

3. A peer-reviewed article is:

4. A qualitative research study focuses on:

5. Provide an example of how a nurse integrates evidence into practice.

6. In the Quality Improvement model, what does PDSA stand for?
    P
    D
    S
    A

7. Provide an at least one example of a patient outcome and measurement.

8. A randomized control trial (RCT) includes which of the following? Select all that apply.
    a. Subjects _____
    b. Experimental therapies _____
    c. A control group _____
    d. Subjective input from the researcher _____
    e. Analysis of the results _____

9. An evidence-based article includes which of the following? Select all that apply.
    a. An abstract _____
    b. The author's biography _____
    c. A literature review _____
    d. The study's design and methods _____
    e. The author's opinions about the subjects _____
    f. A conclusion relevant to the findings _____

Select the best answer for each of the following questions:

10. A nurse recognizes which of the following as a sentinel event?
    1. An error is made and a medication dose is skipped.
    2. A wound infection is noted on a patient who has transferred from a nursing home.
    3. A patient dies within 48 hours of admission to the medical center.
    4. A hip replacement is performed on the wrong leg.

11. Which of the following is the best description of a case control study?
    1. A comparison of one group of subjects to another
    2. A focus on a subgroup with a known condition
    3. A prediction or explanation of phenomena
    4. A description of the responses to an independent variable

CHAPTER 6 • Evidence-Based Practice

STUDY GROUP QUESTIONS

- What is evidence-based practice?
- How does a nurse become involved in the research process?
- What is PICO(T)?
- Where can reliable research-based data be found?
- What databases represent the scientific knowledge of health care?
- What types of evidence or studies are available?
- How are evidence-based findings used in nursing practice?
- How are evidence-based changes communicated and evaluated?
- What is the relationship between evidence-based practice and quality improvement?

Answers available through your instructor.

Critical Thinking 7

CASE STUDIES

1. You receive reports on your patient assignment for the day. You have six patients who require assessment and have orders for treatments and medications.
   a. How can you use critical thinking to approach this multiple patient assignment?
2. As a home care nurse, you have been assigned to visit a patient who requires dressing changes for a foot ulceration. When you arrive in the home, you see that the patient does not have any commercially packaged dressings or saline solution. You have used the last of your supplies and the drive to the office will take more than 1 hour. The dressing that the patient has on her foot is saturated with purulent drainage.
   a. What options are available to you in this situation?
   b. What further investigation about the patient and her living situation may be necessary?

CHAPTER REVIEW

Match the description/definition in Column A with the correct term in Column B.

	Column A	Column B
_____	1. Process of recalling an event to determine its meaning and purpose	a. Scientific method
_____	2. Series of clinical judgments that result in informal or formal diagnoses	b. Decision making
_____	3. End point of critical thinking that leads to problem resolution	c. Intuition
_____	4. Inner sensing that something is so	d. Diagnostic reasoning
_____	5. Process that moves from observable facts from an experience to a reasonable explanation of those facts	e. Reflection

Complete the following:

6. Identify one example of how critical thinking is used in each of the following steps of the nursing process:
   a. Assessment
   b. Nursing diagnosis
   c. Planning
   d. Implementation
   e. Evaluation

7. Identify the level of critical thinking demonstrated by each of the following:
   a. Trusting experts to have the right answers for every problem
   b. Analyzing and examining problems more independently
   c. Making choices without assistance and accepting accountability

8. Identify the elements of the critical thinking model.

9. Identify the attitude of critical thinking demonstrated for each of the following:
   a. Performing a skill safely and effectively
   b. Questioning an order that appears incorrect
   c. Performing a systematic and thorough pain assessment
   d. Developing a unique way to teach the patient how to change a dressing
   e. Admitting to the nurse manager that a medication was given in error

CHAPTER 7 • Critical Thinking

Select the best answer for each of the following questions:

10. In employing critical thinking, the first step that the nurse should use is:
    1. Evaluation
    2. Decision making
    3. Self-regulation
    4. Interpretation
11. Having worked for a number of years in the acute care environment, a nurse achieved the ability to use a complex level of critical thinking. The nurse:
    1. Acts solely on his or her own opinions
    2. Trusts the experts to have the answers to problems
    3. Implements creative and innovative options
    4. Applies rules and principles the same way in every situation
12. Clinical care experiences have recently begun for a student nurse. When beginning to work with patients, the student nurse implements critical thinking in practice by:
    1. Asking for assistance if uncertain
    2. Sharing personal ideas with peers
    3. Acting on independent judgments
    4. Relying on standardized, textbook approaches
13. A nurse has an extremely large patient assignment this evening and begins to feel overwhelmed. Of the following, what is the nurse's priority activity?
    1. Sharing his or her feelings with colleagues
    2. Calling the supervisor and ask for assistance
    3. Reviewing the overall assignment to get his or her bearings
    4. Moving immediately to provide patient care, starting with the room closest to the nurse's station
14. Orientation for new nurses begins. The instructor assembled information on critical thinking and nursing approaches. The instructor recognizes that critical thinkers in nursing:
    1. Make quick, single-solution decisions
    2. Act on intuition instead of experience
    3. Review data in a disciplined manner
    4. Alter interventions for every circumstance
15. A nurse is caring for a patient who is experiencing a respiratory disorder. Intuition is a part of the critical thinking process for the nurse. While caring for the patient, the nurse demonstrates intuition by:
    1. Reviewing care with the patient in advance
    2. Observing communication patterns
    3. Establishing a nursing diagnosis
    4. Sensing that the patient is not doing as well this morning as before
16. Entering a room at 2:00 AM, a nurse notes that the patient is not in bed; the patient is sitting in the chair and states that she is having difficulty sleeping. Employing critical thinking, the nurse responds by:
    1. Assisting the patient back into bed
    2. Asking more about the patient's sleep problem
    3. Positioning the patient and providing a warm blanket
    4. Obtaining an order for a hypnotic medication
17. A nurse has a diverse patient assignment this evening. When reviewing the patients' conditions, the nurse determines that the first individual that should be seen is:
    1. The patient who is hypotensive
    2. The patient receiving a visit from a family member
    3. The patient being treated by the respiratory therapist
    4. The patient waiting for the effects of an analgesic that was given 5 minutes ago
18. In using the critical thinking skill of self-regulation, a nurse will:
    1. Be orderly in data collection
    2. Look at all situations objectively
    3. Use scientific and experiential knowledge
    4. Reflect on his or her own experiences and improve performance
19. During the process of reflection, what is the most appropriate question for a nurse to ask himself or herself?
    1. "What could I have done differently?"
    2. "What's going on right now?"
    3. "How can the patient's status change?"
    4. "What should I do to communicate this information?"
20. A nurse believes that substance abuse is a serious problem with negative consequences for patients and families. The nurse, however, provides excellent care to a patient who is admitted with this problem. The nurse is displaying the critical thinking attitude of:
    1. Integrity
    2. Fairness
    3. Discipline
    4. Perseverance

STUDY GROUP QUESTIONS

- How is critical thinking integrated into nursing practice?
- What attitudes are needed by a nurse in order to be a critical thinker?
- How are the competencies of critical thinking applied in clinical practice?
- Why is critical thinking important throughout the nursing process?

Answers available through your instructor.

Nursing Process

8

CASE STUDIES

1. Mr. B., a 47-year-old male patient, goes to the annual community health fair. During a routine blood pressure screening, it is determined that his blood pressure is significantly above normally expected levels.
   a. What additional assessment data should be obtained from the patient and family?
   b. What limitations exist in this situation for completing an assessment?
2. Mr. B. returns for a follow-up visit at the medical center's adult health clinic. Mr. B. is diagnosed with hypertension and an antihypertensive medication is prescribed, but he appears unsure about how and when he should take the prescription. Mr. B. also identifies that his father died from a heart attack at 54 years old.
   a. Identify the relevant assessment data for this patient.
   b. Based upon this information, identify two nursing diagnoses.
3. During Mr. B.'s appointment at the adult health clinic, he was found to have high blood pressure, and antihypertensive medication was prescribed. Mr. B. did not have any previous knowledge of or experience with either hypertension or hypertensive medication. Mr. B. mentions again that his father died at age 54 years of a heart attack.
   a. Based on the nursing diagnoses that were developed, identify one long-term or short-term goal for each diagnosis and at least one expected outcome for each goal.

Nursing diagnoses	Long-term or short-term goals	Expected outcomes
1.		
2.		

   b. Identify two nursing interventions that may be appropriate in assisting the patient to achieve the expected outcomes and goals.
4. At his next visit to the adult health clinic, Mr. B. tells the nurse that he is taking the antihypertensive medication that was ordered by the physician "when he remembers." He says that he is trying to use the relaxation techniques that he was taught during his last visit, but he does not use them regularly.
   a. What nursing implementation methods should take priority at this time?
   b. What, if any, alterations need to be made in the original plan of care?
5. Mr. B. returns to the adult health clinic for evaluation of his status. His blood pressure is lower than before, but remains slightly above normal limits. He exercises once or twice a week, and states that this is making him feel better. Mr. B. shows the nurse a calendar where he has marked down the times for taking his medication. Mr. B. relates that he has been trying very hard to use the relaxation techniques when he starts to feel anxious or overwhelmed. He identifies that he cannot control all of his "destiny," but he is trying to do things that may help him avoid what happened to his father.
   a. In accordance with previously identified outcomes, what nursing evaluation may be made on this patient's status?
   b. What areas, if any, may require reassessment?

CHAPTER REVIEW

Match the description/definition in Column A with the correct term in Column B.

Column A
1. Unintended effect of a medication, diagnostic test, or intervention
2. Observations or measurements made by the nurse during assessment
3. Comparing data with another source to determine accuracy and relevancy
4. Multidisciplinary, outcome-based care plan
5. Clinical judgment about patient responses to health problems or life processes
6. Information obtained through the senses
7. Activities performed in the course of a normal day
8. Support for why a specific nursing action is chosen
9. Interpretation of cues
10. Information verbally provided by the patient

Column B
a. Subjective data
b. ADLs
c. Adverse reaction
d. Critical pathway
e. Nursing diagnosis
f. Cue
g. Objective data
h. Scientific rationale
i. Inference
j. Validation

CHAPTER 8 • Nursing Process

Complete the following:

11. The three phases of an interview are:

12. Based on the following data clusters, identify possible nursing diagnoses:
    a. Abdominal pain, three loose liquid stools per day, hyperactive bowel sounds:

    b. Fatigue, weakness, tachycardia upon activity, exertional dyspnea:

13. Identify at least one goal, one expected outcome, and one nursing intervention for the following nursing diagnoses:
    a. Deficient knowledge related to the need for postoperative care at home

    Goal:

    Expected outcome:

    Nursing intervention:

    b. Constipation related to lack of physical activity

    Goal:

    Expected outcome:

    Nursing intervention:

14. Identify whether the following are examples of cognitive, interpersonal, or psychomotor skills in patient care:
    a. Preparing and administering an injection
    b. Completing a health history
    c. Providing emotional support to a family member
    d. Changing a surgical dressing
    e. Recognizing the patient's need for nutritional instruction

15. Before implementing standing orders, the nurse should check:

16. The steps of the implementation phase of the nursing process are:

17. During interactions with a patient, a nurse gathers more data and identifies a new patient need. The nurse should:

18. A patient with diabetes mellitus goes to the outpatient center for care. There is a written plan for diet counseling, medication, and follow-up care. These specific procedures are termed a(n) _____ for care.

19. An example of an indirect nursing intervention is:

20. Identify all of the following that typically may be delegated to unlicensed assistive personnel:
    a. Skin care _____
    b. Tracheostomy care _____
    c. Hygienic care _____
    d. Personal grooming _____
    e. Urinary catheterization _____
    f. Administration of IV medications _____
    g. Assistance with ambulation _____

21. Specify how the following patient outcomes may be improved:
    a. Erythema will be less noticeable

    b. Pulse rate will be normal

    c. Patient's calorie intake will increase

22. Identify at least three (3) ways to create a good environment for an interview with a patient.

Select the best answer for each of the following questions:

23. A new graduate is preparing to work with patients on a medical unit. The nursing process is applied as a:
    1. Method for processing the care of many patients
    2. Tool for diagnosing and treating patients' health problems
    3. Guideline for determining the nurse's accountability in patient care
    4. Logical, problem-solving approach to providing patient care

24. Upon admission, the nurse begins to assess the patient. The patient appears uncomfortable, stating that she has severe abdominal pain. The nurse should:
    1. Inquire specifically about the discomfort
    2. Let the patient rest, returning later to complete the assessment
    3. Perform a complete physical examination immediately
    4. Ask the family about the patient's health history

25. The following nursing diagnoses are proposed for patients on the medical unit. The diagnostic statement that contains all of the necessary components is:
    1. Impaired gas exchange related to accumulation of lung secretions
    2. Imbalanced nutrition related to chemotherapy treatment
    3. Complicated grieving
    4. Pain related to abdominal surgery

26. A nurse is working with patients who go to the community center for health screenings and educational sessions. An example of a wellness nursing diagnosis label that is appropriate for this group is:
    1. Risk for impaired skin integrity
    2. Readiness for enhanced family coping
    3. Altered parent-infant attachment
    4. Fluid volume deficit
27. In reviewing the nursing diagnoses written by a new staff member, a supervisor identifies which of the following as a correctly written nursing diagnosis?
    1. Altered respiratory function related to abnormal blood gases
    2. Urinary infection related to long-term catheterization
    3. Deficient knowledge related to need for cardiac monitoring
    4. Pain related to severe arthritis in finger joints
28. A nurse is working with a patient who has the following symptoms: dyspnea, ankle edema, weight gain, abdominal distention, hypertension. The nursing diagnosis that is most appropriate for these signs and symptoms is:
    1. Ineffective tissue perfusion
    2. Disturbed body image
    3. Impaired gas exchange
    4. Excess fluid volume
29. A patient is to have abdominal surgery tomorrow. The nurse determines that an outcome for this patient that meets the necessary criteria is:
    1. Patient will be repositioned every 2 hours.
    2. Patient will express fears about surgery.
    3. Patient will achieve normal elimination pattern before discharge.
    4. Patient will perform active range-of-motion exercises every 2 hours while in bed.
30. There are a number of activities that are to be performed by a nurse during a clinical shift. In deciding to perform a nurse-initiated intervention, the nurse:
    1. Administers oral medications
    2. Orders laboratory tests
    3. Changes a sterile dressing
    4. Teaches newborn hygienic care
31. A nurse implements a preventive nursing action when:
    1. Immunizing patients
    2. Assisting with hygienic care
    3. Inserting a urinary catheter
    4. Providing crisis intervention counseling
32. A nurse has been working with a patient in the rehabilitative facility for 2 weeks. The nurse is in the process of evaluating the patient's progress. During the evaluation phase, the nurse recognizes that:
    1. Nursing diagnoses always remain the same
    2. Time frames for patient outcomes may be adjusted
    3. Evaluative skills differ greatly from those for patient assessment
    4. The number of nursing diagnoses and outcomes is most important
33. An expected outcome for a patient is the following: "Pulse will remain below 120 beats per minute during exercise." If the patient's pulse rate exceeds 120 beats per minute one of every three exercise periods, the nurse appropriately evaluates the patient's goal attainment as:
    1. Patient has achieved desired behavior
    2. Patient requires further evaluation of progress
    3. Patient's response indicates need for elimination of exercise
    4. Patient does not comply with therapeutic regimen
34. The nurse is caring for a patient who has been medically stable. During the change-of-shift report, the nurse is informed that the patient is experiencing a slight arrhythmia. To avoid complications during the implementation of care, the nurse plans to:
    1. Evaluate the patient's vital signs
    2. Ask about the patient's previous diagnoses
    3. Contact the physician immediately
    4. Tell the nursing assistant to perform the usual care for the patient
35. For a patient in the acute care facility, a nurse identifies several interventions. The statement that best communicates the activity of the nurse is to:
    1. Assist with exercises
    2. Take the patient's vital signs
    3. Refer the patient to a therapist
    4. Provide 30 ml of water with the nasogastric tube feedings every 4 hours
36. The nurse is working with a patient who has diabetes mellitus. The nursing diagnosis is "Deficient volume fluid related to osmotic diuresis." An appropriate patient outcome, based on this nursing diagnosis, is:
    1. Patient will have an increased urinary output.
    2. Patient will decrease the amount of fluid intake during a 24-hour period.
    3. Patient will demonstrate a decrease in edema in the lower extremities.
    4. Patient will have palpable peripheral pulses and good capillary refill.
37. A nurse is working with a patient who is experiencing abnormal breath sounds and thick secretions. The nurse identifies a nursing diagnosis of:
    1. Deficient fluid volume
    2. Ineffective airway clearance
    3. Risk for altered mucous membranes
    4. Dysfunctional ventilatory weaning response
38. In completing a health history, a nurse obtains from the patient psychosocial information that includes:
    1. The reason for seeking health care
    2. Past health problems
    3. The primary language spoken
    4. Physical safety status

CHAPTER 8 • Nursing Process

39. A patient tells the nurse that she feels she may not be using the crutches correctly when ambulating. The best way for the nurse to validate this information is to:
   1. Ask the family about the patient's ambulation
   2. Ask the physician how the patient was taught
   3. Discuss the problem with the other staff members
   4. Observe the patient using the crutches

40. An example of the most appropriately written nursing diagnosis is:
   1. Acute pain related to surgery
   2. Shortness of breath related to immobility
   3. Anxiety related to lack of knowledge about cardiac monitoring
   4. Recurrent infection related to improper catheterization procedure

41. In determining which of the following patients on the medical unit to visit first, a nurse selects the patient with which of the following diagnoses?
   1. Imbalanced nutrition: less than body requirements
   2. Ineffective tissue perfusion
   3. Deficient knowledge regarding home care resources
   4. Impaired physical mobility

42. An example of a physician-initiated intervention is:
   1. Teaching a patient about the therapeutic diet
   2. Assessing a patient's skin
   3. Providing emotional support
   4. Preparing a patient for a diagnostic test

STUDY GROUP QUESTIONS

- What is involved in patient assessment, and what priorities does a nurse have in completing an assessment?
- How does the patient assessment fit into the nursing process?
- Why does an error in the assessment phase influence the remaining implementation of the process, and how can a nurse avoid errors?
- What methods may be used to obtain patient data and what type of data is obtained with each method?
- What is involved in a patient interview?
- How can a nurse optimize the environment for a patient interview?
- How can a nurse use different communication strategies to obtain data during patient assessment?
- What is a nursing diagnosis?
- What are the components of a nursing diagnosis?
- How are actual and potential nursing diagnoses different?
- How are medical and nursing diagnoses different?
- What errors are possible in formulating nursing diagnoses, and how may they be avoided?
- Which nursing diagnoses become priorities in planning patient care?
- How are long-term and short-term goals different from each other?
- How are goals and expected outcomes different from each other?
- What are the guidelines for formulating goals and outcomes?
- In selecting nursing interventions, what are three essential nurse competencies?
- How are the three types of nursing interventions different from one another?
- What factors should be considered when selecting nursing interventions?
- What is the purpose of the care plan, and what types are available for use?
- How does a critical pathway differ from a "traditional" care plan?
- How does the consultation process begin, and who and what may be involved in the process?
- What is the focus of the implementation phase of the nursing process?
- What are standing orders and protocols, and how are they used in patient care situations?
- What are the five preparatory nursing activities that are completed before implementing the care plan?
- What are the nursing implementation methods?
- How is nursing implementation communicated to other members of the health care team?
- How is evaluation incorporated into the nursing process?
- How is evaluation used in patient situations and in nursing practice and health care delivery settings?
- What circumstances would lead to a modification of a care plan?

STUDY CHART

Create a study chart to compare the *Steps of the Nursing Process* that identifies the different activities involved in each step.

Answers available through your instructor.

Informatics and Documentation

CASE STUDIES

1. Mrs. Q. has just been transferred to her room from the postanesthesia care unit (PACU) after right hip replacement surgery. She was accompanied by a nurse from PACU. Vital signs were taken upon transfer and found to be within expected limits. A dressing is in place on the patient's right hip. Mrs. Q. does not appear to be having any difficulty at the moment.
    a. What information should be provided by the PACU nurse to the primary nurse on the surgical unit when Mrs. Q. is transferred to her room?
    b. What additional information may Mrs. Q.'s primary nurse want to obtain from the PACU nurse?
2. The primary nurse begins to plan and provide care for Mrs. Q. Upon entering the patient's room, Mrs. Q. is found to be grimacing and moaning in pain. She says that she is having intense pain in her right hip area. The dressing to her hip is dry and intact. Mrs. Q. says that she does not want to move because it really hurts. The primary nurse helps Mrs. Q. to get into a more comfortable position and begins to prepare the pain medication ordered by the physician. The primary nurse administers the pain medication, and, after approximately one-half hour, Mrs. Q. states that the pain has been reduced. Using SOAP or DAR methods, document the nursing interaction with Mrs. Q.
3. Mr. W. has just been diagnosed with type 1 diabetes mellitus and needs to learn how to self-administer his insulin injections.
    a. What information should be included in the patient record regarding the teaching provided to Mr. W. on the self-injection of insulin?

CHAPTER REVIEW

Match the description/definition in Column A with the correct term in Column B.

	Column A		Column B
___	1. An oral or written exchange of information between health care providers	a.	Record
___	2. Information about patients provided only to appropriate personnel	b.	POMR
___	3. Permanent written communication with patient's health care management	c.	Acuity recording
___	4. Structured method of documentation with emphasis on the patient's problems	d.	Report
___	5. Documentation that requires staff to identify interventions and allows patients to be compared with one another	e.	Confidentiality

Complete the following:

6. The following are guidelines for documentation. Indicate the correct action to be taken by the nurse for each guideline.
    a. Never erase entries or use correction fluid, and never use pencil.
    b. Do not write retaliatory or critical comments about patients.
    c. Avoid using generalized, empty phrases.
    d. Do not cross out errors.
    e. Do not leave blank spaces.
    f. Do not speculate or guess.
    g. Do not record: "Physician made error."
    h. Never chart for someone else.
    i. Do not wait until the end of shift to record important information.

7. a. HIPAA (Health Insurance Portability and Accountability Act of 1996) has new regulations that require written consent for disclosure of all patient information. True _____ False _____
   b. Incident or occurrence reports should be documented in the patient's medical record in the nurses' notes section. True _____ False _____

8. Standards for health care agencies and documentation are set by the:

CHAPTER 9 • Informatics and Documentation

9. For each of the following, identify an example of how the patient record is used for:
   a. Communication:
   b. Finance:
   c. Education:
   d. Research:
   e. Auditing/monitoring:

10. Provide an example of a malpractice issue related to charting:

11. Identify the five characteristics of quality documentation:

12. Subjective statements made by the patient are best documented by:

13. Demonstrate how a student nurse should sign a written patient record:

14. Identify what is wrong with the following notations and how they can be corrected:
    a. "Ate some breakfast."
    b. "Voided an adequate amount."
    c. "Provided wound care qd."

15. For telephone reports, identify what the SBAR acronym represents and give an example of each area:
    S:
    B:
    A:
    R:

16. Provide two items that should be included in a discharge summary:

17. Home care documentation is completed both for quality control and as the basis for:

18. Completion of narrative notes only when there are abnormal patient findings is part of the concept of:

19. What are the purposes and advantages of nursing informatics?

20. Identify at least two ways in which electronic records are safeguarded for privacy and security:

21. Identify the four concepts included in informatics:

22. Which of the following are the correct nursing actions for a telephone order? Select all that apply.
    a. Identifying that Mr. J. is in Room 212. _____
    b. Asking the physician to repeat the medication order for Mr. J. three times. _____
    c. Checking that 40 mg of the drug is what should be given. _____
    d. Writing "TO" (telephone order) in the nurse's notes. _____
    e. Asking another nurse to call the physician back to verify the order. _____
    f. Having Mr. J.'s doctor cosign the order within 24 hours. _____

23. What information is usually available to nurses on a clinical information system?

Select the best answer for each of the following questions:

24. A nurse is working in a facility that uses computerized documentation of patient information. To maintain patient confidentiality with the use of computerized documentation, the nurse should:
    1. Delete any and all errors made in the record
    2. Only give his or her password to other nurses working with the patient
    3. Log off the file or computer when not using the terminal
    4. Remove sensitive patient information, such as communicable diseases, from the record

25. The nurses on a medical unit in an acute care facility are meeting to select a documentation format to use. They recognize that less fragmentation of patient data will occur if they implement:
    1. Source records
    2. Focus charting
    3. Charting by exception
    4. Critical pathways

26. While caring for a patient on the surgical unit, a nurse notes that the patient's blood pressure has dropped significantly since the last measurement. The nurse shares this information immediately with the health care provider in a(n):
    1. Flow sheet record
    2. Incident report
    3. Telephone report
    4. Change-of-shift report

27. Documentation of patient care is reviewed during the orientation to the facility. The new graduate nurse understands that the method for written documentation that is acceptable is:
    1. Using red ink to make entries on patients' charts
    2. Charting all of the patient care at the end of the shift
    3. Beginning each entry with the time of the treatment or observation
    4. Leaving space at the end of the notations to allow for additional documentation
28. A nurse has been very busy during the shift to get all of the patient care activities completed. While documenting one of the patient's responses to a pain medication, the nurse mistakenly writes on the wrong patient's chart. The nurse:
    1. Notes the error at the bottom of the page
    2. Erases the error and completes the entry on the correct chart
    3. Uses a dark color marker to completely cover the error
    4. Draws a straight line through the note and initials the error
29. A nurse is caring for a patient who has had abdominal surgery. Accurate and complete documentation of the care provided by the nurse is evident by the following notation:
    1. "Vital signs taken."
    2. "Tylenol with codeine given for pain."
    3. "Provided adequate amount of fluid."
    4. "IV fluids increased to 100 mL per hour according to protocol."
30. A nurse is involved in patient care in an agency that uses military time for documentation. Which of the following represents 4:00 PM?
    1. 0400
    2. 0800
    3. 1400
    4. 1600
31. A nurse would **not** expect to find which of the following in a problem-oriented medical record?
    1. Progress notes
    2. Narrative notes
    3. SOAP notes
    4. PIE notes
32. An appropriate action by a student nurse is demonstrated by:
    1. Accessing records of other students' patients
    2. Writing the patient's name and room number on assignments
    3. Copying patient records for review and preparation of care plans
    4. Reading the patient's record in preparation for clinical care
33. A nurse enters a patient's room and discovers a yellow pill on the bed under the patient's pillow. The patient receives Lasix 40 mg daily. Which of the following notations is appropriate to include on an incident or occurrence report?
    1. "Patient refused to take Lasix at 10 AM."
    2. "Yellow pill found on bed under pillow."
    3. "Lasix not administered by primary nurse."
    4. "Patient did not receive 10 AM diuretic."
34. The nursing information system (NIS) that follows a more traditional format is the:
    1. Protocol design
    2. Critical pathway design
    3. Nursing process design
    4. Medical diagnosis design
35. Which of the following statements made by a new staff nurse during change-of-shift report requires correction?
    1. "The patient is uncooperative about doing his stoma care."
    2. "Oxygen is needed after ambulation. This is a change in priorities."
    3. "Ms. Q is a 62-year-old with diabetes mellitus."
    4. "The abdominal surgical wound is healing slowly, with no drainage noted."

STUDY GROUP QUESTIONS

- What is the purpose of documentation and reporting?
- What are the legal guidelines for documentation?
- How do the guidelines influence nursing documentation and reporting?
- What methods are available for documentation of patient data?
- How do the different types of documentation (for example, SOAP, DAR, and narrative) compare with one another?
- How does written documentation compare with computerized systems, and what are the advantages and disadvantages of each method?
- What types of forms are used for patient documentation?
- How does patient documentation change in different health care settings?
- What information is necessary when doing change-of-shift, telephone, transfer, and incident reports?
- What role do informatics play in heath care?
- How do nurses use information systems?
- What safety measures need to be taken by nurses when accessing electronic records?
- What type of patient information is accessible on electronic systems?

Answers available through your instructor.

10 Communication

CASE STUDY

1. For the following patient situations, identify the communication techniques that may be most effective in establishing a nurse-patient relationship:
   a. An older adult patient who has a moderate hearing impairment
   b. The Russian-speaking parents of a young child who has been taken into the emergency department after a bicycle accident
   c. A young adult patient who is blind and requires daily insulin injections
   d. A 60-year-old Hispanic woman who will be having her first internal pelvic examination

CHAPTER REVIEW

Match the description/definition in Column A with the correct term in Column B.

Column A

_____ 1. Person who initiates interpersonal communication
_____ 2. Information sent or expressed by the sender
_____ 3. Means of conveying messages
_____ 4. Person to whom the message is sent
_____ 5. Indicates whether the meaning of the sender's message was received
_____ 6. Motivates one person to communicate with another
_____ 7. Shades or interpretations of a word's meaning rather than different definitions
_____ 8. Tone of the speaker's voice that may affect a message's meaning
_____ 9. A message within a message that conveys a sender's attitude toward the self and toward the listener
_____ 10. Development of a working, functional relationship by the nurse with the patient, fulfilling the purposes of the nursing process

Column B

a. Therapeutic communication
b. Metacommunication
c. Sender
d. Intonation
e. Feedback
f. Connotations
g. Channels
h. Message
i. Receiver
j. Referent

Complete the following:

11. Determine what level of communication the following examples illustrate:
    a. Talking to oneself

    b. "He looks uncomfortable, and I want to show him that I'm concerned about his discomfort."

    c. The ability to speak to consumers on health-related topics

12. Individuals maintain distances between themselves during interactions. Identify the zone (Intimate, Personal, Social, or Public) that is being used in each of the following examples:
    a. Speaking to a group of students in a classroom

    b. Conducting a small group therapy session

    c. Performing a physical examination

    d. Making patient rounds with a physician

    e. Changing a wound dressing

    f. Testifying at a hearing

    g. Completing a change-of-shift report

13. For an older adult with impaired communication, identify the appropriate communication techniques. Select all that apply.
    a. Maintaining a quiet environment that is free of background noise _____
    b. Shifting from subject to subject during the conversation _____
    c. Letting the person know if you are having difficulty understanding him or her _____

Copyright © 2011, 2007, 2003 by Mosby, Inc., an affiliate of Elsevier Inc. All rights reserved.

d. Using explorative questions to facilitate conversation _____
e. Using long sentences to explain subject matter _____

14. The following are examples of inappropriate communication by a nurse. Specify an effective strategy that should be used to correct the situation.
   a. Calling the patient "Honey"
   b. Reporting to a nursing colleague about the "gallbladder in room 214"
   c. Talking about a patient to other nurses in the elevator
   d. Running into a patient's room to administer medications and then leaving immediately
   e. Informing a patient that the physician will be performing an abdominal hysterectomy and that she should expect a midline incision of approximately 10 centimeters

15. For the following examples, identify a question that the nurse could ask that would be more appropriate and obtain better information from the patient:
   a. "You're feeling okay today, right?"
   b. "You don't take any medication at home, do you?"
   c. "Are you having any lymphedema?"
   d. "The physician will be doing a paracentesis today. He said he explained it to you."

16. Identify the communication strategy that is being used for each of the following examples:
   a. Sitting with a patient who is crying
   b. Showing interest in the patient who is discussing concerns or sharing family information
   c. Saying "Go on" or "Tell me more"
   d. Asking the patient to verify the meaning of statements made
   e. Directing the attention of the patient to a particular idea in the discussion

17. For the nursing diagnosis *impaired verbal communication related to aphasia*, identify at least two nursing interventions to promote communication with the patient.

18. Nurses on a medical unit are discussing issues related to their work schedules. Identify the examples of positive responses:
   a. "There's nothing we can do about the staffing situation." _____
   b. "Don't talk to me like that!" _____
   c. "What do you think we can do to improve this situation?" _____
   d. "I want to hear what your concerns are." _____

19. A nurse takes into account cultural considerations when communicating with patients. Identify the *appropriate* action(s):
   a. Stroking the head of a Southeast Asian patient _____
   b. Assigning a female staff member to care for a female Amish patient _____
   c. Maintaining direct eye contact with a Native American patient _____
   d. Introducing oneself and using the patient's last name _____

20. For the acronym SOLER, identify the skills for attentive listening:
   S:
   O:
   L:
   E:
   R:

21. Identify the nursing actions/responses that occur during the Orientation Phase of the Helping Relationship. Select all that apply.
   a. Achieving a smooth transition for the patient to other caregivers as needed _____
   b. Providing information needed to understand and change behavior _____
   c. Reviewing available data, including the medical and nursing history _____
   d. Expecting the patient to test your competence and commitment _____
   e. Setting the tone for the relationship by adopting a warm, empathetic, caring manner _____
   f. Prioritizing patient problems and identifying patient goals _____

Select the best answer for each of the following questions:

22. A patient tells a nurse that he feels anxious and afraid. The nurse responds by saying, "I will stay here with you." The nurse is using the principle of effective communication known as:
   1. Empathy
   2. Courtesy
   3. Availability
   4. Encouragement

23. A patient states that he believes he may have cancer. The nurse tells him, "I wouldn't be concerned. I'm

sure that the tests will be negative." The response by the nurse demonstrates the use of:
1. Assertiveness
2. False reassurance
3. Professional opinion
4. Hope and encouragement

24. A nurse is assigned to a young adult male patient. Gender sensitivity is demonstrated when the nurse:
1. Uses sexual innuendo
2. Engages in gender-oriented joking
3. Stereotypes male and female roles
4. Uses direct and indirect communication according to gender

25. A patient regularly visits a medical clinic. A nurse establishes a helping relationship with the patient. During the working phase of a helping relationship, the nurse:
1. Encourages and helps the patient to set goals
2. Reminisces about the relationship with the patient
3. Anticipates health concerns or issues
4. Identifies a location for the interaction

26. A nurse is interviewing a patient who is in the outpatient area. The nurse uses paraphrasing communication with the statement:
1. "This is your blood pressure medication. It will help to lower your blood pressure to the level where it should be."
2. "Do you mean that the pain comes and goes when you walk?"
3. "I would like to return to our discussion about your family."
4. "If I understand you correctly, you are primarily concerned about your dizzy spells."

27. A patient tells a nurse that there are other people in the room that are watching her from under the bed. The nurse employs therapeutic communication when he or she:
1. Identifies that there are no people under the bed
2. Tells the patient that he or she will help look for the other people
3. Asks the patient why other people are watching her
4. Reassures the patient that he or she will tell the people to go away

28. While speaking with a female patient, a nurse notes that she is frowning. The nurse wants to find out about possible concerns by:
1. Asking why the patient is unhappy
2. Telling the patient that everything is fine
3. Identifying that the patient is frowning
4. Asking if the patient is angry about the health care problem

29. A patient's condition has deteriorated, and he has been transferred to the intensive care unit. The roommate asks the nurse what is wrong with the patient. The nurse should respond to the roommate by stating:
1. "The patient's condition is no concern of yours."
2. "Everything is fine. Don't worry. He'll be okay."
3. "I recognize your interest in the patient, but I cannot share personal information with you without his permission."
4. "Your roommate's condition worsened overnight, and he had to be moved to the intensive care unit for observation."

30. A patient is experiencing aphasia as a result of a CVA (cerebrovascular accident, or stroke). To promote communication, a nurse plans to:
1. Speak louder
2. Use more questions
3. Use visual clues, such as pictures and gestures
4. Refer to a speech therapist to communicate with the patient

31. A patient is talking endlessly about problems in the past with arthritic pain, but the nurse needs to get specific information for the admission assessment. The nurse's best response is:
1. "You seem to have had difficulty managing the arthritis. What are you doing now for the pain?"
2. "You can tell me more at another time. We need to move on to other information now."
3. "You've given me a lot of information, but I have to ask you something else."
4. "Are you taking medication for the arthritis?"

32. A nurse enters a room and finds the patient crying. The best action by the nurse is to:
1. Ask the patient why he or she is crying
2. Tell the patient that things will get better
3. Let the patient know that you will come back later
4. Sit quietly with the patient

33. A patient has a visual impairment. In communicating with this patient, a nurse should:
1. Use flash cards
2. Use simple sentences
3. Caution the patient before any physical contact
4. Speak very loud and slow

34. A nurse tells the patient's family that recovery may be "difficult." This may lead to an issue with:
1. Pacing
2. Clarity
3. Relevance
4. Connotation

35. A cultural group that may perceive continuous eye contact as intrusive or threatening is:
1. Asian
2. Hispanic
3. African American
4. Northern European

36. A nurse is working with a preschool-age child. An appropriate communication technique to use with an individual in this age-group is to:
    1. Speak loudly and forcibly
    2. Communicate directly with the parents to determine the child's needs
    3. Sit or kneel down to be on the same level as the child
    4. Use medical terms when speaking with the parents so the child will not understand
37. A patient's blood sample was dropped on its way to the lab. The patient asks the nurse why blood needs to be drawn again for the same test. The nurse's best response is:
    1. "One of the vials was dropped and broken by mistake. We will make sure that this sample gets to the lab safely."
    2. "We just have to do the test again."
    3. "Someone didn't do their job right the first time."
    4. "This kind of thing happens. It won't take long."
38. A nurse is evaluating communication skills used during an interaction with a newly admitted patient. Of the statements made, the nurse responded therapeutically with:
    1. "Why aren't you able to keep taking the prescribed medications?"
    2. "We need to move quickly through the rest of the interview because it will be time for your therapy."
    3. "I can understand why you don't like that physician. I think you need to find another one."
    4. "I noticed that you didn't eat any of the lunch. Is there something that is bothering you?"

STUDY GROUP QUESTIONS

- What is therapeutic communication?
- What are the basic elements of communication?
- How do nurses and patients communicate verbally and nonverbally?
- What factors may influence communication?
- How may a patient's physical, psychosocial, and developmental status influence communication with the nurse?
- How is a helping relationship established with a patient?
- What are the principles/techniques of effective communication?
- How are the principles/techniques used by a nurse in a caring relationship?
- How is communication used within the steps of the nursing process?
- What are some of the barriers to effective communication, and how can they be overcome by the nurse?

STUDY CHART

Create a study chart to compare the *Components of Verbal and Nonverbal Communication* that identifies how each may influence the nurse-patient interaction (e.g., intonation).

Answers available through your instructor.

11 Patient Education

CASE STUDY

1. Your patient is a 47-year-old married woman who has gone to the medical clinic for evaluation. She has been diagnosed with hypertension and placed on an antihypertensive medication. She has no previous knowledge or experience with the diagnosis or the medication. There is a family history of coronary disease; her father died of a heart attack at 54 years old.
    a. What information about the patient may affect her motivation to learn?
    b. Formulate a teaching plan for the patient that includes goals and teaching strategies.

CHAPTER REVIEW

Match the description/definition in Column A with the correct term in Column B.

Column A
_____ 1. Expression of feelings, attitudes, opinions, and values
_____ 2. Mental state that allows for focus and comprehension of material
_____ 3. Acquiring skills
_____ 4. Intellectual behaviors, including knowledge and understanding
_____ 5. Desire to learn
_____ 6. Completion of a procedure to show competence.

Column B
a. Cognitive learning
b. Motivation
c. Attentional set
d. Affective learning
e. Return demonstration
f. Psychomotor learning

Complete the following:

7. A mild level of anxiety may motivate learning.
   True _____ False _____
8. From the following, select the appropriate topics for health education related to health maintenance and promotion and illness prevention. Select all that apply.
    a. First aid _____
    b. Occupational therapy _____
    c. Implications of noncompliance with therapy _____
    d. Hygiene _____
    e. Origin of symptoms _____
    f. Immunizations _____
    g. Self-help devices _____
    h. Surgical intervention _____
9. Identify teaching activities for a(n):
    a. Infant
    b. Toddler
    c. Preschooler
    d. School-age child
    e. Older adult

10. A learner may find it difficult to concentrate in the presence of:

11. When selecting an environment for teaching, a nurse needs to consider:

12. Written materials used for teaching a patient with limited health literacy are usually presented at the _____ grade level.

13. Teaching sessions that are usually tolerated best last for _____ minutes. In planning the teaching session, essential information should be taught _____.

14. For the nursing diagnosis *noncompliance with medication regimen related to insufficient knowledge of purpose and actions*, identify possible learning goals and outcomes and nursing interventions.

15. For the following, identify the domain of learning.
    a. Self-injection of insulin
    b. Coping with care of a family member

Copyright © 2011, 2007, 2003 by Mosby, Inc., an affiliate of Elsevier Inc. All rights reserved.

c. Aware of potential complications after a heart attack

d. Response of the family to a member's substance abuse

e. Sterile dressing technique

f. Aware of signs and symptoms of hypoglycemia

16. Identify an instructional technique that may be used in each of the following situations:
    a. A small group of patients in a cardiac rehabilitation group who need dietary information
    b. A patient with a leg cast who will be using crutches
    c. Students learning therapeutic communication skills to be used on a mental health unit

17. Explaining how a test will feel before the procedure is performed is an example of:

18. According to national reports, a total of _____ % of adults in the United States have difficulty reading and understanding health information, including pamphlets and charts.

19. A focused assessment for patient education includes:
    a.
    b.
    c.

Select the best answer for each of the following questions:

20. A nurse is preparing to teach a group of new parents about infant care. The nurse recognizes that learning can be enhanced with:
    1. Previous unfamiliarity with the topic area
    2. Fear of health outcomes
    3. Moderate discomfort
    4. Mild anxiety level

21. The patient who most likely has the greatest motivation to learn is the individual who is:
    1. Waiting for the results of diagnostic tests
    2. Hypertensive, but has no symptoms
    3. Dealing with a family conflict
    4. Recovering from reconstructive surgery

22. While preparing a teaching plan for a group of patients with diabetes, a nurse integrates the basic principle of education that:
    1. Material should progress from complex to simpler ideas
    2. Prolonged teaching sessions improve concentration and attentiveness
    3. Learning is improved when more than one body sense is stimulated
    4. Previous knowledge of a topic area interferes with the acquisition of new information

23. During a teaching session for a patient with heart disease, the nurse uses reinforcement to stimulate learning. An example of reinforcement for this patient is:
    1. Allowing the patient to manage self-care needs
    2. Teaching about the disease process while delivering nursing care
    3. Outlining the exercise plan and providing explicit instructions
    4. Complimenting the patient on his or her ability to identify the action of prescribed medications

24. After approximately 20 minutes have passed in the educational session, the nurse notices that the patient is slightly slumped in the chair and is no longer maintaining eye contact. The nurse should:
    1. Reposition the patient in the chair
    2. Move the patient to a cooler, brighter room
    3. Reschedule the remainder of the teaching for another time
    4. Continue with the teaching session in order to cover the necessary content

25. When preparing to teach the self-injection technique to a patient, the nurse begins with:
    1. Having the patient demonstrate the procedure
    2. Discussing the procedure and the equipment used
    3. Providing written materials and having the patient practice the technique
    4. Demonstrating to the patient how to perform the procedure correctly

26. After teaching a patient about a cerebrovascular accident (CVA/stroke), the nurse prepares to evaluate the patient's psychomotor domain of learning. This is accomplished by:
    1. Observing the patient use a cane to ambulate
    2. Asking the patient about the basic etiology of a stroke
    3. Determining the patient's attitudes about the treatment regimen
    4. Having the patient complete a written schedule for daily activities at home

27. When the teaching session has been completed, a nurse evaluates the patient's cognitive domain of learning to see if there are areas that require additional instruction. The nurse evaluates the patient's ability to:
    1. Perform the range-of-motion exercises independently
    2. Identify the equipment necessary for surgical wound care
    3. Demonstrate the proper use of crutches to ambulate up and down stairs
    4. Discuss concerns about the difficulty in maintaining accurate records of the treatments

28. Which patient appears to be demonstrating the greatest readiness to learn? The patient who says:
    1. "There's nothing wrong with me."
    2. "I think the doctor made a mistake."
    3. "I can manage on my own."
    4. "What do I need to know about this?"
29. A type of reinforcer that works well with children is:
    1. Material
    2. Social
    3. Activity
    4. Negative
30. A nurse recognizes that the most effective teaching strategy for a patient in the acceptance stage is to:
    1. Share small bits of information
    2. Introduce only reality
    3. Provide simple explanations while doing care
    4. Focus on future skills and knowledge

STUDY GROUP QUESTIONS

- What are the standards (e.g., The Joint Commission) for patient education?
- How does patient education promote, maintain, and restore health?
- What are the principles of teaching and learning?
- What factors may influence a patient's ability to learn?
- How does an individual's developmental status influence the selection of teaching methodologies?
- How does the teaching process compare with the communication and nursing processes?
- How does the nurse develop a teaching plan for a patient?
- What teaching approaches and instructional methods may be used by a nurse?
- How is patient education documented?

Answers available through your instructor.

Managing Patient Care 12

CASE STUDIES

1. As a nurse working on a busy surgical unit, this evening you have eight postoperative patients assigned to you.
   a. What types of activities could be delegated to an unlicensed nursing assistant?
   b. What determination do you need to make before safely delegating activities to the nursing assistant?
2. As a nurse on the surgical unit, you will be involved in identifying quality improvement (QI) projects.
   a. What possible areas could be important to the nurses and patients on this unit?
3. A friend tells you that she is interested in becoming a nurse practitioner. She has started to take general courses at a 4-year university that has a nursing program.
   a. What information can you provide to this individual about the preparation for this career role?

CHAPTER REVIEW

Complete the following:

1. Upon completion of a RN or LPN/LVN program, the graduate nurse must pass the:

2. A person who is reasonably independent and self-governing in decision-making and practice is demonstrating:

3. The five rights of delegation are:

4. Provide the correct term for the following definitions:
   a. Duties and activities an individual is employed to perform:
   b. Official power to act:
   c. Being answerable for one's actions:

5. The Standards of Professional Performance and the Standards of Practice were published by the _____.
6. Provide at least one example of how staff members can be actively involved when decentralized decision-making exists on a nursing unit:

Select the best answer for each of the following questions:

7. A student nurse is working with a patient who has begun to have respiratory difficulty. It is the student nurse's initial responsibility to:
   1. Call the pharmacy
   2. Alert the primary nurse
   3. Contact the attending physician
   4. Administer the prescribed medication
8. The nurses on a medical unit are discussing plans to change the focus of the unit to the primary nursing care model. With this model, the assignment for nurse A is:
   1. Mrs. J., Mrs. R., and Mrs. T. for the length of their stays
   2. To receive reports from the nursing assistant on the care of Mrs. J., Mrs. R., and Mrs. T.
   3. Side 1 of the unit in cooperation with nurse B and the nursing assistant
   4. Medication administration for all of the patients on the unit while nurse B does the physical care with the nursing assistant
9. A nurse in the long-term care facility is delegating care to the nursing assistant. It is appropriate for the nurse to delegate the care of the patient who requires:
   1. Catheter care
   2. An admission history
   3. Administration of oral medications
   4. Vital sign measurements after episodes of arrhythmias
10. A student nurse is assigned to care for a patient in the hospital. While taking the patient's vital signs, the student cannot obtain the blood pressure reading after two attempts. The student should:
    1. Keep trying to get the blood pressure measurement
    2. Use the closest measurement to the last reading
    3. Ask another nurse to obtain the blood pressure measurement
    4. Inform the instructor about the difficulty and request assistance

11. A nurse is working with a patient who has just returned from surgery. The nurse has no experience working with the patient's postoperative surgical dressing. During an assessment, the nurse notices that the dressing has come loose and has fallen away from the surgical wound. The patient tells the nurse, "Oh, you can fix it." The nurse:
    1. Asks the patient to help replace the dressing
    2. Replaces the loosened dressing as best as possible
    3. Asks the surgeon to replace the dressing
    4. Covers the wound with a sterile dry dressing until assistance is obtained
12. A nurse has been assigned to work on a very busy medical unit in the hospital. It is important for the nurse to employ time management skills. The nurse implements a plan to:
    1. Have all the patients' major needs met in the morning hours
    2. Anticipate possible interruptions by therapists and visitors
    3. Complete assessments and treatments for each patient at different times each day
    4. Leave each day unstructured to allow for changes in treatments and patient assignments
13. One specific measurement criterion for the standard of "quality of practice" is:
    1. Using creativity to improve nursing care delivery
    2. Discussing concerns with fellow staff members
    3. Attending workshops on new technologies
    4. Speaking on behalf of the patient's family and their concerns
14. A medical unit in an acute care facility is experiencing a staffing shortage. In conjunction with the unit manager, the staff members decide that nurse A will administer all medications, nurse B will complete all treatments, and nurse C will perform vital sign measurements and patient teaching. This is an example of:
    1. Functional nursing
    2. Primary nursing
    3. Total patient care
    4. Team nursing
15. One specific measurement criterion for the standard of practice of "collegiality" is:
    1. Seeking experiences to maintain clinical skills
    2. Contributing to a healthy work environment
    3. Assigning tasks based on patient needs
    4. Serving as a patient advocate
16. A student nurse has a multiple patient assignment. In reviewing the report obtained from the primary nurse, the student should decide to see which patient first? The patient who is:
    1. Experiencing nausea
    2. Asking for a bedpan
    3. Having a severe anxiety attack
    4. Thirsty and wants another drink with breakfast

STUDY GROUP QUESTIONS

- What are the applications of theoretical models in nursing?
- What are the standards of practice and standards of care?
- How do nurse practice acts influence nursing, including entry into practice, licensure, and role?
- What are the different types of nursing education programs and the preparation required of their graduates?
- To whom may a nurse delegate care responsibilities? What types of responsibilities may be delegated legally and safely?
- What does an advanced practice nurse require in education and experience?
- How does the nurse manager function within the health care team?
- How do the different types of nursing care delivery models differ from one another?
- What is quality improvement (QI), and what does it mean to nurses?
- How are QI processes and results communicated to other members of the health care team?
- What are some of the challenges for nurses and nursing in the future?

STUDY CHART

Create a study chart to compare and contrast the different *Nursing Care Delivery Models*.

Answers available through your instructor.

Infection Prevention and Control   13

CASE STUDIES

1. An 86-year-old woman in an extended care facility has a urinary catheter attached to a drainage system.
   a. What precautions should be taken for this patient to prevent a urinary tract infection?
2. Yesterday a 45-year-old man had abdominal surgery. He has a large midline abdominal incision covered by a sterile dressing. He will require dressing changes twice daily.
   a. What precautions should be taken for this patient to prevent wound infection?
3. An 85-year-old man requires isolation precautions. He is oriented to his surroundings and is concerned about whether his family will be able to visit him.
   a. What specific nursing care should be implemented for this patient?

CHAPTER REVIEW

Match the description/definition in Column A with the correct term in Column B.

Column A

____ 1. Arises from microorganisms outside the patient
____ 2. Cellular response to injury or infection
____ 3. Microorganisms that cause another infection because they are resistant to antibiotics
____ 4. Infection that developed that was not present at the time of patient admission
____ 5. Methods to reduce or eliminate disease-producing microorganisms
____ 6. Microorganisms that do not cause disease but help to maintain health
____ 7. Process that eliminates all forms of microbial life
____ 8. Disease-producing microorganism
____ 9. Substance formed through the inflammatory process that may ooze from openings in the skin or mucous membranes
____ 10. Microorganism that grows but does not cause disease
____ 11. Ability of microorganisms to produce disease
____ 12. Being more than normally vulnerable to a disease
____ 13. Alteration of a patient's flora with a resulting overgrowth

Column B

a. Exudate
b. Aseptic technique
c. Health care–associated infection
d. Sterilization
e. Colonization
f. Inflammation
g. Flora
h. Pathogen
i. Endogenous infection
j. Suprainfection
k. Exogenous infection
l. Virulence
m. Susceptibility

Complete the following:

14. Identify whether the following are performed using sterile technique in an acute care environment:
    a. Hand hygiene ____
    b. Postoperative dressing change ____
    c. Urinary catheter insertion ____
    d. Barrier precautions ____
    e. Intramuscular injection ____
15. An outcome for a patient with a 3-cm-diameter wound is:

16. Immunizations are available for which of the following? Select all that apply.

    a. Hepatitis A ____
    b. Diphtheria ____
    c. Rubella ____
    d. Tuberculosis ____
    e. AIDS ____
    f. Varicella ____

17. For the following, select all actions that require that equipment be discarded and/or the sterile field be re-done.
    a. A mask is worn when opening the sterile tray. ____
    b. The sterile dressing package is torn. ____
    c. The tip of the sterile syringe touches the surface of a clean, disposable glove. ____

CHAPTER 13 • Infection Prevention and Control

   d. A sterile basin is held out over the sterile field. _____
   e. A cup on the sterile field is touched with a sterile gloved hand. _____
   f. Sterile dressings are placed within the 1-inch edge of the sterile field. _____
18. Identify specific actions that a nurse can implement to interrupt the chain of infection.
    a. Control or eliminate the infectious agent:
    b. Control or eliminate the reservoir:
    c. Control the portals of exit:
    d. Control transmission:
    e. Control susceptibility of host:
19. What results would be expected for the following laboratory studies in the presence of an infection?
    a. WBC count
    b. Erythrocyte sedimentation rate
    c. Iron level
    d. Neutrophils
    e. Basophils
20. Health care–acquired infections can be reduced by:
21. A patient's gastrointestinal defenses against infection are altered by:
22. Select all the appropriate techniques for isolation precautions.
    a. Wash hands in the clean utility room after patient care. _____
    b. Provide for the patient's sensory needs during care. _____
    c. Prevent visitors from entering the patient's room. _____
    d. Keep face mask below the level of eyeglasses or goggles. _____
    e. Place disposable items in paper bags. _____
    f. Maintain each patient's personal protective equipment (PPE) within the patient's room. _____
    g. Keep PPE at the door to the room or in an anteroom area. _____
23. Handling of biohazardous waste includes:
24. Specify the order in which the following PPE should be applied before entering an isolation room:
    a. Mask _____
    b. Gloves _____
    c. Gown _____
25. If a mask, gown, and gloves are worn into an isolation room, the first item of PPE that is removed when exiting the room is/are the:
26. Select all of the following in which appropriate asepsis has occurred:
    a. Handling a sterile dressing with clean gloves _____
    b. Holding a sterile bowl above waist level using sterile gloves _____
    c. Keeping the hands above the elbows after a surgical scrub _____
    d. Turning away from and placing one's back to the sterile field _____
    e. Talking or coughing over the sterile field _____
    f. Discarding sterile packages that are wet _____
    g. Placing objects to the edge of the sterile field _____
    h. Discarding a small amount of solution before pouring the remainder into a sterile container on the field _____
27. For the nursing diagnosis *impaired skin integrity, related to 2-inch-diameter pressure ulcer on sacrum*, identify a patient goal, objectives, and nursing interventions.
28. Number the flaps on the sterile package in the figure according to which should be opened first, second, and last.

29. Proper disposal of contaminated sharps includes:
30. Provide an example of how the nurse needs to be aware of his or her own breaks in aseptic technique.

31. What equipment is needed to collect a urine specimen from the patient with an indwelling urinary catheter?

32. Select all of the following actions that are appropriate for hand hygiene.
    a. Cleaning under artifical nails _____
    b. Removing rings during washing _____
    c. Leaning against the sink _____
    d. Keeping the water temperature hot _____
    e. Washing the hands for at least 15 seconds _____
    f. Turning off the faucet with the elbows _____
    g. Keeping hands and forearms lower than the elbows during washing _____
    h. Drying from the forearms to the fingers _____

Select the best answer for each of the following questions:

33. At the community health fair, a nurse is asked by one of the residents about the influenza vaccine. The nurse responds to the resident that the influenza vaccine is recommended for individuals who are:
    1. Health care workers
    2. Traveling to other countries
    3. Younger than 6 years of age
    4. Between 40 and 65 years of age

34. A nurse is preparing a room for a patient with tuberculosis. The specific aspect for this tier of Standard Precautions that is different than tier 1 is that the care should include:
    1. A private room with negative air flow
    2. Hand hygiene after gloves are removed
    3. Eye protection if splashing is possible
    4. Disposal of sharps in a puncture-resistant container

35. A nurse is preparing a teaching plan for patients about the hepatitis B virus. The nurse informs them that this virus may be transmitted by:
    1. Mosquitoes
    2. Droplet nuclei
    3. Blood products
    4. Improperly handled food

36. A nurse is working on a unit with a number of patients who have infectious diseases. One of the most important methods for reducing the spread of microorganisms is:
    1. Sterilization of equipment
    2. The use of gloves and gowns
    3. Maintenance of isolation precautions
    4. Hand hygiene before and after patient care

37. The assignment today for a nurse includes a patient with tuberculosis. In caring for a patient on droplet precautions, the nurse should routinely use:
    1. Regular masks and eyewear
    2. Regular masks, gowns, and gloves
    3. Surgical hand hygiene and gloves
    4. Particulate filtration masks and gowns

38. A nurse is caring for a patient who has a large abdominal wound that requires a sterile saline soak and dressing. While performing the care, the nurse drops the saline-soaked 4 × 4 gauze near the wound on the patient's abdomen. The nurse:
    1. Discontinues the procedure
    2. Throws the gauze away and prepares a new 4 × 4 gauze
    3. Picks up the 4 × 4 with sterile forceps and places it on the wound
    4. Rinses the 4 × 4 with saline and places it on the wound using sterile gloves

39. A nurse is checking the laboratory results of a male patient admitted to the medical unit. The nurse is alerted to the presence of an infectious process based on the finding of:
    1. Iron: 80 g/100 mL
    2. Neutrophils: 65%
    3. Erythrocyte sedimentation rate (ESR): 13 mm per hour
    4. White blood cells (WBC): 16,000/mm^3

40. The individual most at risk for a latex allergy is the patient with a history of:
    1. Hypertension
    2. Congenital heart disease
    3. Diabetes mellitus
    4. Cholecystitis

41. A nurse is working with a patient who has a deep laceration to the right lower extremity. To reduce a possible reservoir of infection, the nurse:
    1. Wears gloves and a mask at all times
    2. Isolates the patient's personal articles
    3. Has the patient cover the mouth and nose when coughing
    4. Changes the dressing to the extremity when it becomes soiled

42. A nurse implements droplet precautions for the patient with:
    1. Pulmonary tuberculosis
    2. Varicella
    3. Rubella
    4. Herpes

43. A patient who has had a transplant will require what type of isolation?
    1. Contact
    2. Airborne
    3. Droplet
    4. Protective

44. For a patient with hepatitis A, the nurse is aware that the disease is transmitted through:
    1. Feces
    2. Blood
    3. Skin
    4. Droplet nuclei

45. A sign that is indicative of a systemic infection resulting from a wound is:
    1. Redness
    2. Drainage
    3. Edema
    4. Fever
46. There are small open wounds on the hands of the nurse. The nurse's most appropriate action is:
    1. Asking to work at the nurse's station for the day
    2. Using clean, disposable gloves for patient care
    3. Applying antibacterial ointment before patient contact
    4. Providing patient care as usual and washing the hands more frequently
47. A nurse is aware that older adults are more susceptible to infection as a result of:
    1. Thickening of the dermal and epidermal skin layers
    2. Increased production of T lymphocytes
    3. Increased production of digestive juices
    4. Drying of the oral mucosa

STUDY GROUP QUESTIONS

- What is the nature of the infectious process?
- What are the components of the chain of infection?
- What are the body's normal defenses against infection?
- What is a health care–associated infection, who are the patients at risk, and how can a nurse prevent this infection?
- How is the nursing process applied to infection control in the acute, extended care, and home care environments?
- What nursing measures may be implemented to prevent or control the spread of infection?
- What is included in Standard Precautions?
- What information may be taught to the patient and the patient's family for prevention or control of infectious processes?
- How does the nurse perform the procedures that are important for infection control?

Answers available through your instructor.

CHAPTER 13 • Infection Prevention and Control

Name _____ Date _____ Instructor's Name _____

Procedural Guidelines 13-1: Hand Hygiene

	S	U	NP	Comments

1. Inspect surface of hands for breaks or cuts in skin or cuticles. ___ ___ ___ _____
2. Note condition of nails. Nails should be short, filed, and smooth. Avoid artificial nails and long or unkempt nails that may harbor microbes. Your agency may ban these depending upon its policy. Cover any skin lesions before providing patient care. ___ ___ ___ _____
3. Inspect hands for visible soiling. ___ ___ ___ _____
4. Push wristwatch and long uniform sleeves above wrists. Remove rings before hand washing. ___ ___ ___ _____
5. Perform hand hygiene using antiseptic hand wash or hand rub.
    A. If using antiseptic hand rub, dispense ample amount of product into palm of one hand. ___ ___ ___ _____
    B. Rub hands together, covering all surfaces with antiseptic. ___ ___ ___ _____
    C. Rub hands together until the alcohol is dry. Allow hands to dry before applying gloves. ___ ___ ___ _____
6. If using regular lotion soap or antimicrobial soap and water, stand in front of sink, keeping hands and uniform away from sink surface. (If hands touch sink during hand washing, repeat.)
    A. Turn faucet on or push knee pedals laterally, or press pedals with foot to regulate flow and temperature. ___ ___ ___ _____
    B. Avoid splashing water against uniform. ___ ___ ___ _____
    C. Regulate flow of water so that temperature is warm. ___ ___ ___ _____
    D. Wet hands and wrists thoroughly under running water. Keep hands and forearms lower than elbows during washing. ___ ___ ___ _____
    E. Apply a small amount of soap or antiseptic. Lather thoroughly. Soap granules and leaflet preparations are an option. ___ ___ ___ _____
    F. Perform hand hygiene using plenty of lather and friction for at least 15 seconds. Interlace fingers and rub palms and back of hands with circular motion at least 5 times each. Keep fingertips down. ___ ___ ___ _____
    G. Clean areas under fingernails with the fingernails of other hand and additional soap, or clean with orangewood stick. ___ ___ ___ _____
    H. Rinse hands and wrists thoroughly, keeping hands down and elbows up. ___ ___ ___ _____
    I. Dry hands thoroughly from fingers to wrists and forearms with paper towel, single-use cloth, or warm air dryer. ___ ___ ___ _____
    J. If paper towel is used, discard in proper receptacle. ___ ___ ___ _____
    K. To turn off hand faucet, use clean, dry paper towel, avoiding touching handles with hands. Turn off water with foot or knee pedals (if applicable). ___ ___ ___ _____
    L. Apply lotion to hands. ___ ___ ___ _____

Copyright © 2011, 2007, 2003 by Mosby, Inc., an affiliate of Elsevier Inc. All rights reserved.

CHAPTER 13 • Infection Prevention and Control

Name _____ Date _____ Instructor's Name _____

Procedural Guidelines 13-2: Caring for a Patient on Isolation Precautions

	S	U	NP	Comments
1. Assess isolation indications.	____	____	____	_____
2. Review agency policies and nursing considerations for the specific isolation system.	____	____	____	_____
3. Review nurses' notes or confer with colleagues regarding patient's emotional state and adjustment to isolation.	____	____	____	_____
4. Perform hand hygiene, and prepare all equipment to be taken into patient's room.	____	____	____	_____
5. Prepare for entrance into isolation room.				
A. Apply cover gown, being sure it covers all outer garments. Pull sleeves down to wrists. Tie securely at neck and waist.	____	____	____	_____
B. Apply either surgical mask or respirator around mouth and nose.	____	____	____	_____
C. Apply eyewear or goggles snugly around face and eyes (when needed).	____	____	____	_____
D. Apply clean gloves. Bring glove cuffs over edge of gown sleeves.	____	____	____	_____
6. Enter patient's room. Arrange supplies and equipment.	____	____	____	_____
7. Explain purpose of isolation and necessary precautions to patient and family. Offer opportunity to ask questions. Assess for evidence of emotional problems caused by isolation.	____	____	____	_____
8. Assess vital signs.				
A. If patient is infected or colonized with a resistant organism, equipment remains in room. This includes stethoscope and BP cuff.	____	____	____	_____
B. If you reuse the stethoscope, clean diaphragm or bell with 70% alcohol. Set aside on clean surface.	____	____	____	_____
C. Use disposable thermometer.	____	____	____	_____
9. Administer medications:				
A. Give oral medication in wrapper or cup.	____	____	____	_____
B. Dispose of wrapper or cup in plastic-lined receptacle.	____	____	____	_____
C. Administer injection, being sure to wear gloves.	____	____	____	_____
D. Discard syringe and uncapped needle or sheathed needle into sharps container.	____	____	____	_____
E. Place a reusable syringe (e.g., Carpuject) on clean towel for eventual removal and disinfection.	____	____	____	_____
F. If you do not wear gloves and hands contact contaminated article or body fluids, perform hand hygiene as soon as possible.	____	____	____	_____
10. Administer hygiene encouraging patient to discuss questions or concerns about isolation.				
A. Avoid allowing gown to become wet. Carry washbasin out away from gown, avoid leaning against any wet surface.	____	____	____	_____
B. Remove linen from bed. If excessively soiled, avoid contact with gown. Place in leak-proof linen bag.	____	____	____	_____
C. Change gloves and perform hand hygiene as necessary.	____	____	____	_____
11. Collect specimens:				
A. Place specimen containers on clean paper towel in patient's bathroom.	____	____	____	_____

CHAPTER 13 • Infection Prevention and Control

	S	U	NP	Comments

B. Follow procedure for collecting specimen of body fluids. ___ ___ ___ _____

C. Transfer specimen to container without soiling outside of container. Place container in plastic bag and place label on outside of bag or as per facility policy. ___ ___ ___ _____

D. Perform hand hygiene and reglove if additional procedures are needed. ___ ___ ___ _____

E. Check label on specimen for accuracy. Send to laboratory. Label containers with a biohazard label (see illustration). ___ ___ ___ _____

12. Dispose of linen and trash bags as they become full:
   A. Use sturdy, moisture-impervious single bags to contain soiled articles. Use double bag if outside of bag is contaminated. ___ ___ ___ _____
   B. Tie bags securely in a knot at top. ___ ___ ___ _____
   C. Remove all reusable equipment. Clean any contaminated surfaces (check health care facility or agency policy). ___ ___ ___ _____

13. Resupply room as needed. ___ ___ ___ _____

14. Explain to patient when you plan to return to room. Ask whether patient requires any personal care items, books, or magazines. ___ ___ ___ _____

15. Leave isolation room. The order for removing PPE depends on what was needed for the type of isolation. The sequence listed is based on full PPE being required.
   A. Remove gloves. Remove one glove by grasping cuff and pulling glove inside out over hand. Hold removed glove in glove hand. With ungloved hand, slide finger inside cuff of remaining glove at wrist. Pull glove off over first glove. Discard gloves in proper container. ___ ___ ___ _____
   B. Remove eyewear or goggles by handling at headband or earpieces. Discard in proper container. ___ ___ ___ _____
   C. Untie neck strings and then back strings of gown. Allow gown to fall from shoulders. Remove hands from sleeves without touching outside of gown. Hold gown inside at shoulder seams and fold inside out. Discard in laundry bag if fabric or in trash can if gown is disposable. ___ ___ ___ _____
   D. Remove mask. If mask loops over your ears, remove from ears and pull away from face. For a tie-on mask, untie *bottom* mask strings and then top strings. Hold top strings and pull mask away from face, and drop into trash receptacle. Do not touch outer surface of mask. ___ ___ ___ _____
   E. Perform hand hygiene. ___ ___ ___ _____
   F. Leave room and close door, if necessary. (Close door if patient is on airborne precautions.) ___ ___ ___ _____
   G. Dispose of all contaminated supplies and equipment in a manner that prevents spread of microorganisms to other persons (check agency policy). ___ ___ ___ _____

Name _____ Date _____ Instructor's Name _____

Procedural Guidelines 13-3: Applying a Surgical Type of Mask

	S	U	NP	Comments
1. Find top edge of mask. Pliable metal fits snugly against bridge of nose.	___	___	___	_____
2. Hold mask by top two strings or loops. Tie the two top ties at top of back of head, with ties above ears. (*Alternative:* slip loops over each ear.)	___	___	___	_____
3. Tie two lower strings snugly around neck with mask well under chin.	___	___	___	_____
4. Gently pinch upper metal band around bridge of nose.	___	___	___	_____

NOTE: Change mask if it is wet, moist, or contaminated.

CHAPTER 13 • Infection Prevention and Control

Name _____ Date _____ Instructor's Name _____

Procedural Guidelines 13-4: Putting on Sterile Gloves

	S	U	NP	Comments
1. Consider the procedure you will perform, and consult agency policy on use of gloves.	___	___	___	_____
2. Inspect hands for cuts, open lesions, or abrasions. Cover with an occlusive dressing before gloving.	___	___	___	_____
3. Assess if the patient or health care worker has a known allergy to latex.	___	___	___	_____
4. Determine correct glove size and type of glove you will use.	___	___	___	_____
5. Examine glove package to ensure it is not wet, torn, or discolored.	___	___	___	_____
6. Perform thorough hand hygiene.	___	___	___	_____
7. Remove outer glove package wrapper by carefully separating and peeling apart sides.	___	___	___	_____
8. Grasp inner package and lay it on clean, flat surface just above waist level. Open package, keeping gloves on wrapper's inside surface.	___	___	___	_____
9. Identify right and left gloves. Each glove has a cuff approximately 5 cm (2 inches) wide. Glove dominant hand first.	___	___	___	_____
10. With thumb and first two fingers of nondominant hand, grasp edge of cuff of the glove for the dominant hand. Touch only glove's inside surface.	___	___	___	_____
11. Carefully pull glove over dominant hand, leaving a cuff and being sure the cuff does not roll up wrist. Be sure thumb and fingers are in proper spaces.	___	___	___	_____
12. With gloved dominant hand, slip fingers underneath second glove's cuff. Carefully pull second glove over nondominant hand. Do not allow fingers and thumb of gloved dominant hand to touch any part of exposed nondominant hand. Keep thumb of dominant hand abducted.	___	___	___	_____
13. After second glove is on, interlock hands. Cuffs usually fall down after application. Be sure to touch only sterile sides.	___	___	___	_____

Name _____ Date _____ Instructor's Name _____

Procedural Guidelines 13-5: Opening Wrapped Sterile Items

	S	U	NP	Comments

1. Place sterile kit or package containing sterile items on clean, dry, flat work surface above waist level.
2. Open outside cover, and remove kit from dust cover. Place on work surface.
3. Grasp outer surface of tip of outermost flap.
4. Open outermost flap away from body, keeping arm outstretched and away from sterile field.
5. Grasp outside surface of edge of first side of flap.
6. Open side flap, pulling to side, allowing it to lie flat on table surface. Keep your arm to side and not over sterile surface. Do not allow flaps to spring back over sterile contents.
7. Repeat steps for second side flap.
8. Grasp outside border of last and innermost flap.
9. Stand away from sterile package and pull flap back, allowing it to fall flat on table.
10. Use the sterile inner surface of the package (except for the 1-inch border around the edges) as a field to add additional items. Grasp the 1-inch border to move the field over the work surface.

CHAPTER 13 • Infection Prevention and Control

Name _____ Date _____ Instructor's Name _____

Procedural Guidelines 13-6: Preparation of a Sterile Field

	S	U	NP	Comments
1. Perform hand hygiene.	___	___	___	_____
2. Place pack containing sterile drape on work surface and open.	___	___	___	_____
3. Apply sterile gloves (*optional;* see agency policy).	___	___	___	_____
4. With fingertips of one hand, pick up the folded top edge of the sterile drape along the 1-inch border.	___	___	___	_____
5. Gently lift the drape up from its outer cover and let it unfold by itself without touching any object. Keep it above the waist. Discard the outer cover with the other hand.	___	___	___	_____
6. With the other hand, grasp an adjacent corner of the drape and hold it straight up and away from the body.	___	___	___	_____
7. Holding the drape, first position and lay the bottom half over the intended work surface.	___	___	___	_____
8. Allow the top half of the drape to be placed over the work surface last.	___	___	___	_____
9. Grasp the 1-inch border around the edge to position as needed.	___	___	___	_____

14 Vital Signs

CASE STUDIES

1. You are volunteering at a community health fair. You have been asked to take blood pressure (BP) readings for the residents participating in the event.
   a. What blood pressure readings indicate that follow-up care should be recommended?
   b. What other information may be obtained from a patient while taking the blood pressure reading?
2. You are assigned to an orthopedic unit in the medical center. A patient was involved in an automobile accident and has bilateral casts on the upper arms.
   a. How will you obtain the patient's pulse rate and blood pressure?
3. You have just started your shift at the extended care facility. The nurse reporting off identifies that one of your assigned patents is febrile.
   a. What signs and symptoms do you expect to find with a patient who is febrile?
   b. What interventions are indicated for febrile patients?
4. A postoperative patient is being monitored with pulse oximetry. You are checking the reading, but the device does not appear to be working.
   a. What "troubleshooting" can you perform to determine if the pulse oximeter is working properly?

CHAPTER REVIEW

Match the description/definition in Column A with the correct term in Column B.

Column A

____ 1. Decrease of systolic and diastolic pressures below normal
____ 2. Another word for fever
____ 3. Rate and depth of respirations increase
____ 4. Widening of blood vessels
____ 5. Pulse rate less than 60 beats per minute for an adult
____ 6. 140/90 mm Hg for two or more readings
____ 7. Rate of breathing abnormally rapid
____ 8. Decreased body temperature
____ 9. No respirations for several seconds
____ 10. Rate of breathing abnormally slow
____ 11. Normal breathing
____ 12. Temporary disappearance of sounds between Korotkoff sounds

Column B

a. Tachypnea
b. Bradypnea
c. Hypothermia
d. Apnea
e. Bradycardia
f. Hypotension
g. Hyperventilation
h. Hypertension
i. Vasodilation
j. Febrile
k. Auscultatory gap
l. Eupnea

CHAPTER 14 • Vital Signs

Complete the following:

13. Convert the following temperature readings:
    a. 97° F = _____ ° C
    b. 38.4° C = _____ ° F
    c. 102° F = _____ ° C
    d. 39.4° C = _____ ° F
14. What readings on Fahrenheit and centigrade thermometers should alert the nurse to an alteration in the patient's temperature regulation?

15. Indicate on the model where the following pulses should be palpated:

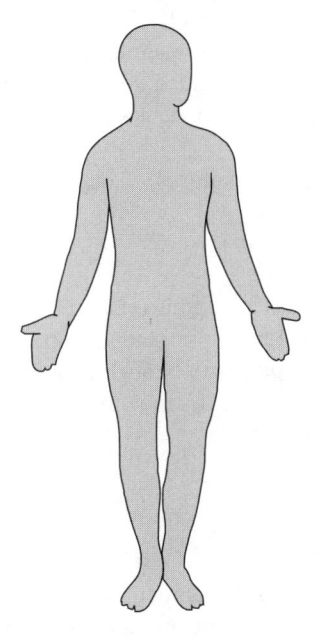

    a. Carotid
    b. Brachial
    c. Radial
    d. Apical
    e. Dorsalis pedis

16. Indicate on the aneroid scale where the following blood pressure reading would be noted:
    a. Korotkoff sounds first heard at 164 mm Hg and inaudible at 92 mm Hg

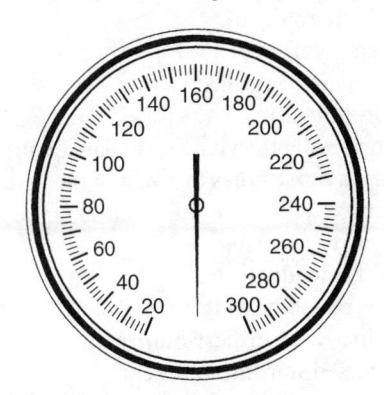

17. Vital sign measurements may not be delegated to unlicensed assistive personnel.
    True _____ False _____
18. Identify the interventions that will reduce body temperature in the following ways:
    a. Conduction:

    b. Convection:

19. A patient is on isolation precautions and temperature measurements are being used to monitor the status of the fever. The thermometer of choice in this situation is a(n):

20. A nurse identifies a pulse deficit. How was this assessed?

21. For a patient who has had a right mastectomy, the nurse should take the blood pressure:

22. Vital signs are usually recorded on the:

23. Decreasing hemoglobin levels will _____ the respiratory rate.
24. To obtain arterial oxygen saturation for an adult patient, the pulse oximeter may be applied to:

25. The expected SpO$_2$ level is:

26. Which of the following are correct for blood pressure measurement? Select all that apply.
    a. The cuff is 40% of the circumference of the limb being used. _____
    b. The bladder encircles 50% of the arm of an adult. _____
    c. The cuff is deflated at a rate of 2 to 3 mm Hg per second. _____
    d. The arm is kept below the level of the heart. _____
    e. The cuff is inflated to 30 mm Hg above the point where the pulse disappears. _____
    f. The systolic blood pressure is identified as the first onset of Korotkoff sounds. _____
    g. A difference of 30 mm Hg is expected between the left and right arm measurements. _____
27. A nurse is preparing to take the patient's oral temperature, but discovers that he has just had a cup of coffee. The appropriate action is to:

28. Identify a situation when a patient's blood pressure may need to be palpated.

29. How are the following vital signs measured differently in children?
    a. Temperature:

    b. Blood pressure:

30. Which of the following are correct techniques for a tympanic temperature measurement? Select all that apply.
    a. Using the right ear if the patient has been lying on his/her left side in bed. _____
    b. Pointing the probe midpoint between the eyebrows and sideburns for children younger than 3 years of age. _____
    c. Pulling the ear pinna backward and down for an adult. _____
    d. Moving the thermometer back and forth a little during the assessment. _____
    e. Fitting the speculum tip loosely into the ear canal _____
    f. Waiting 2 to 3 minutes before repeating the measurement in the same ear. _____

31. A patient's pulse is expected to be increased in the presence of which of the following factors? Select all that apply.
    a. Anxiety _____
    b. Hypothermia _____
    c. Unrelieved severe pain _____
    d. Presence of asthma _____
    e. Hemorrhage _____
    f. Administration of beta blockers _____

Select the best answer for each of the following questions:

32. A nurse is working on a pediatric unit and assessing the vital signs of an infant admitted for gastroenteritis. The nurse expects that the vital signs are normally the following (BP is blood pressure in units of mm Hg, P is pulse rate in units of beats per minute, and R is respirations in units of breaths per minute):
    1. BP = 90/50, P = 122, R = 46
    2. BP = 90/60, P = 80, R = 20
    3. BP = 100/60, P = 140, R = 32
    4. BP = 110/50, P = 98, R = 40

33. While working in an extended care facility, a nurse expects the vital signs of an older adult patient to be:
    1. BP = 98/70, P = 60, R = 12
    2. BP = 120/60, P = 110, R = 30
    3. BP = 140/90, P = 74, R = 14
    4. BP = 150/100, P = 90, R = 25

34. A student nurse is taking vital signs for her assigned patients on the surgical unit. The student is aware that a patient's body temperature may be reduced after:
    1. Exercise
    2. Emotional stress
    3. Periods of sleep
    4. Cigarette smoking

35. While working in an emergency department, a nurse is carefully monitoring the vital signs of the patients who have been admitted. The nurse is alert to the potential for a decrease in a patient's pulse rate as a result of:
    1. Hemorrhage
    2. Hypothyroidism
    3. Respiratory difficulty
    4. Epinephrine (adrenaline) administration

36. A patient is being treated for hyperthermia. The nurse anticipates that the patient's response to this condition will be:
    1. Generalized pallor
    2. Bradycardia
    3. Reduced thirst
    4. Diaphoresis

37. Several friends have gone on a ski trip and have been exposed to very cold temperatures. One of the individuals appears to be slightly hypothermic. The best initial response by the nurse in the ski lodge is to give this individual:
    1. Soup
    2. Coffee
    3. Cocoa
    4. Brandy

38. When checking the temperature of a patient, a nurse notes that he is febrile. An antipyretic medication is ordered. The nurse prepares to administer:
    1. Digoxin
    2. Prednisone
    3. Theophylline
    4. Acetaminophen

39. A nurse has been assigned a number of different patients in the long-term care unit. When taking vital signs, the nurse is alert to the greater possibility of tachycardia for the patient with:
    1. Anemia
    2. Hypothyroidism
    3. A temperature of 95° F
    4. A patient-controlled analgesic (PCA) pump with morphine drip

40. While reviewing the vital signs taken by the aide this morning, a nurse notes that one of the patients is hypotensive. The nurse will be checking to see if the patient is experiencing:
    1. Lightheadedness
    2. A decreased heart rate
    3. An increased urinary output
    4. Increased warmth to the skin

41. Vital sign measurements have been completed on all assigned patients. The nurse will need to immediately report a finding of:
    1. Pulse pressure of 40 mm Hg
    2. Apical pulses of 78, 80, 76 beats per minute
    3. Apical pulse of 82 beats per minute; radial pulse of 70 beats per minute
    4. BP of 140/80 mm Hg left arm, 136/74 mm Hg right arm
42. A nurse is preparing to take vital signs for the patients on the acute care unit. A tympanic temperature assessment is indicated for the patient:
    1. After rectal surgery
    2. Wearing a hearing aid
    3. Experiencing otitis media
    4. After an exercise session
43. Blood pressure monitoring is being conducted on a cardiac care unit. The nurse is determining whether an automatic blood pressure device is indicated for use. This device is selected for the patient with:
    1. An irregular heartbeat
    2. Parkinson disease
    3. Peripheral vascular disease
    4. A systolic blood pressure greater than 140 mm/Hg
44. A 34-year-old patient has gone to a physician's office for an annual physical examination. The nurse is completing the vital signs before the patient is seen by the physician. The nurse alerts the physician to a finding of:
    1. T: 37.6° C
    2. P: 120 beats per minute
    3. R: 18 breaths per minute
    4. BP: 116/78 mm Hg
45. A nurse is assigned to the well-child center that is affiliated with the acute care facility. A mother takes her 1 1/2-year-old son to the center for his immunizations. The nurse assesses the child's pulse rate by checking the:
    1. Radial artery
    2. Apical artery
    3. Popliteal artery
    4. Femoral artery
46. A nurse determines that a patient's pulse rate is significantly lower than it has been during the past week. The nurse reassesses and finds that the pulse rate is still 46 beats per minute. The nurse should first:
    1. Document the measurement
    2. Administer a stimulant medication
    3. Inform the charge nurse or physician
    4. Apply 100% oxygen at maximum flow rate
47. The most important sign of heat stroke is:
    1. Hot, dry skin
    2. Nausea
    3. Excessive thirst
    4. Muscle cramping
48. The most accurate temperature measurement for an adult patient experiencing tachypnea and dyspnea is:
    1. Oral
    2. Rectal
    3. Axillary
    4. Tympanic
49. A nurse should insert a rectal thermometer into the adult patient:
    1. 1/4 to 1/2 inch
    2. 1 to 1 1/2 inches
    3. 1 1/2 to 2 inches
    4. 2 to 2 1/2 inches
50. A patient is determined to have an intermittent fever. This is supported by which of the following observations?
    1. A constant body temperature greater than 38°C (100.4°F)
    2. A fever that spikes and falls but does not return to normal
    3. Long periods of normal temperatures with febrile episodes
    4. Spikes in readings mixed with normal temperatures
51. Which of the following values indicates the correct pulse pressure for a patient with a blood pressure of 170/90?
    1. 80
    2. 170
    3. 260
    4. Value not known based on the information given
52. For a patient who is experiencing a febrile state, the nurse should:
    1. Ambulate the patient frequently
    2. Restrict fluid intake
    3. Keep the patient warm
    4. Provide oxygen as ordered
53. A nurse anticipates that bradycardia will be evident if a patient is:
    1. Exercising
    2. Hypothermic
    3. Asthmatic
    4. Extremely anxious
54. A nurse anticipates that a patient with hypertension will be receiving:
    1. Diuretics
    2. Antipyretics
    3. Narcotic analgesics
    4. Anticholinergics
55. To determine the arterial blood flow to a patient's feet, the nurse should assess the:
    1. Radial artery
    2. Brachial artery
    3. Popliteal artery
    4. Dorsalis pedis artery
56. A nurse anticipates an increase in blood pressure for the patient who is:
    1. Sleeping
    2. Overweight
    3. Taking narcotics
    4. Hemorrhaging

57. Prehypertension is classified as an average of repeated readings of:
    1. Systolic: 120 to 139 mm Hg; diastolic: 80 to 89 mm Hg
    2. Systolic: 140 to 159 mm Hg; diastolic: 90 to 99 mm Hg
    3. Systolic: 160 to 179 mm Hg; diastolic: 90 to 99 mm Hg
    4. Systolic: greater than 180 mm Hg: diastolic; greater than 100 mm Hg

STUDY GROUP QUESTIONS

- What are the guidelines for measurement of vital signs?
- When should vital signs be taken?
- How does the nurse determine what sites and equipment to use for measurement of vital signs?
- What body processes regulate temperature?
- What factors influence body temperature?
- How is the temperature measurement converted from centigrade to Fahrenheit and vice versa?
- What sites and equipment are used for temperature measurement?
- What nursing interventions are appropriate for increases and decreases in a patient's body temperature?
- What factors influence pulse rate?
- What sites may be used for pulse rate assessment?
- How should the stethoscope be used in pulse rate assessment?
- What changes may occur in the pulse rate and rhythm?
- What nursing interventions are appropriate for alterations in pulse rate?
- What is blood pressure?
- What factors may increase or decrease blood pressure?
- What are abnormal alterations in blood pressure?
- What equipment is used for blood pressure measurement?
- What nursing interventions are appropriate for increases and decreases in blood pressure?
- What body processes are involved in respiration?
- How are respirations assessed?
- What alterations may be noted in a patient's respirations?
- How does pulse oximetry function and what is its purpose?
- What are the procedures for assessment of temperature, pulse rate, respirations, blood pressure, and pulse oxygen saturation?
- What should be included in patient and family teaching for measurement and evaluation of vital signs?

STUDY CHART

Create a study chart to compare the *Vital Signs Across the Life Span* that identifies expected temperature, pulse rate, respiration, and blood pressure for each age-group.

Answers available through your instructor.

Name _____ Date _____ Instructor's Name _____

Performance Checklist Skill 14-1: Measuring Body Temperature

	S	U	NP	Comments

Assessment

1. Assess for signs and symptoms of temperature alterations and for factors that influence body temperature.
2. Determine any activity that would interfere with accuracy of temperature measurement. Wait 20 to 30 minutes before measuring oral temperature if patient has smoked or ingested hot or cold liquids or food.
3. Determine appropriate site and measurement device to be used.

Planning

1. Explain route by which you will take temperature and importance of maintaining proper position until reading is complete.

Implementation

1. Perform hand hygiene.
2. Assist patient in assuming comfortable position that provides easy access to route through which you will measure temperature.
3. Obtain temperature reading.
   A. Oral Temperature Measurement With Electronic Thermometer
   (1) Apply disposable gloves *(optional)*.
   (2) Remove thermometer pack from charging unit. Attach oral probe (blue tip) to thermometer unit. Grasp top of probe stem, being careful not to apply pressure on the ejection button.
   (3) Slide disposable plastic probe cover over thermometer probe stem until cover locks in place.
   (4) Ask patient to open mouth; then gently place thermometer probe under tongue in posterior sublingual pocket lateral to center of lower jaw.
   (5) Ask patient to hold thermometer probe with lips closed.
   (6) Leave thermometer probe in place until audible signal indicates completion and patient's temperature appears on digital display; remove thermometer probe from under patient's tongue.
   (7) Push ejection button on thermometer stem to discard plastic probe cover into appropriate receptacle.
   (8) Return thermometer probe stem to storage position of recording unit.
   (9) If gloves worn, remove and dispose of in appropriate receptacle. Perform hand hygiene.
   (10) Return thermometer to charger.

CHAPTER 14 • Vital Signs

	S	U	NP	Comments

B. Rectal Temperature Measurement With Electronic Thermometer

(1) Draw curtain around bed and/or close room door. Assist patient to Sims' position with upper leg flexed. Move aside bed linen to expose only anal area. Keep patient's upper body and lower extremities covered with sheet or blanket.

(2) Apply gloves.

(3) Remove thermometer pack from charging unit. Attach rectal probe (red tip) to thermometer unit. Grasp top of probe stem, being careful not to apply pressure on the ejection button.

(4) Slide disposable plastic probe cover over thermometer probe until it locks in place.

(5) Squeeze liberal portion of lubricant onto tissue. Dip probe cover's end into lubricant, covering 2.5 to 3.5 cm (1 to 1^1/$_2$ inches) for adult.

(6) With nondominant hand, separate patient's buttocks to expose anus. Ask patient to breathe slowly and relax.

(7) Gently insert thermometer probe into anus in direction of umbilicus 3.5 cm (1^1/$_2$ inches) for adult. Do not force thermometer.

(8) Once positioned, hold thermometer probe in place until audible signal indicates completion and patient's temperature appears on digital display; remove thermometer probe from anus.

(9) Push ejection button on thermometer stem to discard plastic probe cover into an appropriate receptacle.

(10) Return thermometer stem to storage position of recording unit.

(11) Wipe patient's anal area with tissue or soft wipe to remove lubricant or feces, and discard tissue. Assist patient in assuming a comfortable position.

(12) Remove and dispose of gloves in appropriate receptacle. Perform hand hygiene.

(13) Return thermometer to charger.

C. Axillary Temperature Measurement With Electronic Thermometer

(1) Draw curtain around bed and/or close room door. Assist patient to supine or sitting position. Move clothing or gown away from shoulder and arm.

(2) Remove thermometer pack from charging unit. Be sure oral probe (blue tip) is attached to thermometer unit. Grasp top of probe stem, being careful not to apply pressure on ejection button.

(3) Slide disposable plastic probe cover over thermometer probe until cover locks in place.

	S	U	NP	Comments

(4) Raise patient's arm away from torso. Inspect for skin lesions and excessive perspiration. Insert probe into center of axilla, lower arm over probe, and place arm across patient's chest.

(5) Once positioned, hold thermometer probe in place until audible signal indicates completion and patient's temperature appears on digital display; remove thermometer probe from axilla.

(6) Push ejection button on thermometer stem to discard plastic probe cover into appropriate receptacle.

(7) Return thermometer stem to storage position of recording unit.

(8) Assist patient in assuming a comfortable position, replacing linen or gown.

(9) Perform hand hygiene.

(10) Return thermometer to charger.

D. **Tympanic Membrane Temperature Measurement With Electronic Tympanic Thermometer**

(1) Assist patient in assuming comfortable position with head turned toward side, away from you. If patient has been lying on one side, use other ear.

(2) Note if there is obvious earwax in the patient's ear canal.

(3) Remove thermometer handheld unit from charging base, being careful not to apply pressure on the ejection button.

(4) Slide disposable speculum cover over tip until it locks into place. Be careful not to touch cover.

(5) If holding handheld unit with right hand, obtain temperature from patient's right ear; left-handed persons obtain temperature from patient's left ear.

(6) Insert speculum into ear canal following manufacturer's instructions for tympanic probe positioning.

   (a) Pull ear pinna backward, up and out for an adult. For children younger than 2 years of age, point covered probe toward midpoint between eyebrow and sideburns.

   (b) Move thermometer in a figure-eight pattern.

   (c) Fit speculum probe snugly into canal, and do not move, pointing tip toward nose.

(7) Once positioned, press scan button on handheld unit. Leave speculum in place until audible signal indicates completion and patient's temperature appears on digital display.

(8) Carefully remove speculum from auditory canal.

	S	U	NP	Comments

(9) Push ejection button on handheld unit to discard speculum cover into appropriate receptacle.

(10) If temperature is abnormal or a second reading is necessary, replace speculum cover and wait 2 minutes before repeating the measurement in the same ear. Measurement can be repeated in other ear or via an alternative measurement site or instrument.

(11) Return handheld unit to charging base.

(12) Assist patient in assuming a comfortable position.

(13) Perform hand hygiene.

Evaluation

1. Inform patient of reading and record measurement.
2. If you are assessing temperature for the first time, establish temperature as baseline if it is within normal range.
3. Compare temperature reading with patient's previous temperature and normal temperature range for patient's age group.
4. Record temperature in patient's record.
5. Report abnormal findings to nurse in charge or physician.

Name _____ Date _____ Instructor's Name _____

Performance Checklist Skill 14-2: Assessing the Radial and Apical Pulses

	S	U	NP	Comments

Assessment

1. Determine need to assess radial and/or apical pulse.
2. Assess for factors that influence pulse rate and rhythm.
3. Determine patient's previous baseline pulse rate (if available) from patient's record.

Planning

1. Explain to patient that you will assess pulse or heart rate.

Implementation

1. Perform hand hygiene.
2. If necessary, draw curtain around bed and/or close door.
3. Obtain pulse measurement.
    A. **Radial pulse**
    (1) Assist patient to assume a supine or sitting position.
    (2) If supine, place patient's forearm straight alongside or across lower chest or upper abdomen with wrist extended straight. If sitting, bend patient's elbow 90 degrees and support lower arm on chair or on your arm. Slightly extend the wrist with palm down until you note the strongest pulse.
    (3) Place tips of first two fingers of your hand over groove along radial or thumb side of patient's inner wrist.
    (4) Lightly compress against radius, obliterate pulse initially, and then relax pressure so pulse becomes easily palpable.
    (5) Determine strength of pulse.
    (6) After you feel pulse regularly, look at watch's second hand and begin to count rate.
    (7) If pulse is regular, count rate for 30 seconds and multiply total by 2.
    (8) If pulse is irregular, count rate for 60 seconds. Assess frequency and pattern of irregularity.
    (9) When pulse is irregular, compare radial pulses bilaterally.
    B. **Apical pulse**
    (1) Perform hand hygiene, and clean earpieces and diaphragm of stethoscope with alcohol swab.
    (2) Draw curtain around bed, and/or close door.
    (3) Assist patient to supine or sitting position. Move aside bed linen and gown to expose sternum and left side of chest.

Copyright © 2011, 2007, 2003 by Mosby, Inc., an affiliate of Elsevier Inc. All rights reserved.

	S	U	NP	Comments

(4) Locate anatomical landmarks to identify the point of maximal impulse (PMI). Find the angle of Louis just below suprasternal notch between the sternal body and manubrium; it feels like a bony prominence. Slip fingers down each side of angle to find the second intercostal space (ICS). Carefully move fingers down the left side of sternum to fifth ICS and laterally to the left midclavicular line (MCL). A light tap felt within an area 1 to 2 cm ($1/2$ to 1 inch) of the PMI is reflected from the apex of the heart.

(5) Place diaphragm of stethoscope in palm of hand for 5 to 10 seconds.

(6) Place diaphragm of stethoscope over PMI at the fifth ICS, at left MCL, and auscultate for normal S_1 and S_2 heart sounds (heard as "lub dub").

(7) When S_1 and S_2 are heard with regularity, use watch's second hand and begin to count rate.

(8) If apical rate is regular, count for 30 seconds and multiply by 2.

(9) Note if heart rate is irregular, and describe pattern of irregularity (S_1 and S_2 occurring early or later after previous sequence of sounds; for example, every third or fourth beat is skipped).

(10) Replace patient's gown and bed linen; assist patient in returning to comfortable position.

(11) Perform hand hygiene.

(12) Clean earpieces and diaphragm of stethoscope with alcohol swab routinely after each use.

Evaluation

1. Discuss findings with patient and record measurement.
2. Compare readings with previous baseline and/or acceptable range of heart rate for patient's age.
3. Compare peripheral pulse rate with apical rate, and note discrepancy.
4. Compare radial pulse equality, and note discrepancy.
5. Correlate pulse rate with data obtained from BP reading and related signs and symptoms.
6. Record pulse rate with assessment site in patient's record.
7. Report abnormal findings to nurse in charge or physician.

Name _____ Date _____ Instructor's Name _____

Performance Checklist Skill 14-3: Blood Pressure Measurement

	S	U	NP	Comments

Assessment
1. Determine need to assess patient's BP. ____ ____ ____ _____
2. Determine best site for BP assessment. ____ ____ ____ _____
3. Determine previous baseline BP (if available) from patient's record. ____ ____ ____ _____

Planning
1. Explain to patient that you will assess BP. Have patient rest at least 5 minutes before measuring lying or sitting BP and 1 minute when standing. Ask patient not to speak when BP is being measured. ____ ____ ____ _____
2. Be sure patient has not ingested caffeine or smoked for 30 minutes before BP assessment. ____ ____ ____ _____
3. Have patient assume sitting or lying position. Be sure room is warm, quiet, and relaxing. ____ ____ ____ _____
4. Select appropriate cuff size. ____ ____ ____ _____
5. Perform hand hygiene, and clean stethoscope earpieces and diaphragm with alcohol swab. ____ ____ ____ _____

Implementation
1. With patient sitting or lying, position patient's forearm or thigh, supported at heart level, if needed, with palm turned up; for thigh, position with knee slightly flexed. If sitting, instruct patient to keep feet flat on floor without legs crossed. ____ ____ ____ _____
2. Expose extremity (arm or leg) fully by removing constricting clothing. ____ ____ ____ _____
3. Palpate brachial artery (arm) or popliteal artery (leg). With cuff fully deflated, apply bladder of cuff above artery. Position cuff 2.5 cm (1 inch) above site of pulsation (antecubital or popliteal space). If there are no center arrows on cuff, estimate the center of the bladder and place this center over artery. Wrap cuff evenly and snugly around extremity.
4. Position manometer vertically at eye level. Make sure observer is no farther than 1 m (approximately 1 yard) away. ____ ____ ____ _____
5. Measure BP.
   A. **Two-Step Method**
      (1) Relocate brachial pulse. Palpate artery distal to the cuff with fingertips of nondominant hand while inflating cuff. Note point at which pulse disappears and continue to inflate cuff to a pressure of 30 mm Hg above that point. Note the pressure reading. Slowly deflate cuff, and note point when pulse reappears. Deflate cuff fully and wait 30 seconds. ____ ____ ____ _____

	S	U	NP	Comments

  (2) Place stethoscope earpieces in ears and be sure sounds are clear, not muffled.

  (3) Relocate brachial artery, and place diaphragm of stethoscope over it. Do not allow chestpiece to touch cuff or clothing.

  (4) Close valve of pressure bulb clockwise until tight.

  (5) Quickly inflate cuff to 30 mm Hg above patient's estimated systolic pressure.

  (6) Slowly release pressure bulb valve and allow manometer needle gauge to fall at rate of 2 to 3 mm Hg per second. Make sure there are no extraneous sounds.

  (7) Note point on manometer when you hear the first clear sound. The sound slowly will increase in intensity.

  (8) Continue to deflate cuff gradually, noting point at which sound disappears in adults. Note pressure to nearest 2 mm Hg. Listen for 20 to 30 mm Hg after the last sound and then allow remaining air to escape quickly.

B. **One-Step Method**

  (1) Place stethoscope earpieces in ears, and be sure sounds are clear, not muffled.

  (2) Relocate brachial artery, and place diaphragm of stethoscope over it. Do not allow chestpiece to touch cuff or clothing.

  (3) Close valve of pressure bulb clockwise until tight.

  (4) Quickly inflate cuff to 30 mm Hg above patient's usual systolic pressure.

  (5) Slowly release pressure bulb valve and allow manometer needle to fall at rate of 2 to 3 mm Hg per second. Note point on manometer when you hear the first clear sound. The sound will slowly increase in intensity.

  (6) Continue to deflate cuff gradually, noting point at which sound disappears in adults. Note pressure to nearest 2 mm Hg. Listen for 20 to 30 mm Hg after the last sound and then allow remaining air to escape quickly.

6. The JNC recommends the average of two sets of BP measurements, 2 minutes apart. Use the second set as the baseline.

	S	U	NP	Comments

7. Remove cuff from extremity unless you need to repeat measurement. If this is the first assessment of patient, repeat procedure on the other extremity.
8. Assist patient in returning to comfortable position, and cover upper arm if previously clothed.
9. Discuss findings with patient as needed.
10. Perform hand hygiene. Clean earpieces, bell, and diaphragm of stethoscope with alcohol.

Evaluation
1. Compare reading with previous baseline and/or acceptable value of BP for patient's age.
2. Compare BP measurements in both arms or both legs.
3. Correlate BP readings with data obtained from pulse assessment and related cardiovascular signs and symptoms.
4. Record BP reading in patient's record.
5. Report abnormal findings to nurse in charge or physician.

Name _____ Date _____ Instructor's Name _____

Performance Checklist Skill 14-4: Assessing Respiration

	S	U	NP	Comments

Assessment

1. Determine need to assess patient's respiration.
2. Assess pertinent laboratory values.
3. Determine previous baseline respiratory rate (if available) from patient's record.
4. Assess respirations after measuring the pulse in an adult.

Planning

1. Be sure patient is in comfortable position, preferably sitting or lying with the head of the bed elevated 45 to 60 degrees.

Implementation

1. Draw curtain around bed and/or close door. Perform hand hygiene.
2. Be sure patient's chest is visible. If necessary, move bed linen or gown.
3. Place patient's arm in relaxed position across the abdomen or lower chest, or place your hand directly over patient's upper abdomen.
4. Observe complete respiratory cycle (one inspiration and one expiration).
5. After you observe cycle, look at watch's second hand and begin to count rate.
6. If rhythm is regular, count number of respirations in 30 seconds and multiply by 2. If rhythm is irregular, less than 12, or greater than 20, count for 1 full minute.
7. Note depth of respirations.
8. Note rhythm of ventilatory cycle.
9. Replace bed linen and patient's gown.
10. Perform hand hygiene.

Evaluation

1. Discuss findings with patient as needed.
2. If you are assessing respirations for the first time, establish rate, rhythm, and depth as baseline if within normal range.
3. Compare respiration with patient's previous baseline and normal rate, rhythm, and depth.
4. Correlate respiratory rate, depth, and rhythm with data from pulse oximetry and arterial blood gases, if available.
5. Record respiratory rate and character in patient's record. Indicate type and amount of oxygen therapy if used by patient during assessment.
6. Report abnormal findings to nurse in charge or physician.

Name _____ Date _____ Instructor's Name _____

Performance Checklist Skill 14-5: Measuring Oxygen Saturation (Pulse Oximetry)

	S	U	NP	Comments

Assessment

1. Determine need to measure patient's oxygen saturation.
2. Assess for factors that normally influence measurement of SpO_2.
3. Review patient's record for health care provider's order. Check agency policy or procedure manual for standard of care for measurement of SpO_2.
4. Determine most appropriate site for sensor probe placement.
5. Determine if patient has a latex allergy.

Planning

1. Determine previous baseline SpO_2 if available) from patient's record.
2. Obtain oximeter and probe and place at bedside.
3. Explain purpose of procedure to patient. Instruct patient to breathe normally.

Implementation

1. Perform hand hygiene.
2. Position patient comfortably. If finger is chosen as monitoring site, support lower arm.
3. If using the finger, remove fingernail polish from finger with acetone.
4. Attach sensor probe to monitoring site.
5. Once sensor is in place, turn on oximeter by activating power. Observe pulse waveform/intensity display and audible beep. Correlate oximeter pulse rate with patient's radial pulse.
6. Inform patient that oximeter will sound if sensor falls off or if patient moves sensor.
7. Leave probe in place until oximeter reaches constant value and pulse display reaches full strength during each cardiac cycle. Read SpO_2 value on digital display.
8. Verify alarm limits and volume for continuous monitoring.
9. Discuss findings with patient as needed.
10. Remove probe and turn oximeter power off for intermittent monitoring.
11. Assist patient in returning to comfortable position.
12. Perform hand hygiene.

Evaluation

1. Compare SpO_2 readings with patient's baseline and acceptable values.
2. Compare SpO_2 with SaO_2 obtained from arterial blood gas measurements if available.
3. Correlate SpO_2 reading with data obtained from respiratory rate, depth, and rhythm assessment.

CHAPTER 14 • Vital Signs

	S	U	NP	Comments
4. During continuous monitoring, assess skin integrity underneath probe at least every 2 hours, based on patient's peripheral circulation.	____	____	____	_____
5. Record SpO$_2$ value in patient's record, indicating type and amount of oxygen therapy used by patient during assessment. Also record any signs and symptoms of oxygen desaturation.	____	____	____	_____
6. Report abnormal findings to nurse in charge or physician.	____	____	____	_____
7. Record patient's use of continuous or intermittent pulse oximetry. Document use of equipment for third-party payers.	____	____	____	_____

Name _____ Date _____ Instructor's Name _____

Procedural Guidelines 14-1: Measuring Orthostatic Blood Pressure

	S	U	NP	Comments

1. With patient supine, take BP measurement in each arm. Select arm with highest systolic reading for subsequent measurements.
2. Leaving BP cuff in place, help patient to sitting position. After 1 to 3 minutes with patient in sitting position, take BP. If orthostatic symptoms occur, such as dizziness, weakness, lightheadedness, feeling faint, or sudden pallor, stop BP measurement and help patient to a supine position.
3. Leaving BP cuff in place, help patient to standing position. After 1 to 3 minutes with patient in standing position, take BP. If orthostatic symptoms occur, stop BP measurement and return patient to a supine position. In most cases, you will detect orthostatic hypotension within 1 minute of standing.
4. Record patient's BP in each position. Note any additional symptoms or complaints.
5. Report findings of orthostatic hypotension or orthostatic symptoms to nurse in charge and physician or health care provider. Instruct patient to ask for assistance when getting out of bed if orthostatic hypotension is present or orthostatic symptoms occur.

Name _____ Date _____ Instructor's Name _____

Procedural Guidelines 14-2: Palpating Systolic Blood Pressure

	S	U	NP	Comments
1. Perform hand hygiene.	___	___	___	_____
2. Apply BP cuff to the extremity selected for measurement.	___	___	___	_____
3. Continually palpate the brachial, radial, or popliteal artery with fingertips of one hand.	___	___	___	_____
4. Inflate the BP cuff 30 mm Hg above the point at which you no longer palpate the pulse.	___	___	___	_____
5. Slowly release valve and deflate cuff, allowing manometer needle to fall at rate of 2 mm Hg/sec.	___	___	___	_____
6. Note point on manometer when pulse is again palpable; this is the systolic BP.	___	___	___	_____
7. Deflate cuff rapidly and completely. Remove cuff from patient's extremity unless you need to repeat the measurement.	___	___	___	_____
8. Perform hand hygiene.	___	___	___	_____

Name _____ Date _____ Instructor's Name _____

Procedural Guidelines 14-3: Automatic Blood Pressure Measurement

	S	U	NP	Comments
1. Determine the appropriateness of using electronic BP measurement.	___	___	___	_____
2. Determine best site for cuff placement.	___	___	___	_____
3. Assist patient to comfortable position, either lying or sitting. Plug in device and place device near patient, ensuring that connector hose between cuff and machine will reach.	___	___	___	_____
4. Locate on/off switch and turn on machine to enable device to self-test computer systems.	___	___	___	_____
5. Select appropriate cuff size for patient extremity and appropriate cuff for machine. Electronic BP cuff and machine are matched by manufacturer and are not interchangeable.	___	___	___	_____
6. Expose extremity for measurement by removing constricting clothing to ensure proper cuff application. Do not place BP cuff over clothing.	___	___	___	_____
7. Prepare BP cuff by manually squeezing all the air out of the cuff and connecting cuff to connector hose.	___	___	___	_____
8. Wrap flattened cuff snugly around extremity, verifying that only one finger fits between cuff and patient's skin. Make sure the "artery" arrow marked on the outside of the cuff is correctly placed.	___	___	___	_____
9. Verify that connector hose between cuff and machine is not kinked. Kinking prevents proper inflation and deflation of cuff.	___	___	___	_____
10. Following manufacturer's directions, set the frequency control of automatic or manual; then press start button. The first BP measurement will pump the cuff to a peak pressure of approximately 180 mm Hg. After this pressure is reached, the machine begins a deflation sequence that determines the BP. The first reading determines the peak pressure inflation for additional measurements.	___	___	___	_____
11. When deflation is complete, digital display will provide the most recent values and flash time in minutes that has elapsed since the measurement occurred.	___	___	___	_____
12. Set frequency of BP measurements and upper and lower alarm limits for systolic, diastolic, and mean BP readings. Intervals between BP measurements are set from 1 to 90 minutes.	___	___	___	_____
13. You are able to obtain additional readings at anytime by pressing the start button.	___	___	___	_____
14. If frequent BP measurements are required, leave the cuff in place. Remove cuff every 2 hours to assess underlying skin integrity, and if possible, alternate BP sites. When you are finished using the electronic BP machine, clean BP cuff according to facility policy.	___	___	___	_____
15. Compare electronic BP readings with auscultatory BP measurements to verify accuracy of electronic BP device.	___	___	___	_____

15 Health Assessment and Physical Examination

CASE STUDIES

1. You are assigned to assist with physical examinations in the outpatient clinic. On the schedule for today are three patients. One of the patients is a 72-year-old Hispanic woman, another is a 16-year-old girl, and the last is a 4-year-old boy.
    a. How can you assist each of these patients to feel more at ease before and during the physical examination?
2. A patient in the physician's office informs you that he is having trouble hearing when other people are speaking to him.
    a. What specific assessments will you perform on this patient?

CHAPTER REVIEW

Match the description/definition in Column A with the correct term in Column B.

Column A	Column B
1. Black, tarry stools	a. Ptosis
2. Fluid accumulation, swelling	b. Alopecia
3. Loss of hair	c. Edema
4. Drooping of eyelid over the pupil	d. Jaundice
5. Tiny, pinpoint red spots on the skin	e. Bruit
6. Curvature of the thoracic spine	f. Melena
7. Yellow-orange discoloration	g. Kyphosis
8. A hardened area	h. Petechiae
9. Blowing, swishing sound in blood vessel	i. Erythema
10. A red discoloration	j. Induration

Complete the following:

11. Identify the five skills used in physical assessment and briefly describe each.

12. Identify the following positions for physical examination.
    a. 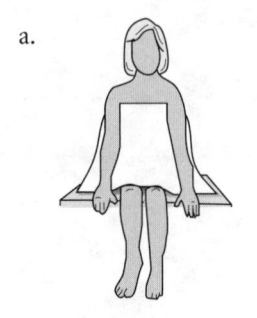
    b. 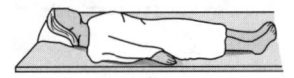
    c. 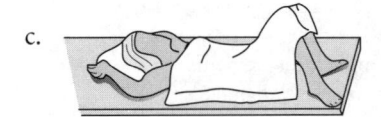
    d. 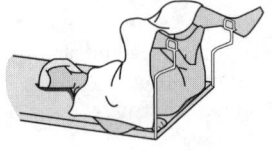
    e.

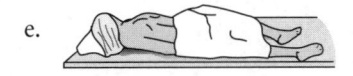

CHAPTER 15 • Health Assessment and Physical Examination

f.

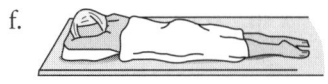

g.

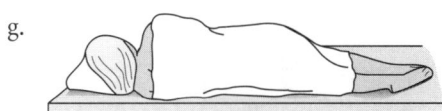

h.

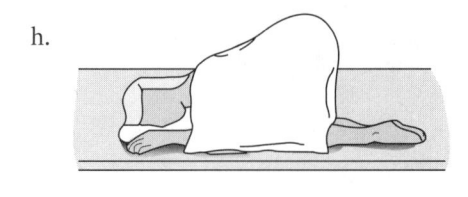

13. Identify which of the pulses is being palpated in each illustration.

a.

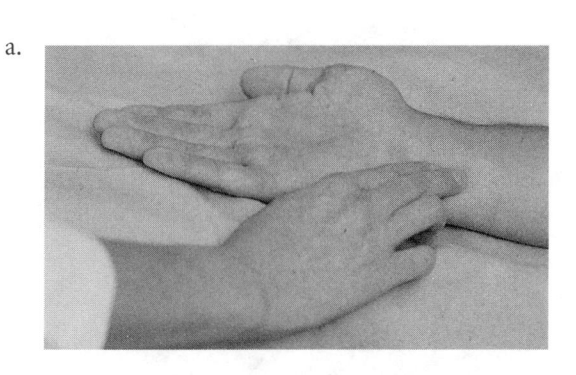

b.

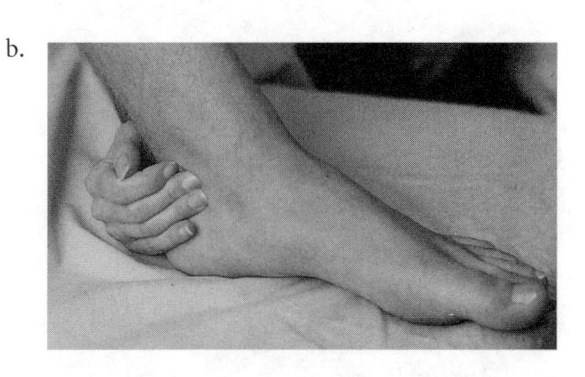

c.

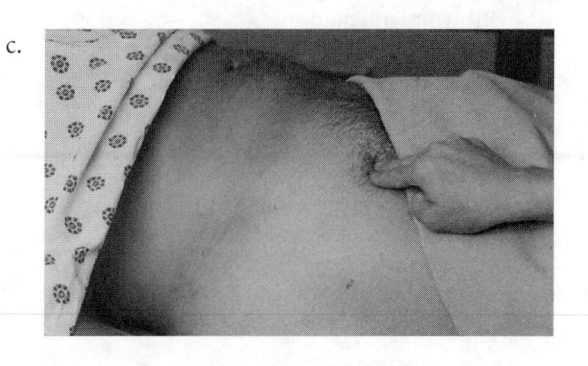

d.

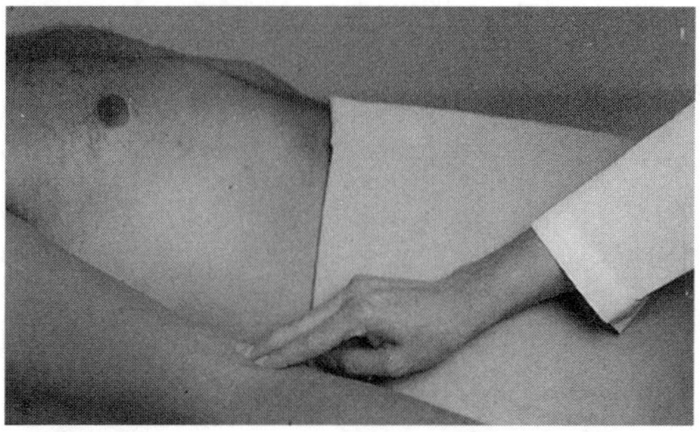

e.

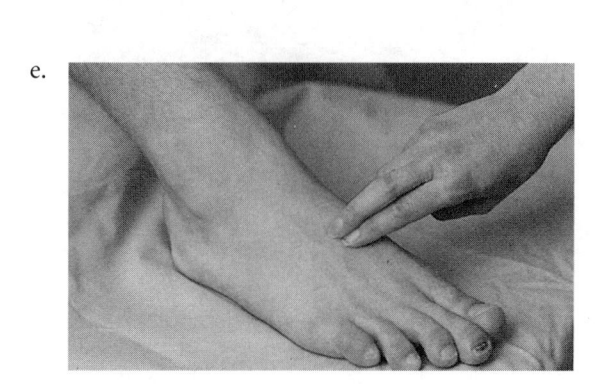

14. Correctly identify the primary skin lesion in each illustration.

a.

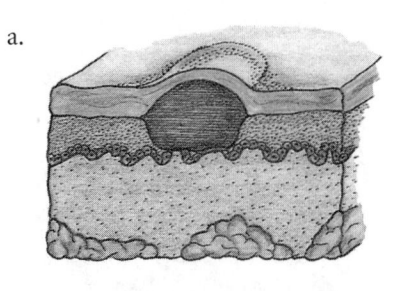

b.

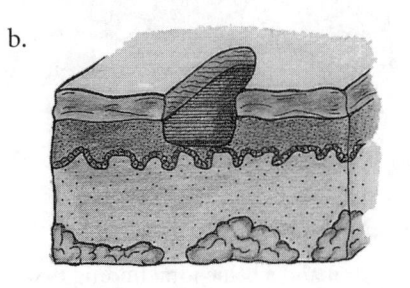

c.

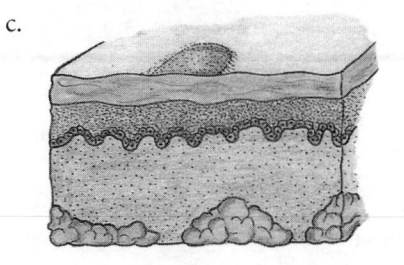

66 CHAPTER 15 • Health Assessment and Physical Examination

d.

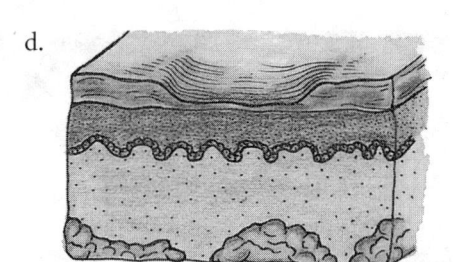

e.

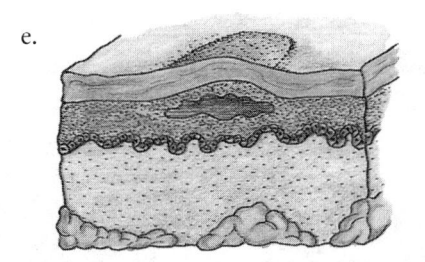

15. Identify on the illustration where the PMI is located.

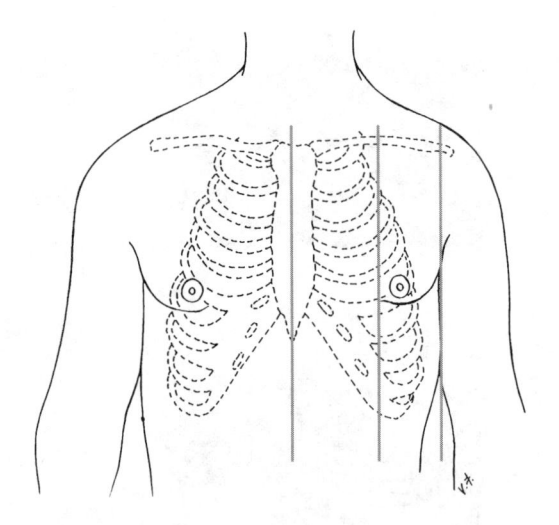

16. Identify a physical and a behavioral finding that may indicate abuse for the following:

	Physical	Behavioral
a. Child sexual abuse	_____	_____
b. Domestic abuse	_____	_____
c. Older adult abuse	_____	_____

17. Identify the abdominal structures that are assessed.

a.

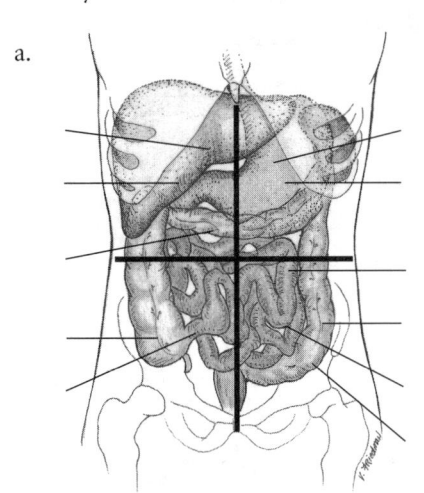

b.

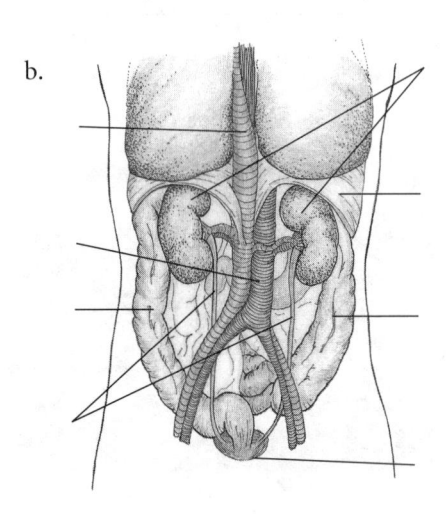

18. Mark each of the following physical assessment findings as either expected or unexpected. For unexpected findings, investigate what may be the possible etiology.

	Expected	Unexpected
a. Skin lifts easily and snaps back	_____	_____
b. Erythema noted over bony prominences	_____	_____
c. Hair evenly distributed over scalp and pubic area	_____	_____
d. Brown pigmentation of nails in longitudinal streaks (dark-skinned patient)	_____	_____
e. Pallor in face and nail beds	_____	_____
f. Clubbing of nails	_____	_____
g. PEERLA	_____	_____
h. Pupils cloudy	_____	_____
i. Yellow discoloration of sclera	_____	_____

Copyright © 2011, 2007, 2003 by Mosby, Inc., an affiliate of Elsevier Inc. All rights reserved.

CHAPTER 15 • Health Assessment and Physical Examination

		Expected	Unexpected
j.	Eardrum translucent, shiny, and pearly gray	_____	_____
k.	Light brown or gray cerumen	_____	_____
l.	Nasal septum midline	_____	_____
m.	Nasal mucosa pale with clear, watery discharge	_____	_____
n.	Sinuses tender to touch	_____	_____
o.	Teeth chalky white, with black discoloration	_____	_____
p.	Tongue medium red, moist, and slightly rough on top	_____	_____
q.	Soft palate rises when patient says "ah"	_____	_____
r.	Uvula reddened and edematous, tonsils with yellow exudate	_____	_____
s.	Thyroid gland small, smooth, and free of nodules	_____	_____
t.	Lungs resonant to percussion	_____	_____
u.	Costal angle greater than 90 degrees between costal margins	_____	_____
v.	Bulging of intercostal spaces	_____	_____
w.	No carotid bruit present	_____	_____
x.	Extra heart sound noted	_____	_____
y.	Jugular vein distention at 45-degree angle	_____	_____
z.	Dependent edema in ankles	_____	_____
aa.	Female breasts smooth, symmetrical, without retraction	_____	_____
bb.	Soft, well-differentiated, moveable lumps in the breasts noted	_____	_____
cc.	Bowel sounds active and audible in all four quadrants	_____	_____
dd.	Bulging flanks	_____	_____
ee.	Flat or concave umbilicus	_____	_____
ff.	Rebound tenderness found	_____	_____
gg.	Perineal skin smooth and slightly darker than surrounding skin	_____	_____
hh.	Bartholin glands palpable with discharge evident	_____	_____
ii.	Glans penis smooth and pink on all surfaces	_____	_____
jj.	Testes smooth and ovoid	_____	_____
kk.	No crepitus found on range of motion	_____	_____
ll.	Hips and shoulders aligned parallel	_____	_____
mm.	Lordosis of spine noted	_____	_____
nn.	Reflexes symmetrical	_____	_____
oo.	Able to recall past events, unable to repeat series of five numbers	_____	_____
pp.	Able to perform rapidly alternating movements	_____	_____

19. A patient has an area of discomfort. The nurse will examine this area:
    a. First
    b. Last
20. When using the stethoscope, high-pitched sounds are heard best with a:
    a. Diaphragm
    b. Bell
21. To inspect an adult patient's ear canal, the nurse pulls the auricle:
    a. Up and back
    b. Down and back
22. The position to place the patient in for a genital examination is:

23. The position to place the patient in for an abdominal examination is:

24. Identify what a nurse is able to assess in a general survey of a patient:

25. A weight gain of 5 lb or 2.2 kg/day indicates:

26. What techniques are appropriate when assessing patients of different ages? Select all that apply.
    a. Speaking privately with adolescents about their concerns _____
    b. Using close-ended questions to increase the speed of the examination _____
    c. Calling children and their parents by their first names _____
    d. Providing time for children to play _____
    e. Performing the examination for an older adult near bathroom facilities _____
    f. Proceeding rapidly through the examination of an older adult to finish it as quickly as possible _____

27. Patients older than 65 years should be instructed to have yearly eye examinations.
    True _____ False _____
28. A nurse is preparing to perform a skin assessment for an average adult patient. Select all of the following techniques that are correct:
    a. Using fluorescent lighting _____
    b. Keeping the room very warm _____
    c. Using disposable gloves to inspect lesions _____
    d. Looking for coloration changes by checking the tongue and nail beds _____
29. During a physical examination, a nurse notes that the patient appears to be very anxious. The nurse should:

30. One example of a test for colorectal cancer is:

31. Select the three best positions that a patient may be placed in for a cardiac assessment:
    a. Prone _____
    b. Supine _____
    c. Lithotomy _____
    d. Sitting _____
    e. Left lateral recumbent _____
    f. Dorsal recumbent _____
    g. Sims _____
32. Identify signs and symptoms that a patient may have if he or she has cardiopulmonary disease.

33. What are the risk factors associated with osteoporosis? Select all that apply.
    a. An active lifestyle _____
    b. Smoking _____
    c. African American background _____
    d. A history of falls _____
    e. A history of Cushing disease _____
    f. Exposure to sunlight _____
    g. A thin, light body frame _____
34. Identify at least two techniques that are used in assessment of the lymph nodes:

Select the best answer for each of the following questions:

35. A nurse is assessing a patient's nail beds. An expected finding is indicated by:
    1. Softening of the nail bed
    2. A concave curve to the nail
    3. Brown, linear streaks in the nail bed
    4. A 160-degree angle between the nail plate and nail
36. A young adult woman arrives at the family planning center for a physical examination. For this patient with mature breasts, the nurse expects to find that the:
    1. Breast tissue is softer
    2. Nipples project and areolae have receded
    3. Areolae are dark and have increased diameter
    4. Breasts are elongated and nipples are smaller and flatter
37. A nurse has checked the medical record and found that a patient has anemia. The presence of anemia is accompanied by the nurse's finding of:
    1. Pallor
    2. Erythema
    3. Jaundice
    4. Cyanosis
38. A patient with asthma has gone to an urgent care center for treatment. On auscultation of the lungs, a nurse hears rhonchi. These sounds are described as:
    1. Dry and grating
    2. Loud, low-pitched, and coarse
    3. High-pitched, fine, and short
    4. High-pitched and musical
39. A patient is admitted to a medical center with a peripheral vascular problem. A nurse is performing the initial assessment of the patient. While assessing the lower extremities, the nurse is alert to venous insufficiency as indicated by:
    1. Marked edema
    2. Thin, shiny skin
    3. Coolness to touch
    4. Dusky red coloration
40. A nurse is performing a complete neurological assessment on a patient after a cerebrovascular accident (CVA/stroke). To assess cranial nerve III, the nurse:
    1. Uses the Snellen chart
    2. Lightly touches the cornea with a wisp of cotton
    3. Whispers into one ear at a time
    4. Measures pupil reaction to light and accommodation
41. Student nurses are practicing neurological assessment and determination of cranial nerve functioning. To assess cranial nerve X, the student nurse should ask the patient to:
    1. Say "ah"
    2. Shrug the shoulders
    3. Smile and frown
    4. Stick out the tongue
42. While completing a physical examination, a nurse assesses and reports that a patient has petechiae. The nurse has found:
    1. Light perspiration on the skin
    2. Moles with regular edges
    3. Thickness on the soles of the feet
    4. Pin-point size, flat, red spots
43. A nurse reviews a chart and sees that a patient who has been admitted to the unit this morning has a hyperthyroid disorder. The nurse anticipates that an examination of the eyes will reveal:
    1. Diplopia
    2. Strabismus
    3. Exophthalmos
    4. Nystagmus

CHAPTER 15 • Health Assessment and Physical Examination

44. In preparation for an examination of the internal ear, a nurse anticipates that the color of the eardrum should appear:
    1. White
    2. Yellow
    3. Slightly red
    4. Pearly gray
45. A patient with a history of smoking and alcohol abuse has gone to a clinic for a physical examination. Based on this history, the nurse is particularly alert during an examination of the oral cavity to the presence of:
    1. Spongy gums
    2. Pink tissue
    3. Thick, white patches
    4. Loose teeth
46. A patient in a physician's office has an increased anteroposterior diameter of the chest. The nurse should inquire specifically about the patient's history of:
    1. Smoking
    2. Thoracic trauma
    3. Spinal surgery
    4. Exposure to tuberculosis
47. When auscultating a patient's chest, a nurse hears what appears to be an S_3 sound. This is an expected finding if the patient is:
    1. 10 years old
    2. 35 years old
    3. 56 years old
    4. 82 years old
48. A patient in a medical center has been prescribed bed rest for a prolonged period of time. There is a possibility that the patient may have developed phlebitis. The nurse assesses for the presence of this condition by:
    1. Palpating the ankles for pitting edema
    2. Checking the popliteal pulses bilaterally
    3. Inspecting the thighs for clusters of ecchymosis
    4. Checking the appearance and circumference of the lower legs
49. When teaching a 45-year-old patient in the gynecologist's office about breast cancer, a nurse includes information on recommendations for screening. The patient is informed that a woman her age should have:
    1. Annual mammograms
    2. Biannual CT scans
    3. Physical examinations every 3 years
    4. Breast self-examinations every 3 months
50. A patient has been experiencing some lightheadedness and loss of balance over the past few weeks. A nurse wants to check the patient's balance while waiting for the patient to have other laboratory tests. The nurse administers the:
    1. Allen test
    2. Rinne test
    3. Weber test
    4. Romberg test
51. Screenings are being conducted at the junior high school for scoliosis. A nurse is observing the students for the presence of:
    1. An S-shaped curvature of the spine
    2. An exaggerated curvature of the thoracic spine
    3. An exaggerated curvature of the lumbar spine
    4. A bulging of the cervical vertebrae and disks
52. While reviewing a medical record, a nurse notes that a patient has suspected pancreatitis. The nurse assesses the patient for:
    1. Positive rebound tenderness
    2. Midline abdominal pulsations
    3. Hyperactive bowel sounds in all quadrants
    4. Bulging of the flanks with dependent distention
53. An 80-year-old woman is being assessed by a nurse in an extended care facility. The nurse is assessing the genitalia of this patient and suspects that there may be a malignancy present. The nurse's suspicion is due to the finding of:
    1. Scaly, nodular lesions
    2. Yellow exudates and redness
    3. Small ulcers with serous drainage
    4. Extreme pallor and edema
54. A screening for osteoporosis is being conducted at an annual health fair. To determine the risk factors for osteoporosis, a nurse is assessing individuals for:
    1. Multiparity
    2. A heavier than recommended body frame
    3. An African American background
    4. A history of dieting and/or alcohol abuse
55. A patient in a rehabilitation facility has experienced a cerebrovascular accident (CVA/stroke) that has left the patient with an expressive aphasia. The nurse anticipates that this patient will:
    1. Be unable to speak or write
    2. Be unable to follow directions
    3. Respond inappropriately to questions
    4. Have difficulty interpreting words and phrases
56. A peripheral pulse that is easily palpable and normal in tension is documented as:
    1. 1+
    2. 2+
    3. 3+
    4. 4+
57. To assess a patient's visual fields, a nurse should:
    1. Ask the patient to read text
    2. Turn the room light on and off
    3. Move a finger at arm's length toward the patient from an angle
    4. Shine a penlight into the patient's eye at an oblique angle
58. A nurse exerts downward pressure on the thigh. This assessment is determining the muscle strength of the:
    1. Triceps
    2. Trapezius
    3. Quadriceps
    4. Gastrocnemius

59. Light palpation involves depressing the part being examined:
    1. ½ inch
    2. 1 inch
    3. 1½ inches
    4. 2 inches
60. A nurse teaches the male patient that he should notify a health care provider if he finds the following during a testicular self-examination:
    1. Small, pea-sized lumps on the front of the testicle
    2. Cordlike structures on the top of the testicles
    3. Loose, deeper color scrotal skin with a coarse surface
    4. Smegma under the foreskin
61. A nurse manager observes a new nurse on the unit performing a patient assessment. The new nurse's assessment should be interrupted if the manager observes the nurse:
    1. Using the pads of the first three fingers to palpate the breast tissue
    2. Auscultating the abdomen continuously for 5 minutes
    3. Palpating both carotid arteries simultaneously
    4. Testing sensory function on random locations with the patient's eyes closed
62. A nurse assesses a patient's skin and documents that vesicles are present. This observation is based on the nurse finding:
    1. Flat, nonpalpable changes in skin color
    2. Palpable, solid elevations smaller than 1 cm
    3. Irregularly shaped, elevated areas that vary in size
    4. Circumscribed elevations of skin filled with serous fluid
63. A nurse is assessing a patient's level of consciousness using the Glasgow Coma Scale. The following findings are documented: Eyes open to speech, responses are oriented, localized pain is noted. The score for this patient is:
    1. 15
    2. 13
    3. 11
    4. 9

STUDY GROUP QUESTIONS

- What are the purposes of the physical examination?
- How is physical assessment integrated into patient care?
- How does a nurse incorporate cultural sensitivity and awareness of ethnic physiological differences into the physical examination?
- What are the physical assessment skills, and what information is obtained through their use?
- How does a nurse prepare a patient and environment for a physical examination?
- What similarities and differences exist in the preparation and procedure for a physical examination of a child, adult, and older adult?
- What information is obtained through a general survey?
- What positions and equipment are used for completion of the physical examination?
- What is the usual sequence for performing the physical examination?
- What are the expected and unexpected findings of a complete physical examination?
- What self-screening procedures may be taught to patients?
- How does a nurse report and record the findings of a physical examination?

STUDY CHART

Create a study chart to compare the *Expected vs. Unexpected Findings in a Physical Examination,* working in sequential order of the exam from the integumentary system through the neurological system.

Answers available through your instructor.

Administering Medications 16

CASE STUDIES

1. A nurse is visiting a patient at home who has poor eyesight and occasional forgetfulness. The patient has four oral medications to take at different times of the day.
    a. What strategies may be implemented to assist this patient in maintaining the medication regimen?
2. A nurse is preparing to give medications in the medical center, but the prescriber's handwriting is difficult to read.
    a. What should the nurse do to prevent medication errors?
3. A patient in a long-term care facility is about to receive her medications, but the nurse notices that she does not have an identification band.
    a. What is the appropriate next action?
4. A nurse is to administer an injection to a 6-year-old child on a pediatric acute care unit.
    a. What safety measures need to be implemented?
5. A nurse is about to prepare a narcotic medication for administration to a patient. The nurse notices that the record shows that 24 tablets should remain in the box but there are only 23 tablets left.
    a. What should the nurse do?
6. A nurse is caring for a patient who requires an antipyretic medication that is ordered for oral administration, but the patient has been experiencing severe nausea.
    a. What should the nurse do?
7. A nurse is visiting a patient who has been recently discharged from the hospital. The patient shows the nurse the number of medications that have been prescribed and tells her that he really does not think he can remember all of the information he was told in the hospital.
    a. What is the nurse's initial action?
    b. What information should be included in a teaching plan for this client?

CHAPTER REVIEW

Match the description/definition in Column A with the correct term in Column B.

	Column A		Column B
___	1. Placing medication under the tongue		a. Parenteral administration
___	2. The effect of two medications combined is greater than each given separately		b. Inhalation
___	3. Secondary effects of medication, such as nausea		c. Instillation
___	4. Unpredictable effect of medications		d. Buccal
___	5. Fluid administered and retained in a body cavity		e. Subcutaneous
___	6. Injection into tissues below the dermis of the skin		f. Intraocular
___	7. Severe allergic response characterized by bronchospasm and laryngeal edema		g. Idiosyncratic reaction
___	8. Inserting medication into the eye		h. Polypharmacy
___	9. Administering medications through the oral, nasal, or pulmonary passages		i. Sublingual
___	10. Patient taking many medications		j. Synergistic effect
___	11. Placing solid medication against the mucous membranes of the cheek		k. Side effects
___	12. Injecting medication into body tissues		l. Anaphylactic reaction

CHAPTER 16 • Administering Medications

Complete the following:

13. Provide an example of how a nurse's professional responsibility in administering medications is controlled or regulated.

14. a. Identify a strategy for a nurse to implement to avoid errors with medications that appear the same.

    b. Specify two acceptable patient identifiers.

15. Provide an example of how each of the following factors can influence the actions of medications.
    a. Dietary factors
    b. Physiological variables
    c. Environmental conditions

16. Identify the four routes for parenteral administration of medications.

17. For the following medication orders, identify the essential component that is missing. (NOTE: All have been correctly signed by the prescriber.)
    a. Apresoline IM stat
    b. Morphine sulfate 10 mg q3-4h
    c. Vancomycin 1 g IV
    d. Lasix 40 mg bid

18. Identify the six guidelines or "rights" that a nurse uses for administering medications.
    1. _____
    2. _____
    3. _____
    4. _____
    5. _____
    6. _____

19. Place the following steps for mixing two types of compatible insulin in one syringe in the correct sequence.
    a. With an insulin syringe, injecting air equal to the dose of cloudy insulin to be administered into the cloudy vial _____
    b. Removing the syringe from the vial of cloudy insulin _____
    c. Placing the needle of the syringe back into the cloudy vial and withdrawing the correct dose _____
    d. Performing hand hygiene _____
    e. With the same syringe, injecting air equal to the dose of clear insulin to be administered into the clear vial and withdrawing the correct dose into the syringe _____
    f. Removing the syringe from the clear insulin and getting rid of air bubbles to ensure accurate dosing _____
    g. Verifying insulin labels before preparing the dose to ensure that the correct type of insulin is going to be given _____
    h. Rolling cloudy insulin between the hands to resuspend the insulin preparation _____
    i. Wiping the tops of both insulin vials with alcohol swabs _____

20. Identify the form of medication for the following.
    a. Solid dose form for oral use; medication in a powder, liquid, or oil form and encased by a gelatin shell:
    b. Solid dose form mixed with gelatin and shaped in form of pellet for insertion into body cavity:
    c. Clear liquid containing water and/or alcohol; designed for oral use; usually has a sweetener added:
    d. Finely divided drug particles dispersed in a liquid medium; when left standing, particles settle to the bottom of the container:
    e. A small, flexible oval consisting of two soft outer layers and a middle layer containing medication:
    f. Drug in liquid suspension applied to protect skin:

21. An example of a commonly abused over-the-counter medication is:

22. Noncompliance with or nonadherence to medication therapy may be related to:

23. Identify at least one strategy to promote medication adherence.

24. For each of the following pairs, identify which of the two has the faster absorption or action in the body:
   a. IV _____ or Oral _____
   b. IM _____ or Subcutaneous _____
   c. Acidic oral medication _____ or Alkaline oral medication _____
   d. Tablets _____ or Solutions _____
   e. Large surface area _____ or Smaller surface area _____
   f. Less lipid soluble _____ or Highly lipid soluble _____
   g. Albumin binding _____ or Nonalbumin binding _____

25. The time that it takes for a medication to reach its highest effective concentration is its:

26. Oral medication is contraindicated for a patient with:

27. What is a potential problem with this medication order? Lasix 40.0 mg

28. Identify the appropriate equivalents for the following:
   a. 1 mL = _____ gtt
   b. 60 mL = _____ ounces
   c. _____ L = 1 quart
   d. 3 g = _____ mg
   e. 0.25 L = _____ mL
   f. _____ mL = 1 teaspoon

29. Identify the five different types of medication orders and provide an example of each:
   1.
   2.
   3.
   4.
   5.

30. Verbal orders are usually required to be signed by the prescriber within what time frame?

31. A nurse calculates the medication order and determines that 6 tablets should be given to the patient for each dose. What should the nurse do first?

32. After a patient is given medications, the patient tells the nurse that the medicine looks different from the previous administrations of the medication. The nurse should:

33. An unopened unit-dose medication that is refused by the patient needs to be discarded.
True _____ False _____

34. Crushed medication should be mixed in a large amount of food to mask the taste.
True _____ False _____

35. A nurse is responsible for administering an incorrect medication or dosage.
True _____ False _____

36. A triple check to compare the medication label to the order should be done:
   1.
   2.
   3.

37. Identify a technique that may be used to facilitate administration of medications to children.
   a. Oral medications:
   b. Injections:

38. Identify a way that a nurse may minimize the discomfort of an injection.

39. How should a medication that is irritating to the tissues be injected?

40. Identify the correct angle for each of the following illustrations, and the type of injection that is being administered.
   a. _____ b. _____ c. _____

CHAPTER 16 • Administering Medications

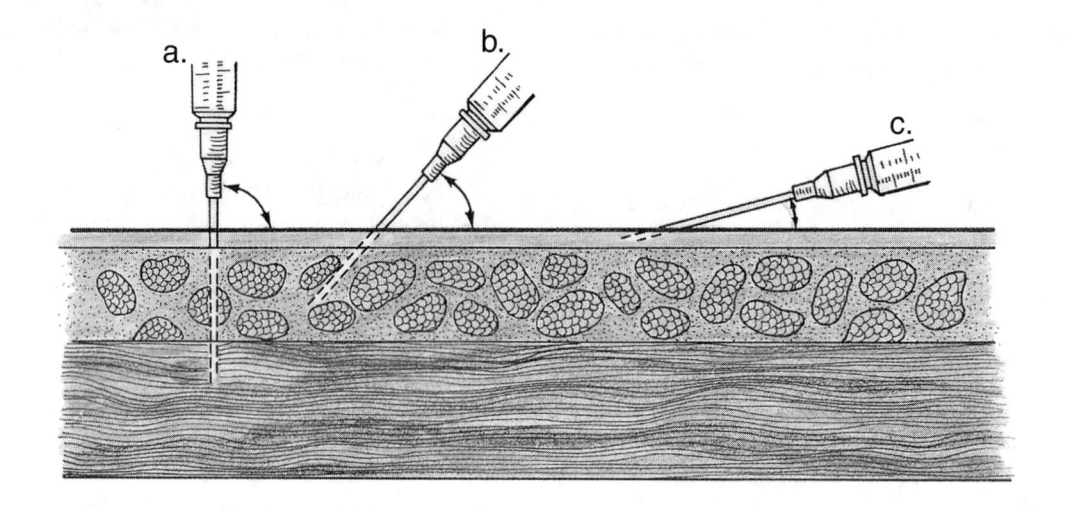

41. Identify three ways in which medication may be administered intravenously.
    1.
    2.
    3.

42. A wireless barcode scanner is usually used to identify:
    a.
    b.
    c.

43. Identify the meaning of the following abbreviations.
    a. ac: _____
    b. bid: _____
    c. prn: _____
    d. q4h: _____
    e. stat: _____

44. Check the orders and calculate the correct dosages for the following medication orders.
    a. Prescriber's order: Synthroid 0.150 mg PO daily
       In stock: Split tablets in a container labeled 75 mcg
       How many tablets should be given?

    b. Prescriber's order: Mellaril 150 mg PO bid
       In stock: Mellaril 50 mg/mL
       How much of the medication should be given?

    c. Prescriber's order: Lasix 20 mg IM stat
       In stock: Lasix 10 mg/mL
       How much medication should be given?

    d. Prescriber's order: Aldomet 250 mg PO bid
       In stock: Tablets labeled 125 mg
       How many tablets should be given?

    e. Prescriber's order: Demerol 75 mg IM prn
       In stock: Demerol 25 mg/0.5 mL
       How much medication should be given?
       Mark the amount to be administered on the syringe.

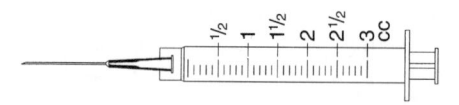

    f. Prescriber's order: Regular insulin 24 units
       In stock: Regular insulin U-100
       How much medication should be administered?
       Mark the amount to be administered on the syringe.

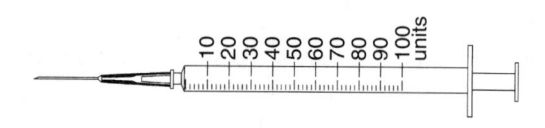

    g. Prescriber's order: cefazolin 500 mg q8h
       In stock: Keflex 250 mg tablets
       How many tablets should be given?

45. Identify an area of patient assessment before administration of a parenteral injection.

CHAPTER 16 • Administering Medications

46. Identify on the figure the sites recommended for subcutaneous injections.

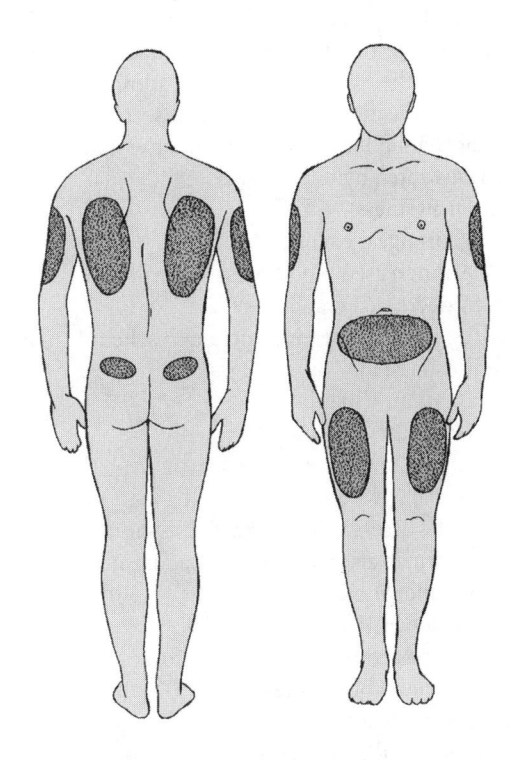

47. Select all of the following actions that are correct for the administration of medications to a patient with dysphagia.
    a. Do not allow the patient to self-administer, even if able. _____
    b. Position the patient upright. _____
    c. Turn the patient's head toward the weaker side to help the patient swallow. _____
    d. Use thinner liquids for the patient to take with the medications. _____
    e. Use a straw for liquids. _____
    f. Crush medication and mix with pureed food, if indicated. _____

48. A priority assessment specifically for the patient receiving medication through a nasogastric tube is for the nurse to:

49. Before administration of a topical medication, the nurse needs to:

50. Identify the following for the administration of ear drops:
    a. Position the patient.
    b. Pull ear pinna backward, up, and out for an adult patient.
    c. Irrigate with _____ mL of _____ temperature fluid.

51. For the use of a metered-dose inhaler:
    a. When the patient has difficulty coordinating the inhaler, a(n) _____ should be used.
    b. The medication order is 2 puffs of the inhaler qid. The canister contains 160 puffs total. How many days will the canister last? _____

52. The patient should be placed in _____ position for the administration of a rectal suppository.

53. Identify the specific assessments that should be done before administration of the following types of medications.
    a. Anticoagulant
    b. Antihypertensive
    c. Analgesic
    d. Cardiotonic

54. Eye drops should be administered directly onto the cornea. True _____ False _____

55. From the following, identify the guidelines that are appropriate for pediatric medication administration. Select all that apply.
    a. Identify the dosage based on the child's weight in pounds. _____
    b. Pediatric doses are usually given in micrograms and small syringes. _____
    c. IM doses are very small and usually do not exceed 1 mL in small children. _____
    d. Most medications are rounded to the nearest tenth. _____
    e. Mentally estimate a patient's dose before beginning the calculation, comparing the answer with the estimate before preparing the medication. _____
    f. Dosage ranges for 24-hour periods are similar to adult dosages. _____

56. Identify the correct sequence of actions for a saline flush.
    a. Pulling back gently on syringe plunger and checking for blood return _____
    b. Cleaning lock's injection port with antiseptic swab _____
    c. Flushing IV site with normal saline by pushing slowly on plunger _____
    d. Removing saline-filled syringe _____
    e. Preparing two syringes filled with 2 to 3 mL of normal saline (0.9%) _____
    f. Inserting syringe with normal saline 0.9% through injection port of IV lock _____

Select the best answer for each of the following questions:

57. A nurse determines the location for an injection by identifying the greater trochanter of the femur,

anterosuperior iliac spine, and iliac crest. The injection site being used by the nurse is the:
1. Rectus femoris muscle
2. Ventrogluteal area
3. Dorsogluteal area
4. Vastus lateralis muscle

58. Upon receiving the assignment for the evening, a nurse notices that two of the patients have the same name. The best way to identify two patients on a medical unit who have the same name is to:
1. Ask the patients their names
2. Verify their names with the family members
3. Check the patients' ID bands
4. Ask another nurse about their identities

59. A nurse is to administer a subcutaneous injection to an average size adult. The nurse selects a:
1. 27-gauge, ½-inch needle and 0.5-mL syringe
2. 25-gauge, ⅝-inch needle and 1-mL syringe
3. 22-gauge, 1-inch needle and 3-mL syringe
4. 20-gauge, 1-inch needle and 3-mL syringe

60. A nurse has administered medications to all assigned patients on the medical unit. Upon assessing the response of the medications given, the nurse is alert to the possibility of a toxic reaction. This is indicated by the patient experiencing:
1. Itching
2. Nausea
3. Dizziness
4. Respiratory depression

61. The nursing staff is completing a review of the procedures used for the storage and administration of narcotics. A nurse implements the required procedure when:
1. Narcotics are kept together with the patient's other medications
2. Small amounts of medication may be discarded without notation
3. The narcotic count is checked daily by the medication nurse
4. A separate administration record is kept in addition to the patient's medication administration record (MAR)

62. An order is written for a patient to receive potassium chloride (KCl) and vitamins intravenously. The nurse goes into the medication room and selects equipment to provide the medication by a(n):
1. IV bolus administration
2. Tandem administration
3. Piggyback administration
4. Large-volume administration

63. While completing an admission assessment, a nurse discovers that a patient is allergic to shellfish. Later that morning when the nurse is preparing medications for this patient, the nurse will withhold medication that contains:
1. Iodine
2. Alcohol
3. Glucose
4. Calcium carbonate

64. A patient in a nurse practitioner's office is receiving penicillin for the first time. The nurse asks the patient to wait in the office following the administration of the medication. The nurse is observing for a possible anaphylactic response that would be demonstrated by:
1. Drowsiness
2. Pharyngeal edema
3. An increased blood pressure reading
4. A decreased respiratory rate

65. A drug that is to be given on a q4h schedule may be administered at:
1. 10 AM and 10 PM
2. 10 AM, 2 PM, and 10 PM
3. 10 AM, 2 PM, 6 PM, and 10 PM
4. 10 AM, 2 PM, 6 PM, 10 PM, and 2 AM

66. A specific assessment that a nurse should make before the administration of an anticoagulant is to check for:
1. An allergy history
2. Evidence of bruising
3. The patient's level of discomfort
4. Increased blood pressure

67. In the event of a mistake in the administration of medications, the first action that a nurse should take is to:
1. Complete an occurrence report
2. Inform the patient of the problem
3. Report the error to the nurse in charge or the physician
4. Provide an appropriate antidote for the medication given

68. When preparing to administer a patient's medications, a nurse notes that the prescriber's order is difficult to read. The nurse should:
1. Check with the patient
2. Call the prescriber
3. Call the pharmacist
4. Check with the charge nurse

69. The subcutaneous site that is most commonly used for heparin injections is the:
1. Abdomen
2. Anterior thigh
3. Scapular region
4. Outer aspect of the upper arm

70. A prescriber indicates to a nurse that a patient will be receiving an intermediate-acting insulin. The nurse anticipates that the patient will receive:
1. Insulin glargine (Lantus)
2. Insulin lispro (Humalog)
3. Isophane insulin suspension (NPH)
4. Protamine zinc insulin suspension (PZI)

71. A charge nurse is evaluating the injection technique of a new staff member. The correct technique for a Z-track injection is noted when the new staff member:
1. Uses the deltoid site
2. Pulls the skin 1 to 1½ inches laterally

3. Removes the needle immediately after the injection
4. Releases the skin before the needle is removed
72. For a subcutaneous injection to an average size adult, which of the following techniques requires correction? The student nurse:
    1. Selects a 25-gauge, ⅝-inch needle
    2. Injects the needle at a 45-degree angle
    3. Recaps the needle after injecting the medication
    4. Does not massage the injection site after administration
73. A nurse is aware that a parenteral administration of a concentrated dose of medication in a small amount of fluid is a:
    1. Bolus injection
    2. Piggyback infusion
    3. Volume control infusion
    4. Mini-infuser administration

STUDY GROUP QUESTIONS

- How are medications named and classified, and what forms of medications are available?
- What legislation and standards guide medication administration?
- How are medications absorbed, distributed, metabolized, and excreted from the body?
- What are the different types of medication actions?
- What are the different routes for medication administration, and what are the advantages, disadvantages, and contraindications for each route?
- What are the systems used for drug measurement, and how are amounts converted within and between the systems?
- How are dosages calculated for oral, parenteral, and pediatric medications?
- What are the roles of the health team members in the administration of medications?
- What are the six "rights" of medication administration?
- What patient assessment data are critical to obtain before administering medications?
- What equipment is used for the administration of medications via different routes?
- What are the sites or body landmarks for parenteral administration?
- What are the procedures for administration of medications?
- How can IV medication be administered?
- How is administration of medications adapted to patients of different ages and levels of health?
- What information is included in patient/family teaching for medication administration?
- How has technology influenced the administration of medications?

STUDY CHART

Create a study chart to compare *Parenteral Medication and Preparation* that identifies the equipment, needle gauge, amount of medication, site to be used, and angle of injection for subcutaneous, intramuscular, and intradermal injections.

Answers available through your instructor.

CHAPTER 16 • Administering Medications

Name _____ Date _____ Instructor's Name _____

Performance Checklist Skill 16-1: Administering Oral Medications

	S	U	NP	Comments

Assessment
1. Check accuracy and completeness of each medical administration record (MAR) or computer printout with prescriber's written medication order.
2. Assess for any contraindications to patient receiving oral medication.
3. Assess risk for aspiration. Assess patient's swallow, cough, and gag reflexes.
4. Assess patient's medical history, history of allergies, medication history, and diet history.
5. Gather and review assessment and laboratory data that influences drug administration.
6. Assess patient's knowledge regarding health and medication usage.
7. Assess patient's preferences for fluids. Maintain ordered fluid restriction (when applicable).

Planning
1. Determine expected outcomes. Clarify order as necessary.
2. Recopy or reprint parts of MAR that are difficult to read.

Implementation
1. Preparing medications
   A. Perform hand hygiene.
   B. If medication cart is used, move it outside patient's room.
   C. Unlock medicine drawer or cart.
   D. Prepare medications for one patient at a time. Keep all pages of MAR or computer printouts for one patient together.
   E. Select correct drug from stock supply or unit-dose drawer. Compare label of medication with MAR or computer printout.
   F. Check expiration date on all medications.
   G. Calculate drug dose as necessary. Double-check calculation.
   H. When preparing narcotics, check record for previous drug count and compare with supply available.
   I. Prepare solid forms of oral medications.
      (1) To prepare tablets or capsules from a floor stock bottle, pour required number into bottle cap and transfer medication to medication cup. Do not touch medication with fingers. Return extra tablets or capsules to bottle. Break medications that need to be broken to administer half the dosage; pills can be broken using a gloved hand, or cut with a pillating device. Make sure these tablets are prescored.
      (2) To prepare unit-dose tablets or capsules, place packaged tablet or capsule directly into medicine cup. (Do not remove wrapper.)
      (3) Place all tablets or capsules to be given to patient at same time in one medicine cup. Place medications requiring preadministration assessments in separate cups.

Copyright © 2011, 2007, 2003 by Mosby, Inc., an affiliate of Elsevier Inc. All rights reserved.

	S	U	NP	Comments

(4) If patient has difficulty swallowing and liquid medications are not an option, use a pill-crushing device, such as a mortar and pestle, to grind pills. If a pill-crushing device is not available, place tablet between two medication cups and grind with a blunt instrument. Mix ground tablet in small amount of soft food (e.g., custard, applesauce).

J. Prepare liquids:
  (1) Gently shake container. Remove bottle cap from container and place cap upside down or open the unit-dose container. If unit-dose container has correct amount to administer, no further preparation is necessary.
  (2) Hold bottle with label against palm of hand while pouring.
  (3) Hold medication cup at eye level and fill to desired level. Make sure scale is even with fluid level at its surface or base of meniscus, not edges. For small doses of liquid medications, draw liquid into a calibrated 10-mL syringe without needle.
  (4) Discard any excess liquid into sink. Wipe lip and neck of bottle with paper towel.
  (5) Administer liquid medications packaged in single-dose cups directly from the single-dose cup. Do not pour them into medicine cups.

K. Compare MAR with prepared drug and container.
L. Return stock containers or unused unit-dose medications to shelf or drawer, and read label again.
M. Do not leave drugs unattended.

1. Administering medications:
  A. Take medications to patient at correct time.
  B. Verify patient's identity by using at least two identifiers.
  C. Compare medication labels with MAR at bedside.
  D. Explain purpose of each medication and its action to patient. Allow patient to ask any questions about drugs.
  E. Assist patient to sitting or Fowler's position. Use side-lying position if sitting is contraindicated.
  F. Administer medication.
    (1) **For tablets:** Patient may wish to hold solid medications in hand or cup before placing in mouth.
    (2) Offer water or juice to help patient swallow medications.
    (3) **For sublingual medications:** Have patient place medication under tongue and allow it to dissolve completely. Caution patient against swallowing tablet whole.
    (4) **For buccal medications:** Have patient place medication in mouth against mucous membranes of the cheek until it dissolves. Avoid administering liquids until buccal medication has dissolved.
    (5) Caution patient against chewing or swallowing lozenges.

	S	U	NP	Comments

 (6) **For powdered medications:** Mix with liquids at bedside, and give to patient to drink.
 (7) Give effervescent powders and tablets immediately after dissolving.
G. If patient is unable to hold medications, place medication cup to the lips and gently introduce each drug into the mouth, one at a time. Do not rush.
H. If tablet or capsule falls to the floor, discard it and repeat preparation.
I. Stay in room until patient has completely swallowed each medication. Ask patient to open mouth if uncertain whether patient has swallowed medication.
J. For highly acidic medications, offer patient nonfat snack if not contraindicated by patient's condition.
K. Assist patient in returning to comfortable position.
L. Dispose of soiled supplies, and perform hand hygiene.
M. Replenish stock such as cups and straws, return cart to medicine room, and clean work area.

Evaluation
1. Evaluate patient's response to medications at times that correlate with the medication's onset, peak, and duration.
2. Ask patient or family member to identify medication name, purpose, action, schedule, and potential side effects.
3. Record administration of medication on MAR or computer printout. Return MAR or computer printout to appropriate file for next administration time.
4. Notify prescriber if patient exhibits a toxic effect or allergic reaction or side effects occur. Withhold further doses.

Name _____ Date _____ Instructor's Name _____

Performance Checklist Skill 16-2: Administering Eye Medications

	S	U	NP	Comments

Assessment
1. Check accuracy and completeness of each MAR or computer printout with prescriber's written medication order.
2. Recopy or reprint any portion of MAR that is difficult to read.
3. Assess condition of external eye structures.
4. Determine whether patient has any known allergies to eye medications. Also ask if patient has allergy to latex.
5. Determine whether patient has any symptoms of visual alterations.
6. Assess patient's level of consciousness and ability to follow directions.
7. Assess patient's knowledge regarding drug therapy and desire to self-administer medication.
8. Assess patient's ability to manipulate and hold equipment necessary for eye medication.

Planning
1. Determine expected outcomes. Clarify order as necessary.
2. Recopy or reprint parts of MAR that are difficult to read.

Implementation
1. Prepare medication.
2. Take medications to patient at correct time and perform hand hygiene.
3. Verify patient's identity by using at least two patient identifiers.
4. Compare label of medication against MAR for third time.
5. Explain procedure to patient regarding positioning and sensations to expect.
6. Arrange supplies and medications at bedside. Apply clean gloves.
7. Gently roll container.
8. Ask patient to lie supine or sit back in chair with head slightly hyperextended.
9. If crust or drainage is present along eyelid margins or inner canthus, gently wash away. Apply damp washcloth or cotton ball over eye for a few minutes to soak crusts that are dried and difficult to remove. Always wipe clean from inner to outer canthus.
10. Hold cotton ball or clean tissue in nondominant hand on patient's cheekbone just below lower eyelid.
11. With tissue or cotton resting below lid, gently press downward with thumb or forefinger against bony orbit.
12. Ask patient to look at ceiling.
13. Administer ophthalmic medication.

	S	U	NP	Comments

A. To instill eye drops:
  (1) With dominant hand resting on patient's forehead, hold filled medication eye dropper or ophthalmic solution approximately 1 to 2 cm (½ to ¾ inch) above conjunctival sac.
  (2) Drop prescribed number of medication drops into conjunctival sac.
  (3) If patient blinks or closes eye or if drops land on outer lid margins, repeat procedure.
  (4) After instilling drops, ask patient to close eye gently.
  (5) When administering drugs that cause systemic effects, apply gentle pressure with your finger and clean tissue on the patient's nasolacrimal duct for 30 to 60 seconds.

B. To instill eye ointment:
  (1) Ask patient to look at ceiling.
  (2) Holding ointment applicator above lower lid margin, apply thin stream of ointment evenly along inner edge of lower eyelid on conjunctiva from inner canthus to outer canthus.
  (3) Have patient close eye and roll eye behind closed eyelid.

C. To administer intraocular disc:
  (1) Application:
    (a) Open package containing the disc. Apply gloves. Gently press your fingertip against the disc so that it adheres to your finger. Position the convex side of the disc on your fingertip.
    (b) With your other hand, gently pull the patient's lower eyelid away from the eye. Ask patient to look up.
    (c) Place the disc in the conjunctival sac so that it floats on the sclera between the iris and lower eyelid.
    (d) Pull the patient's lower eyelid out and over the disc.
  (2) Removal:
    (a) Perform hand hygiene, and put on gloves.
    (b) Explain procedure to patient.
    (c) Gently pull down on the patient's lower eyelid.
    (d) Using your forefinger and thumb of your opposite hand, pinch the disc and lift it out of the patient's eye.

14. If excess medication is on eyelid, gently wipe it from inner to outer canthus.
15. If patient had eye patch, apply clean patch by placing it over affected eye so entire eye is covered. Tape securely without applying pressure to eye.

	S	U	NP	Comments

16. If patient receives more than one eye medication to the same eye at the same time, wait at least 5 minutes before administering the next medication.
17. If patient receives eye medication to both eyes at the same time, use a different tissue or cotton ball with each eye.
18. Remove gloves, dispose of soiled supplies in proper receptacle, and perform hand hygiene.

Evaluation
1. Note patient's response to instillation; ask if any discomfort was felt.
2. Observe response to medication by assessing visual changes and noting any side effects.
3. Ask patient to discuss drug's purpose, action, side effects, and technique of administration.
4. Have patient demonstrate self-administration of next dose.
5. Record drug, administration, and appearance of eye(s).
6. Record and report any undesirable side effects to nurse in charge or physician.

CHAPTER 16 • Administering Medications

Name _____ Date _____ Instructor's Name _____

Performance Checklist Skill 16-3: Using Metered-Dose or Dry Powder Inhalers

	S	U	NP	Comments

Assessment
1. Check accuracy and completeness of each MAR or computer printout with prescriber's written medication order.
2. Assess respiratory pattern and auscultate breath sounds.
3. If previously instructed in self-administration of inhaled medicine, assess patient's technique in using inhaler.
4. Assess patient's ability to hold, manipulate, and depress canister and inhaler.
5. Assess patient's readiness to learn.
6. Assess patient's ability to learn.
7. Assess patient's knowledge and understanding of disease and purpose and action of prescribed medications.
8. Determine drug schedule and number of inhalations prescribed for each dose.

Planning
1. Determine expected outcomes. Clarify order as necessary.
2. Check accuracy and completeness of each MAR or computer printout with prescriber's written medication order.
3. Verify patient's identity by using at least two patient identifiers.
4. Perform hand hygiene, and arrange equipment needed.
5. Provide adequate time for teaching session.

Implementation
1. Prepare medication.
2. Verify patient's identity using at least two patient identifiers.
3. Compare the label of the medication with the MAR one more time at the patient's bedside.
4. Help patient get into a comfortable position, such as sitting in chair in hospital room or sitting at kitchen table in home.
5. Have patient manipulate inhaler, canister, and spacer device. Explain and demonstrate how canister fits into inhaler.
6. Explain what metered dose is, and warn patient about overuse of inhaler and medication side effects.
7. Explain steps for administering inhaled dose of metered-dose inhaler (MDI):
    A. Insert MDI canister into holder.
    B. Remove mouthpiece cover from inhaler.
    C. Shake inhaler strongly five or six times.
    D. Tell patient to sit up or stand and take a deep breath and exhale.
    E. Instruct the patient to position the inhaler in one of two ways:
        (1) Close mouth around MDI with opening toward back of throat.
        (2) Position MDI 2 to 4 cm (1 to 2 inches) from the mouth.
    F. With the inhaler positioned correctly, have patient hold inhaler with thumb at the mouthpiece and the index finger and middle finger at the top.

Copyright © 2011, 2007, 2003 by Mosby, Inc., an affiliate of Elsevier Inc. All rights reserved.

	S	U	NP	Comments

G. Instruct patient to tilt head back slightly, inhale slowly and deeply through mouth, 3 to 5 seconds, while fully pressing down on the canister.
H. Have patient hold breath for approximately 10 seconds.
I. Remove MDI, and exhale through pursed lips.
8. Explain steps to administer MDI using a spacer such as an Aerochamber:
   A. Remove mouthpiece cover from inhaler and spacer.
   B. Insert MDI into end of spacer.
   C. Shake inhaler strongly five or six times.
   D. Have patient take a deep breath and exhale completely before closing mouth around spacer's mouthpiece.
   E. Have patient press medication canister one time, spraying one puff into spacer.
   F. Instruct patient to inhale slowly and deeply through mouth for 3 to 5 seconds.
   G. Hold full breath for approximately 10 seconds.
   H. Remove MDI and spacer before exhaling.
9. Explain steps to administer dry powder inhaler (DPI):
   A. Remove mouthpiece cover. Do not shake DPI.
   B. Hold inhaler upright, and turn wheel to the right and then to the left until you hear a click.
   C. Exhale away from the inhaler.
   D. Position mouthpiece between lips.
   E. Inhale deeply and forcefully through the mouth.
   F. Hold full breath for 5 to 10 seconds.
10. Instruct patient to wait at least 1 minute between inhalations or as ordered by prescriber.
11. Tell patient not to repeat inhaler doses until next scheduled dose.
12. Explain that patient may feel gagging sensation in throat caused by droplets of medication on pharynx or tongue.
13. Instruct patient on cleaning of inhaler in warm water.

Evaluation
1. Ask if patient has any questions.
2. Have patient explain and demonstrate steps in use of inhaler.
3. Ask patient to explain medication schedule, side effects, and when to call health care provider.
4. Ask patient to calculate how many days the inhaler will last.
5. After medication instillation, assess patient's respirations and auscultate lungs.
6. Record patient education and patient's ability to perform self-administration.
7. Record medication administration and patient's response.

Name _____ Date _____ Instructor's Name _____

Performance Checklist Skill 16-4: Preparing Injections From Vials and Ampules

	S	U	NP	Comments

Assessment
1. Check accuracy and completeness of each MAR or computer printout with prescriber's written medication order.
2. Review pertinent information related to medication, including action, purpose, side effects, and nursing implications.
3. Assess patient's body build, muscle size, and weight if giving subcutaneous or intramuscular medication.

Planning
1. Determine expected outcomes. Clarify order as necessary.
2. Recopy or reprint parts of MAR that are difficult to read.

Implementation
1. Perform hand hygiene and assemble supplies.
2. Prepare medication. Check medication order or MAR against label on medication.
   A. **Ampule Preparation:**
      (1) Tap top of ampule lightly and quickly with finger until fluid moves from neck of ampule.
      (2) Place small gauze pad or unopened alcohol pad around neck of ampule.
      (3) Snap neck of ampule quickly and firmly away from hands.
      (4) Draw up medication quickly, using a filter needle long enough to reach bottom of ampule.
      (5) Hold ampule upside down, or set it on a flat surface. Insert filter needle into center of ampule opening. Do not allow needle tip or shaft to touch rim of ampule.
      (6) Aspirate medication into syringe by gently pulling back on plunger.
      (7) Keep needle tip under surface of liquid. Tip ampule to bring all fluid within reach of the needle.
      (8) If you aspirate air bubbles, do not expel air into ampule.
      (9) To expel excess air bubbles, remove needle from ampule. Hold syringe with needle pointing up. Tap side of syringe to cause bubbles to rise toward needle. Draw back slightly on plunger, and then push plunger upward to eject air. Do not eject fluid.
      (10) If syringe contains excess fluid, use sink for disposal. Hold syringe vertically with needle tip up and slanted slightly toward sink. Slowly eject excess fluid into sink. Recheck fluid level in syringe by holding it vertically.
      (11) Cover needle with its safety sheath or cap. Replace filter needle with regular needle.

	S	U	NP	Comments

B. **Vial Containing a Solution:**
   (1) Remove cap covering top of unused vial to expose sterile rubber seal. If a multidose vial has been used before, cap is removed already. Firmly and briskly wipe surface of rubber seal with alcohol swab, and allow it to dry. _____ _____ _____ _____
   (2) Pick up syringe and remove needle cap. Pull back on plunger to draw amount of air into syringe equivalent to volume of medication to be aspirated from vial. _____ _____ _____ _____
   (3) With vial on flat surface, insert tip of needle through center of rubber seal. Apply pressure to tip of needle during insertion. _____ _____ _____ _____
   (4) Inject air into the vial's air space, holding on to plunger. Hold plunger with firm pressure; plunger may be forced backward by air pressure within the vial. _____ _____ _____ _____
   (5) Invert vial while keeping firm hold on syringe and plunger. Hold vial between thumb and middle fingers of nondominant hand. Grasp end of syringe barrel and plunger with thumb and forefinger of dominant hand to counteract pressure in vial. _____ _____ _____ _____
   (6) Keep tip of needle below fluid level. _____ _____ _____ _____
   (7) Allow air pressure from the vial to fill syringe gradually with medication. If necessary, pull back slightly on plunger to obtain correct amount of solution. _____ _____ _____ _____
   (8) When you obtain desired volume, position needle into vial's air space; tap side of syringe barrel carefully to dislodge any air bubbles. Eject any air remaining at top of syringe into vial. _____ _____ _____ _____
   (9) Remove needle from vial by pulling back on barrel of syringe. _____ _____ _____ _____
   (10) Hold syringe at eye level at 90-degree angle to ensure correct volume and absence of air bubbles. Remove any remaining air by tapping barrel to dislodge any air bubbles. Draw back slightly on plunger, then push plunger upward to eject air. Do not eject fluid. _____ _____ _____ _____
   (11) If you need to inject medication into patient's tissue, change needle to appropriate gauge and length according to route of medication. _____ _____ _____ _____
   (12) For multidose vial, make label that includes date of opening vial and your initials. _____ _____ _____ _____

C. **Vial Containing a Powder (Reconstituting Medications):**
   (1) Remove cap covering vial of powdered medication and cap covering vial of proper diluent. Firmly swab both caps with alcohol swab, and allow to dry. _____ _____ _____ _____
   (2) Draw up diluent into syringe. _____ _____ _____ _____
   (3) Insert tip of needle through center of rubber seal of vial of powdered medication. Inject diluent into vial. Remove needle. _____ _____ _____ _____
   (4) Mix medication thoroughly. Roll in palms. Do not shake. _____ _____ _____ _____

CHAPTER 16 • Administering Medications

	S	U	NP	Comments

    (5) Reconstituted medication in vial is ready to be drawn into new syringe. Read label carefully to determine dose after reconstitution. _____ _____ _____ _____

    (6) Draw up reconstituted medication in syringe. _____ _____ _____ _____

3. Dispose of soiled supplies. Place broken ampule and/or used vials and used needle in puncture-proof and leak-proof container. Clean work area, and perform hand hygiene. _____ _____ _____ _____

Evaluation

1. Compare dose in syringe with desired dose. _____ _____ _____ _____

CHAPTER 16 • Administering Medications

Name _____ Date _____ Instructor's Name _____

Performance Checklist Skill 16-5: Administering Injections

	S	U	NP	Comments

Assessment
1. Check accuracy and completeness of each MAR or computer printout with prescriber's written medication order.
2. Assess patient's medical history.
3. Assess patient's history of allergies, and known patient's normal allergic reaction.
4. Observe verbal and nonverbal responses toward receiving injection.
5. Assess for contraindications.
6. Assess patient's knowledge regarding medication to be received.

Planning
1. Determine expected outcomes. Clarify order as necessary.
2. Recopy or reprint parts of MAR that are difficult to read.

Implementation
1. Prepare medication.
2. Take medication to patient at the correct time, and perform hand hygiene.
3. Close room curtain or door.
4. Verify patient's identity by using at least two patient identifiers.
5. Compare the label of the medication with the MAR one more time at the patient's bedside.
6. Explain steps of procedure, and tell patient injection will cause a slight burning or sting.
7. Apply clean disposable gloves.
8. Keep sheet or gown draped over body parts not requiring exposure.
9. Select appropriate injection site. Inspect skin surface over sites for bruises, inflammation, or edema.
    A. **Subcutaneous:** Palpate sites for masses or tenderness. Be sure needle is correct size by grasping skinfold at site with thumb and forefinger. Measure fold from top to bottom.
    B. **IM:** Note integrity and size of muscle, and palpate for tenderness or hardness. Avoid these areas. If injections are given frequently, rotate sites.
    C. **ID:** Note lesions or discolorations of skin. If possible, select site three or four fingerwidths below antecubital space and one handwidth above wrist. If forearm cannot be used, inspect the upper back.
10. Assist patient to comfortable position:
    A. **Subcutaneous:** Have patient relax arm, leg, or abdomen, depending on site chosen for injection.
    B. **IM:** Position patient depending on site chosen.
    C. **ID:** Have patient extend elbow and support it and forearm on flat surface.
    D. Talk with patient about subject of interest.
11. Relocate site using anatomical landmarks.
12. Cleanse site with an antiseptic swab. Apply swab at center of the site, and rotate outward in a circular direction for about 5 cm (2 inches).

Copyright © 2011, 2007, 2003 by Mosby, Inc., an affiliate of Elsevier Inc. All rights reserved.

CHAPTER 16 • Administering Medications

	S	U	NP	Comments

13. Hold swab or gauze between third and fourth fingers of nondominant hand.
14. Remove needle cap by pulling it straight off.
15. Hold syringe between thumb and forefinger of dominant hand.
    A. **Subcutaneous:** Hold as dart, palm down.
    B. **IM:** Hold as dart, palm down.
    C. **ID:** Hold bevel of needle pointing up.
16. Administer injection.
    A. **Subcutaneous:**
       (1) For average-size patient, spread skin tightly across injection site or pinch skin with nondominant hand.
       (2) Inject needle quickly and firmly at 45- to 90-degree angle. Then release skin, if pinched.
       (3) For obese patient, pinch skin at site and inject needle at 90-degree angle below tissue fold.
       (4) Inject medication slowly.
    B. **Intramuscular:**
       (1) Position nondominant hand just below site and pull skin approximately 2.5 to 3.5 cm down or laterally with ulnar side of hand to administer in a Z-track. Hold position until medication is injected. With dominant hand, inject needle quickly at 90-degreee angle into muscle.
       (2) *(Option)* If patient's muscle mass is small, grasp body of muscle between thumb and fingers.
       (3) After needle pierces skin, grasp lower end of syringe barrel with nondominant hand to stabilize syringe. Continue to hold skin tightly with nondominant hand. Move dominant hand to end of plunger. Do not move syringe.
       (4) Pull back on plunger 5 to 10 seconds. If no blood appears, inject medication slowly at a rate of 1 mL per 10 seconds.
       (5) Wait 10 seconds, then smoothly and steadily withdraw needle and release skin.
    C. **Intradermal**
       (1) With nondominant hand, stretch skin over site with forefinger or thumb.
       (2) With needle almost against patient's skin, insert it slowly at a 5- to 15-degree angle until resistance is felt. Then advance needle through epidermis to approximately 3 mm (1/8 inch) below skin surface. Needle tip can be seen through skin.
       (3) Inject medication slowly. Normally, resistance is felt. If not, needle is too deep; remove and begin again.
       (4) While injecting medication, note that small bleb (approximately 6 mm [1/2 inch]) resembling mosquito bite appears on skin surface.
17. After withdrawing needle, apply alcohol swab or gauze gently over site.
18. Apply gentle pressure. Do not massage site. Apply bandage if needed.
19. Assist patient to comfortable position.
20. Discard uncapped needle or needle enclosed in safety shield and attached syringe into puncture- and leak-proof receptacle.
21. Remove disposable gloves, and perform hand hygiene.
22. Stay with patient, and observe for any allergic reactions.

	S	U	NP	Comments

Evaluation
1. Return to room, and ask if patient feels any acute pain, burning, numbness, or tingling at injection site.
2. Inspect site, noting any bruising or induration.
3. Observe patient's response to medication at times that correlate with the medication's onset, peak, and duration.
4. Ask patient to explain purpose and effects of medication.
5. *For ID injections,* use skin pencil and draw circle around perimeter of injection site. Read site within appropriate amount of time, designated by type of medication or skin test given.
6. Correctly record medication administration and patient's response.
7. Report any undesirable effects from medication to nurse in charge or physician.

CHAPTER 16 • Administering Medications

Name _____ Date _____ Instructor's Name _____

Performance Checklist Skill 16-6: Administering Medications by Intravenous Bolus

	S	U	NP	Comments

Assessment
1. Check accuracy and completeness of each MAR or computer printout with prescriber's written medication order.
2. Collect drug reference information necessary to administer drug safely.
3. If you will give drug through existing IV line, determine compatibility of medication with IV fluids and any additives within IV solution.
4. Perform hand hygiene. Assess condition of IV needle insertion site for signs of infiltration or phlebitis.
5. Check patient's medical history and drug allergies.
6. Check date of expiration for medication vial or ampule.
7. Assess patient's understanding of purpose of drug therapy.

Planning
1. Determine expected outcomes. Clarify order as necessary.

Implementation
1. Prepare medication.
2. Take medication to patient at the right time, and perform hand hygiene.
3. Verify patient's identity by using at least two patient identifiers.
4. Compare the label of the medication with the MAR one more time at the patient's bedside.
5. Explain procedure to patient. Encourage patient to report symptoms of discomfort at IV site.
6. Put on disposable gloves.
7. IV push (existing line):
   A. Select injection port of IV tubing closest to patient.
   B. Clean port with antiseptic swab.
   C. Connect syringe to IV line: Insert needleless tip of syringe or small-gauge needle containing drug through center of port.
   D. Occlude IV line by pinching tubing just above injection port. Pull back gently on syringe's plunger to aspirate for blood return.
   E. Release tubing and inject medication within amount of time recommended. Allow IV fluids to infuse when not pushing medication.
   F. Withdraw syringe and recheck fluid infusion rate after injecting medication.
8. IV push (IV lock):
   A. Prepare flush solutions according to hospital policy:
      (1) *Saline flush method (preferred):*
         (a) Prepare two syringes with 2 to 3 mL of normal saline.
      (2) *Heparin flush method (traditional):*
         (a) Prepare one syringe with ordered amount of heparin flush solution.
         (b) Prepare two syringes with 2 to 3 mL of normal saline (0.9%).

	S	U	NP	Comments

B. Administer medication:
   (1) Clean lock's injection port with antiseptic swab.
   (2) Insert syringe with normal saline (0.9%) through injection port of IV lock.
   (3) Pull back gently on syringe plunger and check for blood return.
   (4) Flush IV site with normal saline by pushing slowly on plunger.
   (5) Remove saline-filled syringe.
   (6) Clean lock's injection port with antiseptic swab.
   (7) Insert syringe containing prepared medication through injection port of IV lock.
   (8) Inject medication within amount of time recommended.
   (9) After administering bolus, withdraw syringe.
  (10) Clean lock's injection site with antiseptic swab.
  (11) Flush injection port.
     (a) Attach syringe with normal saline, and inject normal saline flush at the same rate the medication was given.
     (b) *Heparin flush option:* After instilling saline, attach syringe containing heparin flush, inject slowly, and remove syringe.

9. Dispose of uncapped needles and syringes in puncture-proof and leakproof container.
10. Remove gloves, and perform hand hygiene.

Evaluation

1. Observe patient closely for adverse reactions during administration and for several minutes thereafter.
2. Observe IV site during injection for sudden swelling.
3. Assess patient's status after giving medication to evaluate its effectiveness.
4. Ask patient to explain the drug's purpose and side effects.
5. Record medication administration, including drug name, dose, route, and time of administration.
6. Report and record any adverse reactions.

94   CHAPTER 16 • Administering Medications

Name _____ Date _____ Instructor's Name _____

Performance Checklist Skill 16-7: Administering Intravenous Medications by Piggyback, Intermittent Intravenous Infusion Sets, and Mini-Infusion Pumps

	S	U	NP	Comments

Assessment
1. Check accuracy and completeness of each MAR or computer printout with prescriber's written medication order.
2. Determine patient's medical history.
3. Collect information necessary to administer drug safely, including action, purpose, side effects, normal dose, time of peak onset, and nursing implications.
4. Assess compatibility of drug with existing IV solution.
5. Assess patency of patient's existing IV infusion line.
6. Perform hand hygiene. Assess IV insertion site for signs of infiltration or phlebitis: redness, pallor, swelling, or tenderness on palpation.
7. Assess patient's history of drug allergies.
8. Assess patient's understanding of purpose of drug therapy.

Planning
1. Determine expected outcomes. Clarify order as necessary.
2. Collect and organize supplies. Prepare patient by informing patient that medication will be given through IV equipment.

Implementation
1. Assemble medications and supplies at bedside.
2. Compare the label of the medication with the MAR at least two times while preparing supplies.
3. Give medication to patient at the right time, and perform hand hygiene.
4. Verify patient's identity by using at least two patient identifiers.
5. Explain purpose of medication and side effects to patient, and explain that medication is to be given through existing IV line. Encourage patient to report symptoms of discomfort at site.
6. Compare the label of the medication with the MAR one more time.
7. Administer infusion:
   A. Piggyback Infusion
   (1) Connect infusion tubing to medication bag. Allow solution to fill tubing by opening regulator flow clamp. Once tubing is full, close clamp and cap end of tubing.
   (2) Hang piggyback medication bag above level of primary fluid bag. (Use hook to lower main bag.)
   (3) Connect tubing of piggyback infusion to appropriate connector on primary infusion line.
      (a) *Needleless system:* Wipe off needleless port of IV line, and insert tip of piggyback infusion tubing.
      (b) *Stopcock:* Wipe off stopcock port with alcohol swab, and connect tubing. Turn stopcock to open position.

Copyright © 2011, 2007, 2003 by Mosby, Inc., an affiliate of Elsevier Inc. All rights reserved.

CHAPTER 16 • Administering Medications

	S	U	NP	Comments

    (c) *Needle system:* Connect sterile needle to end of piggyback infusion tubing, remove cap, cleanse injection port on main IV line, and insert needle through center of port. Secure by taping connection. ____ ____ ____ _____

  (4) Regulate flow rate of medication solution by adjusting regulator clamp. ____ ____ ____ _____

  (5) After medication has infused, check flow regulator on primary infusion. ____ ____ ____ _____

  (6) Regulate main infusion line desired rate if necessary. ____ ____ ____ _____

  (7) Leave IV piggyback bag and tubing in place for future drug administration or discard in appropriate containers. ____ ____ ____ _____

B. Mini-infusion Administration

  (1) Connect prefilled syringe to mini-infusion tubing. ____ ____ ____ _____

  (2) Carefully apply pressure to syringe plunger, allowing tubing to fill with medication. ____ ____ ____ _____

  (3) Place syringe into mini-infusion pump (follow product directions). Be sure syringe is secure. ____ ____ ____ _____

  (4) Connect mini-infusion tubing to main IV line. ____ ____ ____ _____

    (a) *Needleless system:* Wipe off needleless port of IV tubing, and insert tip of the mini-infusion tubing. ____ ____ ____ _____

    (b) *Stopcock:* Wipe off stopcock port with alcohol swab, and connect tubing. Turn stopcock to open position. ____ ____ ____ _____

    (c) *Needle system:* Connect sterile needle to mini-infusion tubing, remove cap, cleanse injection port on main IV line or saline lock, and insert needle through center of port. Consider placing tape where IV tubing enters port to keep connection secured. ____ ____ ____ _____

  (5) Hang infusion pump with syringe on IV pole alongside main IV bag. Set pump to deliver medication within time recommended. Press button on pump to begin infusion. ____ ____ ____ _____

  (6) After medication has infused, check flow regulator on primary infusion. Regulate main infusion line to desired rate as needed. ____ ____ ____ _____

C. Volume Control Set

  (1) Fill Volutrol with desired amount of fluid (50 to 100 mL) by opening clamp between Volutrol and main IV bag. ____ ____ ____ _____

  (2) Close clamp, and check to be sure clamp on air vent of volume control set chamber is open. ____ ____ ____ _____

  (3) Clean injection port on top of Volutrol with antiseptic swab. ____ ____ ____ _____

  (4) Remove needle cap or sheath, and insert syringe needle through port; then inject medication. Gently rotate Volutrol between hands. ____ ____ ____ _____

  (5) Regulate IV infusion rate to allow medication to infuse in time recommended. ____ ____ ____ _____

  (6) Label Volutrol with name of drug, dosage, total volume including diluent, and time of administration. ____ ____ ____ _____

  (7) Dispose of uncapped needle or needle enclosed in safety shield and syringe in appropriate container. ____ ____ ____ _____

Copyright © 2011, 2007, 2003 by Mosby, Inc., an affiliate of Elsevier Inc. All rights reserved.

CHAPTER 16 • Administering Medications

	S	U	NP	Comments

Evaluation
1. Observe patient for signs of adverse reactions. ___ ___ ___ _____
2. During infusion, periodically check infusion rate and condition of IV site. ___ ___ ___ _____
3. Ask patient to explain purpose and side effects of medication. ___ ___ ___ _____
4. Record drug, dose, route, and time administered. ___ ___ ___ _____
5. Record volume of fluid in medication bag or volume control set. ___ ___ ___ _____
6. Report any adverse reactions to nurse charge or physician. ___ ___ ___ _____

CHAPTER 16 • Administering Medications

Name _____ Date _____ Instructor's Name _____

Procedural Guidelines 16-1: Administering Medications through an NG Tube, G-Tube, J-Tube, or Small-Bore Feeding Tube

	S	U	NP	Comments
1. Check accuracy and completeness of each MAR or computer printout with prescriber's written mediation order.	___	___	___	_____
2. Investigate and use alternative routes of medication administration if possible.	___	___	___	_____
3. Avoid complicated medication regimens that frequently interrupt enteral feedings.	___	___	___	_____
4. Prepare medication. Check label of medication with MAR two times.	___	___	___	_____
5. Be sure the medication is compatible with the enteral feeding before administering medications. If the medication is incompatible with the feeding, stop the feeding 30 minutes to 1 hour before giving the medication. Never add medications directly to the tube feeding.	___	___	___	_____
6. Administer medications in a liquid form when possible to prevent obstruction of the tube.	___	___	___	_____
7. Before crushing medications, be sure they should be crushed. Do not crush buccal, sublingual, enteric-coated, or sustained-release medications.	___	___	___	_____
8. Take medications to patient at correct time, and perform hand hygiene.	___	___	___	_____
9. Verify patient's identity by using at least two patient identifiers.	___	___	___	_____
10. Compare label of medications against MAR one more time at patient's bedside.	___	___	___	_____
11. Explain procedure to patient, and educate patient about medications.	___	___	___	_____
12. Dissolve crushed tablets, gelatin capsules, and powders in 15 to 30 mL of warm water.	___	___	___	_____
13. Do not give whole or undissolved medications through the feeding tube.	___	___	___	_____
14. Put on clean, disposable gloves.	___	___	___	_____
15. Verify placement of any tube that enters the mouth or nose using pH testing.	___	___	___	_____
16. Assess gastric residual.	___	___	___	_____
17. Flush tube with 30 mL warm water.	___	___	___	_____
18. Draw up each medication in syringe. Do **not** mix medications together.	___	___	___	_____
19. Connect syringe with medication to nasogastric tube, G-tube, J-tube, or small-bore feeding tube.	___	___	___	_____
20. Administer medication by either pushing the medication through the tube with the syringe or by allowing medication to flow into body freely by using gravity. Administer each medication separately.	___	___	___	_____
21. Once you have given all medications, flush tube once more with 30 to 60 mL warm water.	___	___	___	_____
22. Clean area, and put supplies away.	___	___	___	_____
23. Remove gloves, and perform hand hygiene.	___	___	___	_____
24. Document administration of medications on MAR.	___	___	___	_____
25. Continually evaluate the patient's response to medication therapy. If the patient does not achieve the desired effect, a different medication or route of administration may be indicated because of problems with drug bioavailability when given by the enteral route.	___	___	___	_____

Copyright © 2011, 2007, 2003 by Mosby, Inc., an affiliate of Elsevier Inc. All rights reserved.

Name _____ Date _____ Instructor's Name _____

Procedural Guidelines 16-2: Administering Nasal Instillations

	S	U	NP	Comments

1. Check accuracy and completeness of each MAR or computer printout with prescriber's original medication order. ___ ___ ___ _____
2. Determine which sinus is affected by referring to medical record. ___ ___ ___ _____
3. Assess patient's history of hypertension, heart disease, diabetes mellitus, and hyperthyroidism. ___ ___ ___ _____
4. Using a penlight, inspect condition of nose and sinuses. Palpate sinuses for tenderness. ___ ___ ___ _____
5. Assess patient's knowledge regarding use of nasal instillations and technique for instillation and willingness to learn self-administration. ___ ___ ___ _____
6. Prepare medication. ___ ___ ___ _____
7. Take medications to patient at correct time, and perform hand hygiene. ___ ___ ___ _____
8. Verify patient's identity by using at least two patient identifiers. ___ ___ ___ _____
9. Compare MAR with medication labels at bedside. ___ ___ ___ _____
10. Explain procedure to patient regarding positioning and sensations to expect. ___ ___ ___ _____
11. Arrange supplies and medications at bedside. Apply gloves if patient has nasal drainage. ___ ___ ___ _____
12. Gently roll or shake container. ___ ___ ___ _____
13. Instruct patient to clear or blow nose gently unless contraindicated. ___ ___ ___ _____
14. Administer nasal drops:
    A. Assist patient to supine position and position head properly. ___ ___ ___ _____
        (1) For access to posterior pharynx, tilt patient's head backward. ___ ___ ___ _____
        (2) For access to ethmoid or sphenoid sinus, tilt head back over edge of bed or place small pillow under patient's shoulders and tilt head back. ___ ___ ___ _____
        (3) For access to frontal or maxillary sinus, tilt head back over edge of bed or pillow with head turned toward side to be treated. ___ ___ ___ _____
    B. Support patient's head with nondominant hand. ___ ___ ___ _____
    C. Instruct patient to breathe through mouth. ___ ___ ___ _____
    D. Hold dropper 1 cm (½ inch) above nares, and instill prescribed number of drops toward midline of ethmoid bone. ___ ___ ___ _____
    E. Have patient remain in supine position 5 minutes. ___ ___ ___ _____
    F. Offer facial tissue to blot runny nose, but caution patient against blowing nose for several minutes. ___ ___ ___ _____
15. Administer nasal spray:
    A. Assist patient to supine position and position head slightly tilted forward. ___ ___ ___ _____
    B. Help patient place spray nozzle into appropriate nares, pointing the nozzle to the side of the nose and away from the center of the nose. ___ ___ ___ _____
    C. Have patient spray medication into the nose while inhaling. ___ ___ ___ _____
    D. Help patient take nozzle out of nose, and instruct patient to breathe out through the mouth. ___ ___ ___ _____
    E. Offer facial tissue, but caution patient against blowing nose for several minutes. ___ ___ ___ _____

	S	U	NP	Comments
16. Assist patient to a comfortable position after drug is absorbed.	____	____	____	_____
17. Dispose of soiled supplies in proper container, and perform hand hygiene.	____	____	____	_____
18. Document administration of medications on MAR.	____	____	____	_____
19. Observe patient for onset of side effects 15 to 30 minutes after administration. Ask if patient is able to breathe through nose after decongestant administration. May be necessary to have patient occlude one nostril at a time and breathe deeply.	____	____	____	_____
20. Evaluate patient's response to medication at times that correlate with the medication's onset, peak, and duration. Evaluate patient for both desired effect and adverse effects.	____	____	____	_____

CHAPTER 16 • Administering Medications

Name _____ Date _____ Instructor's Name _____

Procedural Guidelines 16-3: Administering Ear Medications

	S	U	NP	Comments

1. Check accuracy and completeness of each MAR or computer printout with prescriber's written medication order. Check patient's name, drug name and dosage, route of administration, and time for administration.
2. Prepare medication. Be sure to compare the label of the medication with the MAR at least two times during medication preparation.
3. Take medication to patient at correct time, and perform hand hygiene.
4. Verify patient's identity by using at least two patient identifiers.
5. Compare the label of the medication with the MAR one more time at the patient's bedside.
6. Explain procedure to patient regarding positioning and sensations to expect.
7. Teach patient about medication.
8. *Administer ear drops:*
   A. Place patient in side-lying position if not contraindicated by patient's condition, with ear to be treated facing up. The patient may also sit in a chair or at the bedside.
   B. Straighten ear canal by pulling auricle down and back for children or upward and outward for adults.
   C. Instill prescribed drops holding dropper 1 cm (½ inch) above ear canal.
   D. Ask patient to remain in side-lying position for 2 to 3 minutes. Apply gentle massage or pressure to tragus of ear with finger.
   E. If you place a cotton ball into the outermost part of the ear canal, do not press cotton ball into the canal. Remove cotton after 15 minutes.
9. *Administer ear irrigations:*
   A. Assess the tympanic membrane, or review medical record for history of eardrum perforation, which contraindicates ear irrigation.
   B. Assist patient into sitting or lying position with head tilted or turned toward affected ear. Place towel under patient's head and shoulder, and have patient hold basin under affected ear.
   C. Fill irrigation syringe with solution (approximately 50 mL) at room temperature.
   D. Gently grasp auricle, and straighten ear by pulling it down and back for children or upward and outward for adults.
   E. Slowly instill irrigating solution by holding tip of syringe 1 cm (½ inch) above opening of ear canal. Allow fluid to drain out during instillation. Continue until you cleanse the canal or use all solution.
10. Clean area, and put supplies away.
11. Remove gloves, and perform hand hygiene.
12. Document medication administration on MAR.
13. Evaluate patient's response to the medication.

Name _____ Date _____ Instructor's Name _____

Procedural Guidelines 16-4: Administering Vaginal Medications

	S	U	NP	Comments
1. Check accuracy and completeness of each MAR or computer printout with prescriber's written medication order.	___	___	___	_____
2. Prepare medication.	___	___	___	_____
3. Take medication to patient at the correct time, and perform hand hygiene.	___	___	___	_____
4. Verify patient's identity by using at least two patient identifiers.	___	___	___	_____
5. Compare label of medication against the MAR one more time at the patient's bedside.	___	___	___	_____
6. Explain procedure to patient regarding positioning and sensations to expect. Be sure patient understands the procedure if she plans to self-administer medication. Teach patient about the medication.	___	___	___	_____
7. Close room door or pull curtain to provide privacy.	___	___	___	_____
8. Put on clean gloves.	___	___	___	_____
9. Be sure there is adequate lighting to visualize vaginal opening. Assess vaginal area, noting the appearance of any discharge and the condition of the external genitalia. Cleanse area with towel or washcloth if needed.	___	___	___	_____
10. *Administer vaginal suppository:*				
A. Remove suppository from wrapper and apply liberal amount of sterile water-based lubricating jelly to smooth or rounded end. Lubricate gloved index finger of dominant hand.	___	___	___	_____
B. With nondominant gloved hand, gently separate and hold labial folds.	___	___	___	_____
C. With dominant gloved hand, gently insert rounded end of suppository along posterior wall of vaginal canal entire length of finger (7.5 to 10 cm [3 to 4 inches]).	___	___	___	_____
D. Withdraw finger and wipe away remaining lubricant from around vaginal opening and labia.	___	___	___	_____
11. *Administer cream or foam:*				
A. Fill cream or foam applicator following package directions.	___	___	___	_____
B. With nondominant gloved hand, gently separate and hold labial folds.	___	___	___	_____
C. With dominant gloved hand, gently insert applicator about 5 to 7.5 cm (2 to 3 inches). Push applicator plunger to deposit medication into vagina.	___	___	___	_____
D. Withdraw applicator and place on paper towel. Wipe off residual cream from labia or vaginal opening.	___	___	___	_____
12. Dispose of supplies, remove gloves, and perform hand hygiene.	___	___	___	_____
13. Instruct patient to remain on back for at least 10 minutes.	___	___	___	_____
14. Document medication administration on MAR.	___	___	___	_____
15. If applicator is used, while wearing gloves wash with soap and warm water, rinse, and store for future use.	___	___	___	_____
16. Offer perineal pad to patient when she begins to ambulate.	___	___	___	_____
17. Evaluate patient's response to medication.	___	___	___	_____

CHAPTER 16 • Administering Medications

Name _____ Date _____ Instructor's Name _____

Procedural Guidelines 16-5: Administering Rectal Suppositories

	S	U	NP	Comments
1. Check accuracy and completeness of each MAR or computer printout with prescriber's written medication order.	___	___	___	_____
2. Prepare medication.	___	___	___	_____
3. Take medication to patient at the correct time, and perform hand hygiene.	___	___	___	_____
4. Verify patient's identity by using at least two patient identifiers.	___	___	___	_____
5. Compare the label of the medication with the MAR one more time at the patient's bedside.	___	___	___	_____
6. Explain procedure to patient regarding positioning and sensations to expect. Be sure patient understands the procedure if he or she plans to self-administer medication. Teach patient about the medication.	___	___	___	_____
7. Close room door or pull curtain to provide privacy.	___	___	___	_____
8. Put on clean gloves. NOTE: If patient has a latex allergy, use latex-free gloves.	___	___	___	_____
9. Assist patient to the Sims' position. Keep patient draped with only anal area exposed.	___	___	___	_____
10. Be sure there is adequate lighting to visualize anus. Assess external condition of anus and palpate rectal walls as needed. Dispose of gloves in proper receptacle if soiled.	___	___	___	_____
11. Apply disposable gloves if gloves were thrown away in previous step.	___	___	___	_____
12. Remove suppository from wrapper and lubricate rounded end with sterile water-soluble lubricating jelly. Lubricate index finger of dominant hand with water-soluble jelly.	___	___	___	_____
13. Ask patient to take slow deep breath through mouth and relax anal sphincter.	___	___	___	_____
14. Retract buttocks with nondominant hand. Using dominant hand, insert suppository gently through anus, past internal sphincter and against rectal wall, 10 cm (4 inches) in adults, or 5 cm (2 inches) in children and infants. You may need to apply gentle pressure to hold buttocks together momentarily.	___	___	___	_____
15. Withdraw finger and wipe anal area with tissue.	___	___	___	_____
16. Dispose of supplies, remove gloves, and perform hand hygiene.	___	___	___	_____
17. Instruct patient to remain on side for at least 5 minutes.	___	___	___	_____
18. If suppository is a laxative or stool softener, place call light within reach of the patient.	___	___	___	_____
19. Document medication administration on MAR.	___	___	___	_____
20. Evaluate patient's response to medication.	___	___	___	_____

Name _____ Date _____ Instructor's Name _____

Procedural Guidelines 16-6: Mixing Two Kinds of Insulin in One Syringe

	S	U	NP	Comments
1. Check accuracy and completeness of each MAR or computer printout with prescriber's written medication order.	___	___	___	_____
2. Verify insulin labels carefully against the MAR before preparing the dose to ensure that you give the correct type of insulin.	___	___	___	_____
3. Perform hand hygiene.	___	___	___	_____
4. If patient takes insulin that is cloudy, roll the bottle of insulin between the hands to resuspend the insulin preparation.	___	___	___	_____
5. Wipe off tops of both insulin vials with alcohol swab.	___	___	___	_____
6. Verify insulin dosages against MAR a second time.	___	___	___	_____
7. If mixing rapid- or short-acting with intermediate- or long-acting insulin, take insulin syringe and aspirate volume of air equivalent to dose to be withdrawn from intermediate- or long-acting insulin first. If two intermediate- or long-acting insulins are mixed, it makes no difference which vial you prepare first.	___	___	___	_____
8. Insert needle and inject air into vial of intermediate- or long-acting insulin. Do not let the tip of the needle touch the insulin.	___	___	___	_____
9. Remove the syringe from the vial of insulin without aspirating medication.	___	___	___	_____
10. With the same syringe, inject air, equal to the dose of rapid- or short-acting insulin, into the vial and withdraw the correct dose into the syringe.	___	___	___	_____
11. Remove the syringe from the rapid- or short-acting insulin, and get rid of air bubbles to ensure accurate dosing.	___	___	___	_____
12. After verifying insulin dosages with MAR a third time, determine what point on the syringe scale combined units of insulin measure by adding the number of units of both insulins together.	___	___	___	_____
13. Place the needle of the syringe back into the vial of intermediate- or long-acting insulin. Be careful not to push plunger and inject insulin in syringe into the vial.				
A. Invert the vial, and carefully withdraw the desired amount of insulin into syringe.	___	___	___	_____
B. Withdraw needle, and check fluid level in syringe. Keep needle of prepared syringe sheathed or capped until ready to administer medication.	___	___	___	_____
C. Dispose of soiled supplies in proper receptacle and perform hand hygiene.	___	___	___	_____

17 Fluid, Electrolyte, and Acid-Base Balances

CASE STUDIES

1. The patient is diagnosed with heart failure and will be taking Digoxin and Lasix on a daily basis.
   a. What patient teaching is indicated in relation to possible fluid and electrolyte imbalances?
2. You are working with two patients today. One of the patients is unconscious, and is experiencing a period of prolonged immobility. The other patient has a long history of alcoholism. You are alert to possible alterations in fluid and electrolyte imbalance.
   a. What specific signs and symptoms may these patients exhibit as a result of their present conditions?
3. An adult male patient has come to the outpatient clinic for an examination. During the initial interview, the patient tells you that he has smoked 2½ packs of cigarettes each day for the last 25 years.
   a. What physical signs do you anticipate finding because of the patient's history?
   b. What acid-base imbalance is this patient most likely to experience?
4. Following a motor vehicle accident, the patient had traumatic injuries and a significant hemorrhage. He will be receiving blood transfusions.
   a. What are the priority assessments that should be completed prior to administration of the blood?
   b. What safety measures should be implemented to reduce the possibility of complications?

CHAPTER REVIEW

Match the description/definition in Column A with the correct term in Column B.

	Column A	Column B
_____	1. Positively charged electrolytes	a. Anions
_____	2. Having the same osmotic pressure	b. Diffusion
_____	3. Movement of water across a semipermeable membrane	c. Filtration
_____	4. Movement of molecules from an area of higher concentration to an area of lower concentration	d. Active transport
_____	5. Negatively charged electrolytes	e. Cations
_____	6. Movement of solutes out of a solution with greater hydrostatic pressure	f. Isotonic
_____	7. Number of molecules in a liter of solution	g. Hypotonic
_____	8. Having a lower osmotic pressure	h. Osmosis
_____	9. Movement of molecules to an area of higher concentration	i. Osmolarity

Complete the following:

10. Identify the following terms:
    a. All fluids outside of the cell:

    b. Fluid between the cells and outside the blood vessels:

    c. All fluids within the cell:

11. Identify if the following electrolytes are cations or anions and whether they are primarily extracellular or intracellular:
    a. Sodium

    b. Potassium

    c. Calcium

    d. Magnesium

e. Chloride

f. Bicarbonate

12. Acid-base balance in the body is regulated by:

13. What two age-groups are most susceptible to fluid and acid-base imbalances?

14. Identify whether the following solutions are isotonic, hypertonic, or hypotonic:
    a. Dextrose 5% in water (D_5W)
    b. 0.45% sodium chloride (0.45% NS)
    c. 0.9% sodium chloride (0.9% NS)
    d. Lactated Ringer's (LR)
    e. Dextrose 5% in 0.45% sodium chloride ($D_5\frac{1}{2}$ NS)

15. Identify three types of medications that may cause fluid, electrolyte, or acid-base imbalances.

16. Specify two possible nursing diagnoses for patients experiencing fluid, electrolyte, or acid-base imbalances.

17. Identify the sites for an IV infusion.

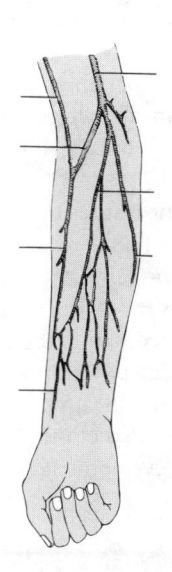

18. A patient who is NPO and receiving intravenous fluids needs to have _____ added to the solution.

19. Identify the signs and symptoms that are associated with phlebitis at an IV site.

20. A patient with a peripherally inserted central catheter (PICC) line develops a fever and increased white blood cell (WBC) count. The nurse anticipates that the health care provider will order:

21. The patient had a rapid infusion of IV fluids and has developed crackles in the lungs, shortness of breath, and tachycardia. The nurse should:

22. Transfusion of a patient's own blood is termed:

23. Identify the electrolyte imbalance that is associated with each of the following test results:
    a. Serum sodium level—125 mEq/L
    b. Serum potassium level—5.8 mEq/L
    c. Serum calcium level—3.7 mEq/L
    d. Serum magnesium level—1.2 mEq/L

24. Calculate the following IV infusion rates:
    a. IV 500 mL of D_5W to infuse in 5 hours; drop factor = 15 gtt/mL. How many gtt/min should infuse?
    b. IV 1000 mL of NS to infuse in 8 hours; drop factor = 10 gtt/mL. How many gtt/min should infuse?
    c. IV 200 mL of NS to infuse in 4 hours; drop factor = 60 gtt/mL. How many gtt/min should infuse?
    d. IV 2 L of D_5W to infuse in 18 hours. How many ml/hour should be set on the infusion pump?

25. Identify the following hormones that control fluid balance:
    a. Pituitary
    b. Adrenal

26. If a hypotonic solution is given intravenously to a patient, the fluid will move into the cells.
    True _____ False _____

27. Arterial pH is an indirect measurement of:

28. Oxygen moves into the lungs via the process of:

29. An average adult's daily intake of fluid is approximately _____ mL.
30. The nurse is going to perform a venipuncture in order to initiate IV therapy. Place the following steps in the correct order.
    a. Prepare the IV infusion tubing and solution ____
    b. Re-apply the tourniquet ____
    c. Perform hand hygiene ____
    d. Cleanse the site ____
    e. Select a large-enough vein ____
31. The nurse is calculating the patient's intake and output for the last 8 hours. During this time, the patient consumed 1 cup of gelatin, 1/2 cup of juice, 1 cup of water, and 1 cup of tea. The IV infusion started with 750 mL in the bag, with 125 mL remaining at the end of the shift. The urinary output was 340 mL and there was 30 mL of drainage from the nasogastric tube.
    Cup = 8 oz
    What is the patient's intake and output?

    I = _____   O = _____

32. Which of the following is/are most likely to lead to a fluid volume deficit? Select all that apply.
    a. Vomiting ____
    b. Heart failure ____
    c. Corticosteroid administration ____
    d. Fever ____
    e. Increased sodium intake ____
    f. Diuretic administration ____

Select the best answer for each of the following questions:

33. The patient has hypernatremia with a fluid deficit. The nurse anticipates finding:
    1. Dry, sticky mucous membranes
    2. Orthostatic hypotension
    3. Abdominal cramping
    4. Diarrhea
34. The patient who is experiencing a gastrointestinal problem has had periods of prolonged vomiting. The nurse is observing the patient for signs of:
    1. Metabolic acidosis
    2. Metabolic alkalosis
    3. Respiratory acidosis
    4. Respiratory alkalosis
35. The nurse is working with a patient who has had emphysema for many years. The nurse believes that the patient has uncompensated respiratory acidosis. This belief is a result of an analysis of the patient's blood gas values that reveals:
    1. pH = 7.35, Pa_{CO_2} = 40 mm Hg, HCO_3^- concentration = 22 mEq/L
    2. pH = 7.40, Pa_{CO_2} = 45 mm Hg, HCO_3^- concentration = 28 mEq/L
    3. pH = 7.30, Pa_{CO_2} = 50 mm Hg, HCO_3^- concentration = 24 mEq/L
    4. pH = 7.45, Pa_{CO_2} = 55 mm Hg, HCO_3^- concentration = 18 mEq/L
36. The patient has been admitted to the medical center for stabilization of congestive heart failure. The physician has prescribed Lasix (a diuretic) for the patient. This patient should be observed for:
    1. Diarrhea
    2. Edema
    3. Dysrhythmia
    4. Hyperactive reflexes
37. The patient has a potassium level above the normal value. The nurse anticipates that treatment for this patient with hyperkalemia will include:
    1. Fluid restrictions
    2. Foods high in potassium
    3. Administration of diuretics
    4. IV infusion of calcium
38. The patient has lost a large amount of body fluid. In assessment of this patient with hypovolemia (fluid volume deficit, FVD), the nurse expects to find:
    1. Oliguria
    2. Hypertension
    3. Periorbital edema
    4. Neck vein distention
39. The nurse is determining the care that is to be provided to the patients on the medical unit. There are a number of patients who have the potential for a fluid and electrolyte imbalance. A nurse-initiated (independent) intervention for these patients is:
    1. Administration of IV fluids
    2. Monitoring of intake and output
    3. Performance of diagnostic tests
    4. Dietary replacement of necessary fluids/electrolytes
40. For a patient who is experiencing a fluid volume excess, the nurse plans to determine the fluid status. The best way to determine the fluid balance for the patient is to:
    1. Obtain diagnostic test results
    2. Monitor IV fluid intake
    3. Weigh the patient daily
    4. Assess vital signs
41. The patient is admitted to the trauma unit following an accident while using power tools at home. The patient experienced significant blood loss and required a large infusion of citrated blood. The nurse assesses this patient for the development of:
    1. Urinary retention
    2. Poor skin turgor
    3. Increased blood pressure reading
    4. Positive Trousseau's sign
42. The patient is experiencing a severe anxiety reaction and the respiratory rate has increased significantly.

Nursing intervention for this patient who may develop respiratory alkalosis is:
1. Placing the patient in a sitting position
2. Providing the patient with nasal oxygen
3. Having the patient breathe into a paper bag
4. Having the patient cough and deep breathe

43. A patient with normal renal function is to be maintained NPO. An IV of 1000 mL of D_5W is ordered to infuse over 8 hours. The nurse should:
1. Infuse the IV at a faster rate
2. Add multivitamins to the solution
3. Provide oral fluids as a supplement
4. Question the prescriber about adding potassium to the IV

44. A patient with an IV infusion may develop phlebitis. The nurse recognizes this condition by the presence at the IV infusion site of:
1. Pallor
2. Swelling
3. Redness
4. Cyanosis

45. The patient has had an IV line inserted. Upon observation of the IV site, the nurse notes that there is evidence of an infiltration. The nurse should first:
1. Slow the infusion
2. Discontinue the infusion
3. Change the IV bag and tubing
4. Contact the prescriber immediately

46. The nurse is reviewing the hospital policy for maintenance of IV infusions. The current guidelines for changing IV tubing (non–blood administration sets) are based on the IV tubing remaining sterile for:
1. 24 hours
2. 36 hours
3. 48 hours
4. 72 hours

47. The patient has just started to receive the blood transfusion. The nurse is performing the patient assessment and notes the patient has chills and flank pain. The nurse stops the infusion and then:
1. Calls the physician
2. Administers epinephrine
3. Collects a urine specimen
4. Sets up a piggyback IV infusion with 0.9% saline

48. A patient who has been admitted with a renal dysfunction is demonstrating signs and symptoms of a fluid volume excess (hypervolemia). Upon completing the patient assessment, the nurse anticipates finding:
1. Poor skin turgor
2. Decreased blood pressure
3. Neck vein distention
4. Increased urine specific gravity

49. The nurse is assisting the patient with a fluid volume deficit to select an optimum replacement fluid. The nurse suggests that the patient drink:
1. Tea
2. Milk
3. Coffee
4. Fruit juice

50. A patient with congestive heart failure and fluid retention is placed on a fluid restriction of 1000 mL/24 hours. On the basis of guidelines for patients with restrictions, for the time period from 7:00 AM to 3:30 PM the nurse plans to provide the patient:
1. 250 mL
2. 400 mL
3. 500 mL
4. 750 mL

51. The patient has come to the orthopedist's office for treatment of osteoporosis. The nurse is explaining to the patient some of the possible complications from this disorder that may affect fluid and electrolyte balance. The nurse informs the patient to report:
1. Low back pain
2. Tingling in the fingers
3. Muscle twitching
4. Positive Trousseau's sign

52. The patient has a history of alcoholism and is admitted to the medical center in a malnourished state. The nurse specifically checks the lab values for:
1. Hypercalcemia
2. Hyponatremia
3. Hyperkalemia
4. Hypomagnesemia

53. The patient who is most prone to respiratory acidosis is the individual who is experiencing:
1. A narcotic overdose
2. An anxiety reaction
3. Renal failure
4. Asthma

54. Older adults have a greater risk of fluid imbalance as a result of:
1. Increased thirst response
2. Decreased glomerular filtration
3. Increased body fluid percentage
4. Increased basal metabolic rate

55. An example of a type of medication that can lead to metabolic alkalosis is a:
1. Narcotic
2. Diuretic
3. Potassium supplement
4. Nonsteroidal anti-inflammatory drug

56. A moderate to severe fluid volume excess is indicated with a weight change of:
1. 1% to 2%
2. 3% to 4%
3. 5% to 8%
4. 9% to 12%

57. An appropriate technique when initiating an intravenous infusion is to:
1. Use hard, stiff veins
2. Shave the arm hair with a razor
3. Use the proximal site in the dominant arm

4. Apply the tourniquet 4 to 6 inches above the selected site
58. A unit of packed cells or whole blood usually transfuses over:
   1. 1/2 hour
   2. 1 hour
   3. 2 hours
   4. 5 hours
59. An individual with type O blood is able to receive:
   1. Type A or type B
   2. Type AB
   3. Type O
   4. All types
60. A specific technique for initiating intravenous therapy for an older adult is to:
   1. Select sites in the hands
   2. Use the largest possible IV cannula gauge
   3. Insert at a decreased angle of 5 to 15 degrees
   4. Set the IV flow rate at 150 to 200 mL/hour
61. The patient lost 4 pounds since last week as a result of taking Lasix. This is approximately:
   1. 1/2 L of fluid
   2. 1 L of fluid
   3. 2 L of fluid
   4. 4 L of fluid

STUDY GROUP QUESTIONS

- How are body fluids distributed in the body?
- What is the composition of body fluids?
- How do fluids move throughout the body?
- How is the intake of body fluids regulated?
- What are the major electrolytes, and what is their function in the body?
- How is acid-base balance maintained?
- What are the major fluid, electrolyte, and acid-base imbalances and their causes?
- What signs and symptoms will the patient exhibit in the presence of a fluid, electrolyte, or acid-base imbalance?
- What diagnostic tests are used to determine the presence of imbalances?
- What information is critical to obtain in a patient assessment in order to determine the presence of a fluid, electrolyte, or acid-base imbalance?
- What health deviations increase a patient's susceptibility to an imbalance?
- What nursing interventions should be implemented for patients with various fluid, electrolyte, and acid-base imbalances?
- What information should be included in patient/family teaching for prevention of imbalances, or restoration of fluid, electrolyte, or acid-base balance?
- What are the nursing responsibilities associated with the initiation and maintenance of IV therapy?
- What are the responsibilities of the nurse with regard to blood transfusions?

STUDY CHARTS

Create study charts to compare:
a. *Electrolyte Imbalances and Patient Responses,* including etiology, diagnostic test results, patient assessment, and nursing interventions for sodium, potassium, calcium, and magnesium imbalances
b. *Acid-Base Imbalances and Patient Responses,* including etiology, diagnostic test results, patient assessment, and nursing interventions both for metabolic acidosis and alkalosis and for respiratory acidosis and alkalosis

Answers available through your instructor.

CHAPTER 17 • Fluid, Electrolyte, and Acid-Base Balances

Name _____ Date _____ Instructor's Name _____

Performance Checklist Skill 17-1: Initiating Intravenous (IV) Therapy

	S	U	NP	Comments

Assessment
1. Review health care provider's order for type and amount of IV fluid and rate of administration.
2. Assess for clinical factors that will be affected by IV fluid administration.
3. Assess patient's previous experience with IV therapy and preference for location of IV.
4. Obtain information from drug reference books or pharmacist about composition of IV fluids, purposes of administration, potential incompatibilities, most appropriate type of catheter for administration, and possible side effects for which to monitor.
5. Determine if patient is to undergo any planned surgeries or is to receive blood infusion later.
6. Assess for risk factors.
7. Assess laboratory data and patient's history of allergies.
8. Assess patient's understanding of purpose of IV therapy.

Planning
1. Collect and organize equipment.
2. Check patient's identity using at least two patient identifiers.
3. Prepare patient and family by explaining the procedure, its purpose, and signs and symptoms of complications.
4. Assist patient to comfortable sitting or supine position. Position yourself at same level as the patient.

Implementation
1. Perform hand hygiene.
2. Organize equipment on clean, clutter-free area.
3. Change patient's gown to the more easily removed gown with snaps at the shoulder, if available.
4. Open sterile packages using sterile aseptic technique.
5. Prepare IV infusion tubing and solution.
   A. Check IV solution, using six rights of medication administration. Make sure prescribed additives, such as potassium and vitamins, have been added. Check solution for color, clarity, and expiration date. Check bag for leaks, preferably before reaching the bedside.
   B. Open infusion set, maintaining sterility of both ends of tubing. Many sets allow for priming of tubing without removal of end cap.
   C. Place roller clamp about 2 to 5 cm (1 to 2 inches) below drip chamber, and move roller clamp to "off" position.
   D. Remove protective covering from IV tubing port on plastic IV solution bag.
   E. Insert infusion set into fluid container. Remove protector cap from tubing insertion spike, not touching spike, and insert spike into opening of IV bag. Cleanse rubber stopper on bottled solution with antiseptic, and insert spike into black rubber stopper of IV bottle.
   F. Prime infusion tubing by filling with IV solution:
      (1) Compress drip chamber and release.
      (2) Allow it to fill one-third to one-half full.
   G. Remove protector cap on end of tubing (some tubing can be primed without removal), and slowly release roller clamp to allow fluid to travel from drip chamber through tubing to needle adapter. Return roller clamp to "off" position after tubing is primed.

Copyright © 2011, 2007, 2003 by Mosby, Inc., an affiliate of Elsevier Inc. All rights reserved.

	S	U	NP	Comments

H. Be certain tubing is clear of air and air bubbles. To remove small air bubbles, firmly tap IV tubing where air bubbles are located. Check entire length of tubing to ensure that all air bubbles are removed. If you use a multiple-port tubing, turn ports upside down and tap to fill and remove air.

I. Replace cap protector on end of tubing.

6. *Option:* Prepare saline lock for infusion.

   A. If a loop or short extension tubing is needed because of an awkward VAD site placement, use sterile technique to connect the IV plug to the loop of short extension tubing. Inject 1 to 3 mL of saline through the plug and through the injection cap or short extension tubing.

7. Identify accessible vein for placement of VAD. Apply tourniquet around arm above antecubital fossa or 4 to 6 inches (10 to 15 cm) above proposed insertion site. Do not apply tourniquet too tightly to avoid injury or bruising to skin. Tourniquet may be applied on top of a thin layer of clothing such as a gown sleeve. *Optional:* Apply BP cuff. Inflate to level just below patient's diastolic pressure (less than 50 mm Hg).

8. Select the vein for VAD insertion.

   A. Use the most distal site in the nondominant arm, if possible.

   B. Avoid areas that are painful to palpation.

   C. Select a vein large enough for VAD.

   D. Choose a site that will not interfere with patient's activities of daily living (ADLs) or planned procedures.

   E. Using your index finger, palpate the vein by pressing downward and noting the resilient, soft, bouncy feeling as you release pressure.

   F. If possible, place extremity in dependent position.

   G. Select well-dilated vein. Methods to foster venous distention include:

   (1) Stroking the extremity from distal to proximal below the proposed venipuncture site.

   (2) Applying warmth to the extremity for several minutes, for example, with a warm washcloth.

   H. Avoid sites distal to previous venipuncture site, veins in antecubital fossa or inner wrist, sclerosed or hardened veins, infiltrate site or phlebitic vessels, bruised areas, and areas of venous valves.

   I. Avoid fragile dorsal veins in older adult patients and vessels in an extremity with compromised circulation.

9. Release tourniquet temporarily and carefully. *Option:* Assess if application of local anesthetic needed.

10. Apply disposable gloves. Wear eye protection if splash or spray of blood is possible.

11. Place adapter end of infusion set nearby on sterile gauze or sterile towel.

12. If area of insertion appears to need cleansing, use soap and water first. Use antiseptic swab to cleanse insertion site; allow the agent to dry.

13. Reapply tourniquet 4 to 5 inches (10 to 12.5 cm) above anticipated insertion site. Check presence of distal pulse.

14. Perform venipuncture. Anchor vein below site by placing thumb over vein and by stretching the skin against the direction of insertion 1½ to 2 inches (4 to 5 cm) distal to the site. Warn patient of a sharp, quick stick.

CHAPTER 17 • Fluid, Electrolyte, and Acid-Base Balances

	S	U	NP	Comments

A. *Over-the-needle catheter (ONC with safety device)*: Insert with bevel up at 5- to 15-degree angle slightly distal to actual site of venipuncture in the direction of the vein.

B. *Winged needle*: Hold needle at 5- to 15-degree angle with bevel up slightly distal to actual site of venipuncture.

15. Observe for blood return through flashback chamber indicating that bevel of needle has entered vein. Lower catheter until almost flush with skin. Advance catheter 1/4 inch into vein and then loosen stylet. Continue to hold skin taut and advance catheter into vein until hub rests at venipuncture site. *Do not reinsert the stylet once it is loosened.* Advance the catheter while the safety device automatically retracts the stylet. Advance a winged needle until hub rests at venipuncture site. (NOTE: Techniques will vary with each IV device.)

16. Stabilize catheter with one hand, and release tourniquet or BP cuff with other. Apply gentle but firm pressure with index finger of nondominant hand 3 cm (1¼ inches) above the insertion site. Keep catheter stable with index finger.

17. Quickly connect end of the infusion tubing set or the prepared saline lock to end of cannula. Do not touch point of entry of connection. Secure connection.

18. Begin infusion by slowly opening the slide clamp or adjusting the roller clamp of the IV tubing or flush injection cap of lock.

19. Observe site for swelling.

20. Secure cannula (follow agency policy).

21. Regulate IV rate.

    A. *Manufactured catheter stabilization device*: Wipe selected area with single-use skin protectant, and allow to dry. Slide device under catheter hub, and center hub over device. Holding catheter in place, peel off half of liner, press to adhere to skin. Repeat on other side. Holding catheter in place, pull tab out from center of device to create opening; insert catheter into slit (see illustration). Cover insertion site with a transparent or sterile gauze dressing.

    B. *Transparent dressing*: Secure with nondominant hand while preparing to apply dressing.

    C. *Sterile gauze dressing*: Place narrow piece (½ inch) of sterile tape over catheter hub. If sterile tape is not available, apply nonsterile tape around catheter hub or stabilization device. Place tape only on the catheter, never over the insertion site. Secure site to allow easy visual inspection. Avoid applying tape around the arm.

22. Apply sterile dressing over site.

    A. **Transparent Dressing:**

    (1) Carefully remove adherent backing. Apply one edge of dressing, and then gently smooth remaining dressing over IV site, leaving connection between IV tubing and catheter hub uncovered. Remove outer covering, and smooth dressing gently over site.

    (2) Take 1-inch piece of tape, and place it over extension tubing or administration set. Do not apply tape over transparent dressing.

    (3) Apply chevron, and place over tape.

    B. **Sterile Gauze Dressing:**

    (1) Place a 2 × 2 gauze pad over insertion site and catheter hub. Secure all edges with tape. Do not cover connection between IV tubing and catheter hub.

Copyright © 2011, 2007, 2003 by Mosby, Inc., an affiliate of Elsevier Inc. All rights reserved.

CHAPTER 17 • Fluid, Electrolyte, and Acid-Base Balances

	S	U	NP	Comments

    (2) Fold a 2 × 2 gauze in half and cover with a 1-inch-wide tape extending about an inch from each side. Place under the tubing/catheter hub junction.

23. Curl a loop of tubing alongside the arm and place a second piece of tape over the tubing and secure.
24. For IV fluid administration, recheck flow rate to correct drops per minute.
25. Label dressing agency per policy.
26. Dispose of used stylet or other sharps in appropriate sharps container. Discard supplies. Remove gloves and perform hand hygiene.
27. Instruct patient how to change position in and out of bed without dislodging VAD.

Evaluation

1. Observe peripheral IV access. Peripheral IV access should be changed every 72 hours or per health care provider's orders, or more frequently if complications occur.
2. Observe patient every 1 to 2 hours.
   A. Check if correct amount of IV solution has infused by comparing time tape on IV bag or by checking EID record.
   B. Count drip rate (if gravity drip) or check rate on infusion pump.
   C. Check patency of VAD.
   D. Observe patient during compression of vessel for signs of discomfort.
   E. Inspect insertion site, and note color. Inspect for presence of swelling, infiltration and phlebitis. Palpate temperature of skin above dressing.
3. Observe patient to determine response to therapy and document.
4. Record IV insertion, type of fluid, insertion site by vessel, flow rate, size, and type of catheter or needle, and when infusion was begun.
5. Report type of fluid, flow rate, status of venipuncture site, amount of fluid remaining in present solution, expected time to hang next IV bag or bottle, and any side effects.

CHAPTER 17 • Fluid, Electrolyte, and Acid-Base Balances

Name _____ Date _____ Instructor's Name _____

Performance Checklist Skill 17-2: Regulating Intravenous Flow Rate

	S	U	NP	Comments

Assessment
1. Check patient's medical record for correct solution and additives. Follow six rights of medication administration.
2. Perform hand hygiene. Observe for patency of VAD and IV tubing.
3. Assess patient's knowledge of how positioning of IV site affects flow rate.
4. Inspect IV site, and assess patient's perception of pain at venipuncture site.
5. Observe for patency of VAD and IV tubing.
6. Identify patient risk for fluid imbalance (e.g., neonate, history of cardiac or renal disease, electrolyte imbalance).

Planning
1. Collect and organize equipment.
2. Check patient's identification using two identifiers. Explain procedure.
3. Have paper and pencil available to calculate flow rate.
4. Acquire calibration (drop factor) of infusion set.
5. Calculate flow rate in mL/hr and gtts/min.

Implementation
1. Read physician's or health care provider's orders, and follow six rights for correct solution and proper additives.
2. Obtain IV fluid/medication and tubing.
3. Confirm hourly rate and place marked adhesive tape or commercial fluid indicator tape on IV bottle or bag next to volume markings.
4. *For gravity transfusion:* Confirm hourly rate and minute rate calculated in planning.
5. Regulate flow rate by counting drops in drip chamber for 1 minute by watch; then adjust roller clamp to increase or decrease rate of infusion.
6. *For infusion using EID:* Follow manufacturer's guidelines for setup of EID:
   A. Place electronic eye on drip chamber. If gravity controller is used, ensure that IV container is 36 inches above IV site.
   B. Insert tubing into chamber of control mechanism, according to manufacturer's directions.
   C. Turn on power button, select required drops per minute or volume per hour, close door to control chamber, and press the start button.
   D. Open regulator clamp completely while EID is in use.
   E. Monitor infusion rates and IV site for complications according to agency policy. Use watch to check rate of infusion, even when using EID.
   F. Assess patency of system when alarm sounds.
7. *For smart pump:*
   A. Place pump module into the computer.
   B. Insert the IV tubing into the pump module, and close the door.
   C. Computer screen will need the patient unit to be identified.

	S	U	NP	Comments

    D. From the list on screen, choose the medication and concentration.

    E. If the programming does not match the database, a visual and audible alarm sounds.

    F. If an alarm sounds, the pump will automatically turn off. You must reprogram it within the facility's database.

    G. Reconfirm that the medication is infusing at the ordered rate.

8. *For a volume-control device*:

    A. Place volume-control device between IV container and insertion spike of infusion set using aseptic technique (see illustration).

    B. Place no more than 2 hours' worth of fluid into device by opening clamp between IV bag and device.

    C. Assess system at least hourly; add fluid to volume control device. Regulate flow rate.

9. Instruct patient about the purpose of the alarms, to avoid raising hand or arm that affects flow rate, and to avoid touching the control clamp.

Evaluation

1. Monitor IV infusion at least every hour, noting volume of IV fluid infused and rate.
2. Observe patient for signs of overhydration or dehydration to determine response to therapy and restoration of fluid and electrolyte balance.
3. Evaluate for signs of complications with IV flow rate: infiltration, inflammation at site, occluded VAD, or kink or obstruction in infusion tubing.

CHAPTER 17 • Fluid, Electrolyte, and Acid-Base Balances

Name _____ Date _____ Instructor's Name _____

Performance Checklist Skill 17-3: Changing Intravenous Solution and Tubing

	S	U	NP	Comments

Assessment
1. Check health care provider's orders for type of fluid, infusion rate, and medication additives. Follow six rights of medication administration.
2. Note date and time when IV tubing and solution were last changed.
3. Determine the compatibility of all IV fluids and additives by consulting appropriate literature or the pharmacy.
4. Determine patient's understanding of need for continued IV therapy.
5. Assess patency of current IV access site.
6. Assess IV insertion site for swelling, coolness to touch, or tenderness around site.
7. Assess IV tubing for puncture, contamination, or occlusions.

Planning
1. Collect appropriate equipment. Have next solution prepared at least 1 hour before needed. If solution is prepared in pharmacy, ensure it has been delivered to the patient's hospital unit. Allow solution to warm to room temperature if it has been refrigerated. Check that solution is correct and properly labeled. Check solution expiration date.
2. Check patient's identification by using at least two patient identifiers.
3. Prepare to change solution when about 50 mL of fluid remains in container.
4. Coordinate tubing changes with bag changes whenever possible.
5. Prepare patient and family by explaining the procedure, its purpose, and expectations of patient.

Implementation
1. Perform hand hygiene.
2. Open new infusion set, and connect add-on pieces (e.g., filters, extension tubing). Keep protective coverings over infusion spike and distal adapter. Secure all connections.
3. Change new solution with existing tubing:
    A. If using plastic bag, remove protective cover from IV tubing port. If using glass bottle, remove metal cap and metal and rubber disks.
    B. Position roller clamp to stop flow rate.
    C. Remove tubing from EID (if used). Remove old IV fluid container from IV pole. Hold container with tubing port pointing upward.
    D. Quickly remove spike from old solution bag or bottle and, without touching tip, insert spike into new bag or bottle.
    E. Hang new solution container on IV pole.
    F. Check for air in tubing. If bubbles form, they can be removed by closing the roller clamp, stretching the tubing downward, and tapping the tubing with the finger. For a larger amount of air, swab port below the air, allow to dry, and insert needleless syringe into the port. Aspirate air into the syringe.

116 CHAPTER 17 • Fluid, Electrolyte, and Acid-Base Balances

	S	U	NP	Comments

    G. Make sure drip chamber is one-third to one-half full. If the drip chamber is too full, pinch off tubing below the drip chamber, invert the container, squeeze the drip chamber, release, turn the solution container upright, and unpinch the tubing.

4. *To change IV tubing without new solution:*
    A. Open new infusion set and connect filter and/or extension tubing, keeping protective coverings over infusion spike and end of tubing.
    B. Apply clean, disposable gloves.
    C. If VAD is not visible, remove dressing. Hold VAD securely with nondominant hand. Do not remove tape securing VAD to skin.
    D. For IV without injection cap:
      (1) Move roller clamp on new IV tubing to "off" position.
      (2) Slow rate of infusion by regulating drip rate on old tubing. Be sure rate is at KVO.
      (3) With old tubing in place, compress drip chamber and fill chamber.
      (4) Remove old tubing from solution and hang or tape the drip chamber on IV pole 36 inches above IV site.
      (5) Place insertion spike of new tubing into old solution bag opening and hang solution bag on IV pole.
      (6) Compress and release drip chamber on new tubing; slowly fill drip chamber one-third to one-half full.
      (7) Slowly open roller clamp, remove protective cap from needle adapter (if necessary), and flush tubing with solution. Replace cap.
      (8) Turn roller clamp on old tubing to "off" position.
      (9) Stabilize hub of catheter or needle, and apply pressure over vein just above insertion site. Apply gloves. Gently disconnect old tubing. Maintain stability of hub and quickly insert adapter of new tubing or saline lock into hub.
    E. For intermittent saline lock:
      (1) If a loop or short extension tubing is needed, swab injection cap with antiseptic swab. Insert syringe with 1 to 3 mL of saline, and inject through the injection cap into the loop or tubing.
      (2) Position roller clamp of existing tubing to "off" position and disconnect tubing from injection cap.
      (3) Take existing IV solution off IV pole.
      (4) Prime tubing by spiking IV solution bag.
      (5) Swab injection port of IV with alcohol and allow to dry.
5. Open roller clamp on new tubing. Allow solution to run rapidly for 30 seconds.
6. Regulate IV drip rate according to health care provider's orders, and monitor rate hourly.
7. Place a piece of tape or preprinted label with the date and time of tubing change and attach to tubing below the level of drip chamber.
8. If necessary, apply new dressing. Secure tubing to extremity with tape.
9. Discard old tubing in proper container.
10. Remove and dispose of gloves. Perform hand hygiene.

Copyright © 2011, 2007, 2003 by Mosby, Inc., an affiliate of Elsevier Inc. All rights reserved.

	S	U	NP	Comments

Evaluation
1. Evaluate flow rate and observe connection site for leakage.
2. Observe patient for signs of overhydration or dehydration.
3. Check IV system for patency and signs symptoms of infiltration or phlebitis.
4. Record changing of tubing and solution on patient's record.

CHAPTER 17 • Fluid, Electrolyte, and Acid-Base Balances

Name _____ Date _____ Instructor's Name _____

Performance Checklist Skill 17-4: Changing a Peripheral Intravenous Dressing

	S	U	NP	Comments

Assessment
1. Determine when dressing was last changed.
2. Observe present dressing for moisture and intactness.
3. Observe IV system for proper functioning or complications: current flow rate, presence of kinks in infusion tubing or VAD. Palpate the VAD through the intact dressing for subjective complaints of pain or burning.
4. Inspect exposed VAD site for inflammation and swelling.
5. Monitor body temperature.
6. Assess patient's understanding of the need for continued IV infusion.

Planning
1. Explain procedure and purpose to patient and family. Explain that affected extremity must be held still and describe length of procedure.
2. Collect equipment.

Implementation
1. Perform hand hygiene. Apply clean gloves and mask.
2. Verify patient's identity using two identifiers.
3. Remove tape, gauze, and/or transparent dressing from old dressing one layer at a time by pulling toward the insertion site, leaving tape that secures VAD intact. Be cautious if catheter tubing becomes tangled between two layers of dressing. When removing transparent dressing, hold catheter hub and tubing with nondominant hand.
4. Observe insertion site for signs and/or symptoms of infection: redness, swelling, and exudate.
5. If IV is infusing properly, gently remove tape securing VAD. Stabilize VAD with one hand. Use adhesive remover to cleanse skin and remove adhesive residue, if needed.
6. Clean insertion site with antiseptic swab using circular friction motion from insertion site outward.
7. Allow antiseptic to dry.
8. *Option:* Apply skin protectant solution (e.g., Skin-Prep, No Sting Barrier Film) to the area where you will apply the tape or transparent dressing. Allow to dry.
9. While securing catheter, apply sterile dressing over site.
   A. *Manufactured catheter stabilization device*: Wipe selected area with single-use skin protectant, and allow to dry. Slide device under catheter hub, and center hub over device. Holding catheter in place, peel off half of liner, press to adhere to skin. Repeat on other side. Holding catheter in place, pull tab out from center of device to create opening; insert catheter into slit (see illustration). Cover insertion site with a transparent or sterile gauze dressing.
   B. *Transparent dressing:* Secure with nondominant hand while preparing to apply dressing.
   C. *Sterile gauze dressing:* Place narrow piece (½ inch) of sterile tape over catheter hub. If sterile tape is not available, apply nonsterile tape around catheter hub or stabilization device. Place tape only on the catheter, never over the insertion site. Secure site to allow easy visual inspection. Avoid applying tape around the arm.

	S	U	NP	Comments

10. Remove and discard gloves.
11. Label dressing per agency policy.
12. Anchor IV tubing with additional pieces of tape if necessary. When using transparent dressing, avoid placing tape over dressing.
13. Discard equipment, and perform hand hygiene.

Evaluation
1. Observe function, patency, and IV flow rate after changing dressing.
2. Inspect condition of site.
3. Monitor patient's body temperature.
4. Record and report dressing change and observation of IV system.

18 Caring in Nursing Practice

CASE STUDY

1. The daughter of a patient in an extended care facility has traveled from another state to visit. When she arrives with her husband and teenage son, she finds that her mother has deteriorated dramatically from the last time she spoke with her. The patient, in the terminal stages of liver disease, is now only minimally responsive with episodes of agitation and disorientation. The family, especially the daughter, is emotionally distraught.
    a. What can be done by the nurse to demonstrate caring for this patient's family?

CHAPTER REVIEW

Complete the following:

1. Match the theorist with the theoretical concept:
   Patricia Benner and Judith Wrubel
   Jean Watson
   Madeleine Leininger
   Kristen Swanson
   a. Five processes and subdimensions _____
   b. Transpersonal caring _____
   c. Caring is primary _____
   d. Transcultural caring _____

2. For the following nursing behaviors, identify an example of a clinical intervention.
   a. Providing presence

   b. Comforting/touch

   c. Listening

   d. Knowing the patient

3. A patient is to have an IV line inserted. The nurse demonstrates caring behaviors by:

Select the best answer for each of the following questions:

4. A nurse is discussing with her peers how much a patient matters to her. She states that she does not want the patient to suffer. The nurse is implementing the theory described by:
   1. Patricia Benner
   2. Jean Watson
   3. Kristen Swanson
   4. Madeleine Leininger

5. A patient was admitted to the hospital to have diagnostic tests to rule out a cancerous lesion in the lungs. The nurse is sitting with the patient in the room awaiting the results of the tests. The nurse is demonstrating the caring behavior of:
   1. Knowing
   2. Comforting
   3. Providing presence
   4. Maintaining belief

6. A nurse manager would like to promote more opportunities for the staff on the busy unit to demonstrate caring behaviors. The manager elects to implement:
   1. More time off for the staff
   2. A strict schedule for patient treatments
   3. Staff selection of patient assignments
   4. Staff appointment to hospital committees

7. A new graduate is looking at theories of caring. He selects Leininger's theory because it is most agreeable with his belief system. Leininger defines caring as a(n):
   1. New consciousness and moral idea
   2. Nurturing way of relating to a valued other
   3. Central, unifying domain necessary for health and survival
   4. Improvement in the human condition using a transcultural perspective

8. A nurse is working with a patient who has been admitted to the oncology unit for treatment of a cancerous growth. This nurse is applying Swanson's theory of caring and demonstrating the concept of maintaining belief when:
   1. Performing the patient's dressing changes
   2. Providing explanations about the medications
   3. Keeping the patient draped during the physical exam
   4. Discussing how the radiation therapy will assist in decreasing the tumor's size

9. A new graduate is assigned to a surgical unit where there are a large number of procedures to be performed during each shift. This nurse demonstrates a caring behavior in this situation by:
    1. Avoiding situations that may be uncomfortable or difficult
    2. Attempting to do all the treatments independently and quickly
    3. Seeking assistance before performing new or difficult skills
    4. Telling patients that he or she is a new graduate and unfamiliar with all the procedures
10. An example of the caring process of "enabling" is:
    1. Performing a catheter insertion quickly and well
    2. Reassuring the patient that the lab results should be fine
    3. Providing pain medication before a procedure
    4. Assisting a patient during the birth of a child
11. A subdimension of Swanson's process of caring—"doing for others as he/she would do for self"—involves:
    1. Being there
    2. Performing skillfully
    3. Generating alternatives
    4. Offering realistic optimism
12. In the Caring Assessment Tool (CAT), an example of mutual problem solving with a patient is when a nurse:
    1. Discusses health issues with the patient and family
    2. Pays attention to the patient
    3. Provides privacy for the patient
    4. Includes the family members in the patient's care
13. A nurse attempts to understand the specific cultural concerns of a patient and how they relate to his illness. What caring factor is applied?
    1. Attentive reassurance
    2. Encouragement
    3. Provision of basic human needs
    4. Appreciation of unique meanings
14. Additional teaching is required if a nurse observes a nursing assistant working with an older adult patient and:
    1. Has the patient select the clothes to wear
    2. Addresses the patient as "Honey"
    3. Carefully organizes the patient's personal items
    4. Combs and styles the patient's hair

STUDY GROUP QUESTIONS

- What is "caring" in the nursing profession?
- What are the major theories of caring and the key concepts in each one?
- How is caring perceived by patients?
- What are caring behaviors?
- How can a nurse demonstrate caring to patients and families?

Answers available through your instructor.

19 Cultural Diversity

CASE STUDY

1. For the following situations, identify how a nurse should approach the patient and significant others in order to recognize cultural concerns and health care needs:
   a. The male patient comes from a culture with a matriarchal organization.
   b. Large numbers of family members surround the patient on the acute care unit.
   c. Dietary practices of the patient prohibit the eating of meat or meat products.
   d. A traditional healer makes calls to the patient's home between the patient's visits to the physician.
   e. The patient and her family speak another language.

CHAPTER REVIEW

Match the description/definition in Column A with the correct term in Column B.

Column A
____ 1. Process of adapting to and adopting a new culture
____ 2. Shared identity related to social and cultural heritage
____ 3. Tendency to categorize people into particular patterns without further assessment
____ 4. Attitudes associating negative characteristics to people perceived to be different from oneself
____ 5. Integrated patterns of human behavior, including language, customs, and beliefs
____ 6. Common biological characteristics shared by a group of people
____ 7. Cognitive stance or perspective about phenomena characteristic of a particular cultural group
____ 8. Giving up ethnic identity in favor of the dominant culture
____ 9. Holding one's own way of life as superior to others
____ 10. Distinct discipline focused on the comparative study of cultures to understand similarities

Column B
a. Culture
b. Race
c. Ethnicity
d. Ethnocentrism
e. Acculturation
f. Assimilation
g. Prejudices
h. Worldview
i. Transcultural nursing
j. Stereotyping

Complete the following:

11. Subcultures have the same life patterns, values, and norms as the dominant culture.
    True _____ False _____

12. How is a culture that uses folk healers more likely to approach illness causation and treatment? Select all that apply.
    a. Causation is magic/religious based. _____
    b. Treatment is organ specific. _____
    c. Practitioners are sought who have uniform qualifications and follow universalistic standards. _____
    d. Group reliability and interdependence are important. _____
    e. Healing may be learned through apprenticeship. _____
    f. Regular pharmaceutical agents are used exclusively. _____

13. Identify two possible nursing diagnoses that may be related to a patient's cultural needs.

14. Provide an example for how the nurse may develop each of the following.
    a. Cultural awareness
    b. Cultural skills

Copyright © 2011, 2007, 2003 by Mosby, Inc., an affiliate of Elsevier Inc. All rights reserved.

15. A nurse anticipates that a patient who has a present time orientation will arrive at the clinic for his or her appointment:
    a. Early _____
    b. On time _____
    c. Late _____

16. Which of the following is/are correct statements concerning cultural beliefs of pregnancy and childbirth? Select all that apply.
    a. Hindu women are encouraged to eat "hot" foods when pregnant. _____
    b. Arab women seek out male practitioners. _____
    c. Hispanic women tend to avoid early baby showers. _____
    d. Filipino and South Asian women tend to endure labor without complaining or asking for medication. _____
    e. Orthodox Jewish fathers play an active role in the delivery room. _____

17. A nurse may anticipate that decision making for African or Asian patients near death will be made by family members.
    True _____ False _____

18. Identify an example of a question a nurse could use to elicit specific cultural information from a patient.

19. Identify cultural patterns of communication that may influence the nurse-patient interaction.

20. What are some common cultural practices associated with pregnancy and childbirth?

Select the best answer for each of the following questions:

21. A nurse is meeting a patient for the first time for the admission interview. There are eight family members sitting around the patient's bed. After introductions, the most appropriate nursing action is to:
    1. Ask the family members to leave immediately
    2. Proceed with the admission interview
    3. Come back at another time
    4. Ask the patient if he or she wants a family member present

22. A nurse is seeing patients in the outpatient clinic who are Asian American. A patient from this cultural group who incorporates traditional health practices may use a(n):
    1. Herbalist
    2. Curandero
    3. Root worker
    4. Medicine man

23. A nurse recognizes that physiological characteristics of cultural groups may affect overall health and that there may be an increased prevalence of particular disease processes within certain groups. In working with Native American people, the nurse is alert to the signs and symptoms that may indicate:
    1. Cancer of the esophagus
    2. Diabetes mellitus
    3. Parasites
    4. Sickle cell anemia

24. The community center where a nurse volunteers has a culturally diverse population. The nurse wants to promote communication with all the patients from different cultures. A beneficial technique for the nurse is to:
    1. Explain nursing terms that are used
    2. Use direct and consistent eye contact with all patients
    3. Call patients by their first names to establish rapport
    4. Wait for responses to all questions that are asked

25. A patient expresses to the nurse that traditional Western or American practices are used in the home for health promotion. The nurse expects that the patient will use:
    1. Acupuncture
    2. Guided imagery
    3. Aromatic therapy
    4. Over-the-counter medications

26. When working with an interpreter for a patient who speaks another language, the nurse should:
    1. Direct questions to the interpreter
    2. Expect word for word translation
    3. Ensure that the interpreter speaks the patient's dialect
    4. Ask the interpreter to evaluate the patient's nonverbal behaviors

27. When asking a patient specifically about his or her social organization, a nurse will focus on the patient's:
    1. Position in the family hierarchy
    2. Preferred manner of communication
    3. Age at the time of immigration
    4. Dietary practices

28. A nurse is working with a patient who is Muslim. There are foods that are prohibited (Haram), and the nurse recognizes that this will include:
    1. Pork
    2. Fish
    3. Fresh fruit
    4. Vegetables

29. An Orthodox Jewish patient has just died. The nurse anticipates:
    1. A request for an autopsy
    2. Preparation for cremation
    3. Refusal to move the body
    4. Scheduling for immediate burial

30. When working with patients of other cultures, a nurse anticipates that a curandero may be sought for a patient who is:
    1. Hispanic
    2. Chinese
    3. African
    4. Korean

STUDY GROUP QUESTIONS

- What is culture?
- What are the major ethnocultural groups in the country/community, their health and illness beliefs and practices, and their traditional remedies?
- How can a nurse promote communication with individuals who are from other cultures and/or individuals who speak different languages?
- How can a nurse identify and respond to a patient's cultural needs?
- What information may be obtained from a cultural assessment?
- What nursing approaches may be successful in assisting multicultural patients in health care settings?
- What resources are available to assist a nurse in learning about and working with patients from other cultures?

Answers available through your instructor.

Spiritual Health

20

CASE STUDY

1. A nurse is working with a patient in an acute care facility who practices Buddhism.
   a. What information should be obtained in relation to the patient's spiritual practices?
   b. What adaptations may need to be made by the nurse, the other members of the health care team, and the acute care facility to meet the patient's spiritual needs?

CHAPTER REVIEW

Match the description/definition in Column A with the correct term in Column B.

	Column A	Column B
___	1. Does not believe in the existence of a supreme spiritual being or god	a. Faith
___	2. Cultural or institutional religion	b. Hope
___	3. Awareness of one's inner self and a sense of connection to a higher being	c. Connectedness
___	4. Multidimensional concept that gives comfort while a person endures hardship and challenges	d. Atheist
___	5. Awareness of that which cannot be seen or known in ordinary ways	e. Spirituality
___	6. Belief that ultimate reality is unknown or unknowable	f. Self-transcendence
___	7. Having close spiritual relationships with oneself, others, and a god or other spiritual being	g. Agnostic

Complete the following:

8. Identify general nursing interventions for promotion of spiritual health.

9. An example of a nursing intervention for a patient who has had a near death experience is:

10. Identify two possible nursing diagnoses relating to spirituality or spiritual health.

11. Identify what each letter in the BELIEF assessment tool acronym designates:
    B:
    E:
    L:
    I:
    E:
    F:

12. Formulate a question that may be asked to determine a patient's spiritual belief system.

13. There is an order for whole blood replacement for a patient. Before the blood administration, a nurse will check to see if the patient is a member of what religion(s)?

14. Provide at least two examples of rituals associated with spirituality.

15. Religious or spiritual practices may have an impact upon the provision of healthcare to a patient. For an individual who is of the Islamic faith, which of the following may need to be considered by a nurse and other health care providers? Select all that apply.
    a. Organ donation will be approved. ___
    b. Women prefer female providers/examiners. ___
    c. Euthanasia is practiced. ___
    d. Time will need to be set aside during the day for prayer. ___
    e. Faith healing may be used. ___
    f. Blood products and medicines may be refused. ___

Copyright © 2011, 2007, 2003 by Mosby, Inc., an affiliate of Elsevier Inc. All rights reserved.

Select the best answer for each of the following questions:

16. A patient is admitted to a medical center for surgery to repair a fractured hip. Upon reviewing the patient's admission history, a nurse finds that the patient attends religious services routinely. The nurse supports the patient's spiritual needs by stating:
    1. "Do you really go to services often?"
    2. "Don't worry. God will take care of you."
    3. "I'll call your minister and have him stop by to see you."
    4. "Is there any way that I may be able to help you with your spiritual needs?"
17. A patient who is of the Jewish faith is admitted to the long-term care facility. A nurse seeks to provide support of the usual health practices that are part of this religion. The nurse learns that one component of usual Jewish tradition states:
    1. No euthanasia should be used.
    2. A faith healer will be involved.
    3. Modern medical treatment should be refused.
    4. Physical exams should be performed only by individuals of the same sex.
18. While caring for a patient in the intensive care unit, the patient has a cardiac arrest. The patient is successfully resuscitated. After this near death experience, the patient is progressing physically, but appears withdrawn and concerned. The nurse assists the patient by stating:
    1. "The experience that you had is easy to explain and understand."
    2. "That was a very close call. It must be very frightening for you."
    3. "Other people have had similar experiences and worked through their feelings."
    4. "If you would like to talk about your experience, I will stay with you."
19. For a patient with a diagnosis of a chronic disease, a nurse wishes to encourage feelings of hope. The nurse recognizes that hope provides:
    1. A meaning and purpose for the patient
    2. An organized approach to dealing with the disease process
    3. A connection to the cultural background of the patient
    4. A binding relationship with the divine being of the patient's religion
20. A nurse is reviewing the plan of care for a 66-year-old home care patient who is experiencing the beginning stages of Alzheimer disease. Several nursing diagnoses have been identified from the initial home visit and assessment. The nurse believes that the patient may need to be assessed for spiritual needs based on the diagnosis of:
    1. Impaired memory
    2. Altered health maintenance
    3. Ineffective individual coping
    4. Altered thought process
21. According to Erikson's stages of psychosocial development, with regard to spiritual beliefs it is expected that a 6-year-old child will:
    1. Begin to ask about a god or supreme being
    2. Have spiritual well-being provided by the parents
    3. Interpret meanings literally
    4. Begin to learn the difference between right and wrong
22. A nurse recognizes that a group whose members may reject modern medicine based on religious beliefs is:
    1. Hindu
    2. Islamic
    3. Catholic
    4. Navajo
23. According to Erikson's stages of psychosocial development, with regard to spiritual beliefs it is expected that a middle-age person will begin to:
    1. Reflect on inconsistencies in religious stories
    2. Form independent beliefs and attitudes
    3. Review value systems during a crisis
    4. Sort fantasy from fact

STUDY GROUP QUESTIONS

- What is spirituality and how does it relate to an individual's health status?
- What are the concepts of spirituality/spiritual health?
- What spiritual or religious problems may arise during patient care?
- How can a nurse assess a patient's spirituality/spiritual health?
- What is the role of a nurse in promoting spiritual health?
- How can a nurse avoid imposing his or her own beliefs on a patient?
- What are the differences and similarities in spiritual practices and health beliefs between the major religious sects?
- How is hope related to spirituality?

Answers available through your instructor.

Growth and Development 21

CASE STUDIES

1. A student nurse with an inpatient pediatric unit in a medical center has three patients—an infant, a 5-year-old child, and a 16-year-old adolescent.
   a. How should the nurse promote growth and developmental needs for these patients in the acute care environment?
2. A patient in the extended care facility is an 86-year-old woman who is occasionally disoriented to time, place, and person.
   a. How should a nurse approach this patient to assist her in meeting her developmental needs?
3. A student nurse is working as a summer camp nurse with children 8 to 10 years old. It is the nurse's turn to select diversional activities for a group.
   a. What types of games or activities are appropriate for this age-group?
4. A nurse is teaching the parents of adolescents the signs that may indicate a potential suicidal tendency in their children.
   a. What signs/behaviors will the nurse identify for these parents?

CHAPTER REVIEW

Match the description in Column A with the correct theorist in Column B.

	Column A		Column B
_____	1. Development of cognition	a.	Freud
_____	2. Psychosexual focus	b.	Erikson
_____	3. Based on human needs	c.	Maslow
_____	4. Moral development	d.	Piaget
_____	5. Psychosocial development	e.	Kohlberg

Complete the following:

6. An example of a teratogen is:

7. The leading cause of death in the toddler and preschool age-groups is:

8. Select the age-group (infant, toddler, preschool age, school age, adolescent, young adult, middle-aged adult, or older adult) in which each of the following behaviors is evident or usually begins:
   a. Toilet training _____
   b. Tripling of birth weight _____
   c. Use of script handwriting _____
   d. Separation anxiety _____
   e. Moving away from the family _____
   f. Parallel play _____
   g. Search for personal identity _____
   h. Menopause _____
   i. Speaking in short sentences _____
   j. More graceful running and jumping _____
   k. Development of fears _____
   l. Presbycusis _____
   m. Loss of primary teeth _____
   n. Development of primary and secondary sexual characteristics _____
   o. Low risk of chronic illness _____
   p. Diminished skin turgor and appearance of wrinkles _____
   q. Socioeconomic stability _____
   r. Recognition of objects by their outward appearance _____

9. To promote awareness of time, place, and person in an extended care environment, a nurse implements:

10. Prescriptive use or administration of more medication than indicated clinically is termed:

Copyright © 2011, 2007, 2003 by Mosby, Inc., an affiliate of Elsevier Inc. All rights reserved.

11. Identify safety concerns in the home environment for the following age-groups:
    a. Toddler
    b. Older adult

12. What are the expected physical assessment findings for a middle-aged adult? Select all that apply.
    a. Abnormal visual fields and ocular movements _____
    b. Palpable lateral thyroid nodes _____
    c. Pulse rate of 60 to 100 beats per minute _____
    d. Decreased strength of abdominal muscles _____
    e. Responsive sensory system _____
    f. Diminished motor responses _____

13. Identify a topic area that is age appropriate for a group of older adults in a senior housing development.

Select the best answer for each of the following questions:

14. A nurse is assigned to prepare a teaching plan for a group of preschool age children. For this age-group, the nurse includes:
    1. Appropriate use of medications
    2. Cooking safety including use of the stove
    3. Information on prevention of obesity and hypertension
    4. Guidelines for crossing the street or actions to take during a fire

15. Children who are admitted to a hospital may be afraid about the hospitalization. To reduce the fear of school age children in an acute care environment, a nurse:
    1. Restrains them for all assessments and procedures
    2. Shows them the equipment that is to be used for procedures
    3. Provides in-depth information on how procedures are done
    4. Tells them that everything will be all right and the procedures will not hurt

16. During a clinical rotation a student nurse is observing children in a day care center. The student is asked to assist with the activities for the preschool age children. Children in this age-group are usually able to:
    1. Make detailed drawings
    2. Skip, throw, and catch balls
    3. Easily hold a pencil and print letters
    4. Use a vocabulary of more than 8000 words

17. A parent of an infant asks a nurse what the infant should be able to do at the end of the first year. The nurse identifies that the infant will be able to:
    1. Participate in simple games, such as peek-a-boo
    2. Use symbols to represent objects or persons
    3. Differentiate strangers from family members
    4. Recognize his or her own name

18. Parents of a 6-month-old infant are asking about the usual activities that can be expected of a child this age. A nurse informs the parents that a major milestone in gross motor development for a 6-month-old infant is:
    1. Banging hand-held blocks together
    2. Pulling self to a standing position
    3. Sitting up independently
    4. Crawling on the abdomen

19. A nurse is working with a group of young adults at the community center. There are many discussions about life and health issues. The nurse is aware that a health-related concern for young adults is that:
    1. Attachment needs must be enhanced.
    2. "Labeling" may alter their self-perceptions.
    3. Adaptation to chronic disease is developing.
    4. Fast-paced lifestyles may place them at risk for illnesses or disabilities.

20. A nurse is seeking to evaluate the effectiveness of information provided to the parents of an infant. The nurse determines that teaching has been successful when the parents:
    1. Place small pillows in the infant's crib
    2. Position the infant on the stomach for sleeping
    3. Purchase a crib with slats that are less than 2 inches apart
    4. Prop up a bottle for the infant to suck on while falling asleep

21. When presenting a program for a group of individuals in their middle-aged adult years, a nurse informs the members to expect the following physical change:
    1. A decrease in skin turgor
    2. An increased breast size
    3. Palpable lateral thyroid lobes
    4. A visual acuity that is greater than 20/50

22. Parents of a 3½-year-old boy are concerned when, after hospitalization, the boy begins to suck his thumb again. The boy had not sucked his thumb for over a year. A nurse informs the parents that:
    1. Their physician must be informed about this behavior.
    2. The child was probably not ready to stop this behavior previously.
    3. The child is feeling neglected by his parents and they should spend more time with him.
    4. The behavior should be ignored as it is common for a child to regress when anxious.

23. An adolescent girl has gone to a family planning center for information about birth control. The patient asks a nurse what she should use to avoid getting pregnant. The nurse responds:
    1. "Are your parents aware of your sexual activity?"
    2. "You've been using some kind of protection before, right?"
    3. "What are your friends doing to protect themselves?"
    4. "What can you tell me about your past sexual experiences?"

24. A patient has gone to an outpatient obstetric clinic for a routine checkup. The patient asks a nurse what is happening with the baby now that she is in her second trimester. The nurse informs the patient that:
    1. The heartbeat can be heard.
    2. The fingers and toes are well-developed.
    3. The organ systems are just beginning to develop.
    4. The brain is undergoing a tremendous growth spurt.
25. For a patient in a nursing center, the nurse suspects the potentially reversible cognitive impairment of:
    1. Delirium
    2. Dementia
    3. Depression
    4. Disengagement

STUDY GROUP QUESTIONS

- What are the principles of growth and development?
- How can growth and development be influenced both internally and externally?
- What are the differences and similarities of the major developmental theorists?
- How can a nurse apply the different developmental theories to patient situations?
- What are the major physical, psychosocial, and cognitive changes that occur throughout the life span?
- What are the specific health needs for each developmental stage?
- How does the approach of a nurse differ for individuals in each developmental stage to meet their developmental needs?
- What are the different teaching/learning needs of each developmental stage?

STUDY CHART

Create a study chart to compare *Growth and Development Across the Life Span* that identifies the physical abilities, psychosocial/cognitive activities, and health promotion behaviors and strategies for each age-group from infancy to older adulthood.

Answers available through your instructor.

22 Self-Concept and Sexuality

CASE STUDIES

1. A 22-year-old man is admitted to a rehabilitation facility. He was seriously injured in an automobile accident and now is paraplegic. Although medically stable, it appears that he is having difficulty dealing with his physical limitations. The patient speaks frequently about his girlfriend and his involvement in athletics and other social activities.
   a. What self-concept and sexuality issues are involved in this situation?
   b. Formulate a plan of care for this patient.
2. A nurse suspects that a patient is the victim of sexual abuse.
   a. What behaviors may the patient be exhibiting that would lead to this assessment?
   b. What questions should the nurse ask to get more information from the patient about the possible abuse?

CHAPTER REVIEW

Match the description/definition in Column A with the correct term in Column B.

Column A

_____ 1. Set of conscious and unconscious feelings and beliefs about oneself
_____ 2. Set of behaviors that have been approved by family, community, and culture as appropriate in particular situations
_____ 3. Clear, persistent preference for persons of one sex
_____ 4. Emotional evaluation of self-worth
_____ 5. Experiences and attitudes related to appearance and physical abilities
_____ 6. Sense of femaleness or maleness
_____ 7. Irrational fear of homosexuality
_____ 8. Persistent individuality and sameness of a person over time and in various circumstances

Column B

a. Sexuality
b. Self-concept
c. Homophobia
d. Self-esteem
e. Sexual orientation
f. Role
g. Identity
h. Body image

Complete the following:

9. Identify at least two examples of the following.
   a. Positive influences on self-concept
   b. Stressors to self-concept

10. Which of the following behaviors may indicate an altered self-concept? Select all that apply.
    a. Eye contact maintained _____
    b. Straight posture _____
    c. Hesitant speech _____
    d. Overly angry response _____
    e. Independence _____
    f. Passive attitude _____
    g. Able to make decisions _____
    h. Unkempt appearance _____

11. For the following patients, identify the potential concerns related to self-concept and sexuality.
    a. A woman who has had a mastectomy
    b. A woman who is undergoing chemotherapy for cancer and who has a young child at home
    c. A 7-year-old child who has been severely burned
    d. A middle-aged adult man who has had a heart attack

12. A way in which a nurse may promote self-concept in an acute care setting is by:

13. An example of an alteration in sexual health is:

14. Specify an area for patient education to promote sexual health.

Copyright © 2011, 2007, 2003 by Mosby, Inc., an affiliate of Elsevier Inc. All rights reserved.

15. For the nursing diagnosis *situational low self-esteem* related to being unable to successfully pass a required college course, identify a patient goal/outcome and nursing interventions.

16. The capacity for sexuality diminishes significantly in older adults.
    True _____ False _____

17. Cultural background does not directly influence self-concept.
    True _____ False _____

18. The best method of birth control to reinforce with patients is the least expensive selection.
    True _____ False _____

19. An example of an intervention that a nurse may implement to promote self-concept for an older adult is:

Select the best answer for each of the following questions:

20. A nurse recognizes that which of the following age-groups are most vulnerable to identity stressors?
    1. Infancy
    2. Preschool
    3. Adolescence
    4. Middle-aged adulthood

21. An adolescent has gone to the nurse's office in a school to discuss some personal issues. The nurse wishes to determine the sexual health of this adolescent. The nurse begins by asking:
    1. "Do you use contraception?"
    2. "Have you already had sexual relations?"
    3. "Are your parents aware of your sexual activity?"
    4. "Do you have any concerns about sex or your body's development?"

22. During an interview and physical assessment of a female patient in the clinic, a nurse finds that the patient has multiple lacerations and bruises and that she has experienced headaches and difficulty sleeping. The nurse suspects:
    1. Sexual dysfunction
    2. Emotional conflict
    3. Sexually transmitted disease
    4. Physical and/or sexual abuse

23. A patient has gone to a family planning center for assistance in selecting a birth control method. She asks the nurse about contraception that requires a prescription. The nurse responds by discussing:
    1. Condoms
    2. Abstinence
    3. Spermicides
    4. Birth control pills

24. A patient is admitted to a coronary care unit after an acute myocardial infarction. He tells the nurse, "I won't be able to do what I used to at the hardware store." The nurse recognizes that the patient is experiencing a problem with the self-concept component of:
    1. Role
    2. Identity
    3. Self-esteem
    4. Body image

25. An adolescent patient has just been diagnosed with scoliosis and will need to wear a corrective brace. She tells the nurse angrily, "I don't know why I have to have this stupid problem!" The nurse responds most appropriately by saying:
    1. "Tell me what you do when you get angry and upset."
    2. "Don't be angry. You'll be getting the best care available."
    3. "You'll heal quickly and the brace can come off pretty soon."
    4. "It's okay to be angry around your friends, but try not to be upset around your parents."

26. During an initial assessment at an outpatient clinic, a nurse wants to determine a patient's perception of identity. The nurse asks the patient:
    1. "What is your usual day like?"
    2. "How would you describe yourself?"
    3. "What activities do you enjoy doing at home?"
    4. "What changes would you make in your personal appearance?"

27. A patient has been in the rehabilitation facility for several weeks after a cerebral vascular accident (CVA/stroke). During the hospitalization, a nurse has identified that the patient has become progressively more depressed about his physical condition. Although the patient is able, he will not participate in personal grooming and now is refusing any visitors. At this point, the nurse intervenes by:
    1. Telling the patient to think more positively about the future
    2. Helping the patient to get washed and dressed every day
    3. Leaving the patient to complete activities of daily living independently
    4. Contacting the physician to discuss a psychological consultation

28. A nurse is working with a patient who has had a colostomy. The patient asks about resuming a sexual relationship with a partner. The nurse begins by determining:
    1. The patient's knowledge about sexual activity
    2. How the patient has dealt with other life changes in the past
    3. The partner's feelings about the colostomy
    4. How comfortable the patient and the partner are in communicating with each other

29. A nurse who is using Erikson's theory expects that a 5-year-old boy will begin to:
    1. Accept body changes and maturation
    2. Incorporate feedback from peers into his personality
    3. Distinguish himself from the environment around him
    4. Identify with a specific gender group
30. A patient asks a nurse about a prescription for tadalafil (Cialis). The nurse recognizes, however, that this drug is contraindicated for the patient who is taking:
    1. Antibiotics
    2. Beta blockers
    3. Antihistamines
    4. Nonsteroidal antiinflammatory agents
31. A nurse is aware that which of the following strategies is appropriate for teaching a patient for promotion of a positive sexual experience?
    1. Encouraging the use of only one position for intercourse
    2. Instructing couples to work harder at the beginning of intercourse
    3. Discussing side effects of medications that may alter responsiveness
    4. Emphasizing a shorter period of foreplay
32. Correction is required if a new nurse in the women's clinic is observed:
    1. Closing the door during an examination
    2. Determining the patient's cultural beliefs
    3. Identifying physiological changes for the patient
    4. Discussing findings with the patient in the examination room
33. Which of the following is anticipated as a sexual change related to the aging process?
    1. Increased vaginal secretions
    2. Decreased time for ejaculation to be achieved
    3. Decreased time for maintenance of an erection
    4. Increased orgasmic contractions
34. During an initial assessment at an outpatient clinic, a nurse wants to determine a patient's level of self-esteem. The nurse asks the patient:
    1. "What is your usual day like?"
    2. "How do you feel about yourself?"
    3. "What hobbies do you enjoy doing at home?"
    4. "What changes would you make in your personal appearance?"

STUDY GROUP QUESTIONS

- What are the components of self-concept?
- What stressors may influence an individual's self-concept?
- How may a nurse promote an individual's self-concept in different health care settings?
- What is sexuality and how does it develop throughout the life span?
- How can sexual health be defined?
- What are some of the current issues related to sexuality and sexual health?
- How may sexual health be altered?
- What health-related factors may influence sexual function?
- How are self-concept and sexuality related?
- How can a nurse determine an individual's self-concept and sexual health?
- What adaptations may be made by a nurse in approaching different age-groups for the assessment and promotion of self-concept and sexual health?
- How can a nurse apply critical thinking and nursing processes to the areas of self-concept and sexuality?
- What resources are available to assist individuals to promote optimum self-concept and sexual health?
- How can a nurse make the patient feel more at ease when completing an assessment of sexual health?

STUDY CHART

Create a study chart on *Stressors Affecting Self-Concept* that identifies how the components of self-concept may be influenced and nursing interventions that may be implemented to promote a patient's self-concept.

Answers available through your instructor.

Family Context in Nursing 23

CASE STUDY

1. A 65-year-old man has been admitted to the coronary care unit in a medical center. The patient experienced a myocardial infarction (heart attack) while working late in his store. His wife, who accompanied him to the medical center, not only has been the "homemaker" for the family for more than 25 years but also has assisted in the family business run by her husband. They have two children who live on their own. Their son lives with a male roommate in a homosexual relationship, while their younger daughter is married and has two children of her own. The patient and his wife speak readily about the younger daughter, but avoid talking about her older brother.
   a. What factors related to family roles and function are involved in this situation?
   b. What stage of the family life cycle is this family in currently?
   c. What strategies may a nurse use to promote communication in this family?
   d. How may the role of the patient and his wife influence the health education plan?
   e. Identify a family-oriented nursing diagnosis for this situation.

CHAPTER REVIEW

Match the family stages in Column A with the key principle identified for that stage in Column B.

Column A (Family Stages)   *Column B (Key Principles)*
_____ 1. Unattached young adult   a. Increasing flexibility of family's boundaries to include children's independence
_____ 2. Newly married couple   b. Accepting parent-offspring separation
_____ 3. Family with adolescents   c. Accepting shifting of generational roles
_____ 4. Family with young adults d. Committing to a new system
_____ 5. Family in later life   e. Accepting a multitude of exits from and entries into the family system

Complete the following:

6. Identify the major concerns that may influence families today.

7. For families providing care for a family member:
   a. Identify possible indicators of caregiver stress.
   b. Identify a nursing diagnosis for a family coping with the difficult care of an older adult parent in the home.

8. Which of the following are correct statements regarding today's society? Select all that apply.
   a. Families are larger. _____
   b. Divorce rates have tripled since the 1950s. _____
   c. Fewer people are living alone. _____
   d. From the 1970s to the 1990s, the number of single-parent families has doubled. _____
   e. Less than one third of gay male couples live together. _____
   f. Father-only families have increased. _____
   g. The fastest growing age-group is 65 years and older. _____

9. Identify an effect that inadequate functioning may have on a family.

10. What questions may be asked to determine the influence of culture on a family?

11. Provide examples of health promotion interventions for a family.

Select the best answer for each of the following questions:

12. A nurse is working with a family in which the parents, both previously divorced, have brought a total of three unrelated children together. This type of family structure is classified as:
    1. Nuclear
    2. Extended
    3. Blended
    4. Multi-adult

13. A community health nurse has been assigned to work with a patient who is being discharged from a psychiatric facility. The nurse recognizes when dealing with the family that:
    1. All family members do not need to understand and agree to the plan of care.
    2. Health behaviors of the family do not influence the health of individual family members.
    3. A nurse needs to change the structure of the family to meet the needs of the patient.
    4. Health promotion behaviors need to be tied to the developmental stage of the family.

14. Preparation for working with families includes understanding the life cycle stage that the patient is experiencing. A nurse is working with a family that is in the "launching children and moving on" stage. It is expected that a family in this stage may also need to deal with:
    1. A review of life events
    2. Determining career goals
    3. The death of an older parent
    4. Development of intimate peer relationships

15. A nurse is working with a family that has been taking care of a parent with Alzheimer's disease for several years in their home. A nursing diagnosis of *risk for caregiver role strain* is identified. The nurse initially plans for:
    1. Respite care
    2. More medication for the parent
    3. Placement in a long-term care facility
    4. Consultation with a family therapist

16. After initial assessment of a family, a nurse determines that this is a healthy family. This assessment is based on the finding that:
    1. The family responds passively to stressors.
    2. Change is viewed negatively and strongly resisted.
    3. The family structure is flexible enough to adapt to crises.
    4. Minimum influence is exerted by the members upon their environment.

17. An older adult patient who had surgery is going to be discharged tomorrow. The patient has a visual deficit and will need dressing changes twice a day. To meet this specific need, the nurse first:
    1. Refers the patient to an adult day care center
    2. Arranges for a private duty nurse to take care of the patient 24 hours a day
    3. Informs the patient that the dressing changes will have to be managed independently
    4. Investigates the availability of a family member or neighbor to perform the dressing changes

18. A nurse is working in the community with an adult woman who is newly diagnosed with diabetes mellitus. The patient is married, has two school age children, and works part-time. The nurse is focused on assisting the patient to learn to manage the diabetes. At this point, the nurse is viewing the family as:
    1. Patient
    2. Context
    3. Process
    4. Caregiver

19. The concept of a family being able to transcend divorce and remarriage is termed:
    1. Family resiliency
    2. Family diversity
    3. Family durability
    4. Family functioning

20. To determine family form and membership, a nurse asks the patient:
    1. "How are financial decisions made?"
    2. "Who drives the children to school?"
    3. "Where do you go on vacation?"
    4. "Who do you consider your family?"

STUDY GROUP QUESTIONS

- What are the attributes of a family?
- What are the different family forms?
- What are the current issues/trends influencing families?
- How do the structure and function of a family influence family relationships?
- How does communication affect family relationships?
- How are the nursing approaches to the family as patient and the family as context similar/different?
- How may critical thinking and nursing processes be applied to family nursing?
- What specific assessments should a nurse make in relation to a family?
- How does a nurse plan for the educational needs of a patient within a family?
- What must a nurse consider to meet the health needs of patients within families?
- How are psychosocial/cultural factors involved in family processes and the nursing approach to families?
- What resources are available within the health care setting and community to assist and support family functioning?

Answers available through your instructor.

Stress and Coping 24

CASE STUDY

1. A young adult woman is preparing to be married in a few months. She has also received a recent job promotion that requires many additional hours to be spent at work. She is seen in a nurse practitioner's office for vague symptoms.
    a. What possible signs and symptoms may be demonstrated if this patient is experiencing a stress reaction?
    b. Identify a possible nursing diagnosis for this patient.
    c. What relaxation techniques may be presented to this patient?

CHAPTER REVIEW

Complete the following:

1. Evaluating an event for its personal meaning is called:

2. Which of the following are correct statements about stress? Select all that apply.
    a. Increased self-confidence results in decreased tension. _____
    b. The emotional concern of others can increase negative effects. _____
    c. Shorter, less intense stressors increase the stress response. _____
    d. The same event can cause different stress levels in different people. _____
    e. The greater the perceived magnitude of the stressor, the greater the stress response. _____
    f. Stress is decreased if a person is unable to anticipate the occurrence of an event. _____
3. A priority nursing intervention for safety for a patient under extreme stress is to determine:

4. Depression in later adulthood is a common problem. True _____ False _____
5. An example of a positive benefit of exercise for stress reduction is:

6. For the following, select the type of stress-producing factor that is indicated: *Situational, Maturational, Sociocultural, Posttraumatic stress disorder*
    a. Divorce _____
    b. Poverty _____
    c. Rape _____
    d. Immigration status _____
    e. Job change _____
    f. Adolescent identity crisis _____
    g. Hypertension _____
    h. Children moving away from home _____
    i. September 11, 2001 _____
    j. Homelessness _____
7. Identify an indicator of stress for each of the following areas:
    a. Cognitive
    b. Cardiovascular
    c. Gastrointestinal
    d. Behavioral
    e. Neuroendocrine

Select the best answer for each of the following questions:

8. A patient has been hospitalized with a serious systemic infection. If the patient is in the resistance stage of the general adaptation syndrome and moving toward recovery, the nurse expects that the patient will demonstrate a:
    1. Stabilization of hormone levels
    2. Greater degree of tissue damage
    3. Reduction in cardiac output
    4. Greater involvement of the sympathetic nervous system
9. While working in a psychiatric emergency department, a nurse is alert to patients who are having severe difficulty in coping. A priority for the nurse is the safety of the patient and others; therefore, the nurse asks patients:
    1. "How can we help you?"
    2. "Are you thinking of harming yourself?"
    3. "What physical symptoms are you having?"
    4. "What happened that is different in your life?"
10. As a result of a patient's health problem, the family is experiencing economic difficulty and demonstrating signs of crisis. As part of crisis intervention, a nurse:
    1. Refers the patient for financial assistance
    2. Recommends inpatient psychiatric therapy

CHAPTER 24 • Stress and Coping

3. Plans to teach the family about long-term health needs
4. Has the patient avoid discussions about personal feelings and emotions

11. A nurse working for the surgical unit notes that a patient has been exhibiting nervous behavior the evening before a surgical procedure. To assess the degree of stress that the patient is experiencing, the nurse asks:
    1. "Would you like me to call your family for you?"
    2. "How dangerous do you think the surgery will be?"
    3. "You seem anxious. Would you like to talk about the surgery?"
    4. "How would you like to speak with another patient who has had the procedure already?"

12. A nurse notes that a patient is experiencing a stress reaction. To determine how the patient may cope with the event, the nurse should ask:
    1. "Are you taking any hypnotics?"
    2. "What do you think caused your stress?"
    3. "How long have you felt this way?"
    4. "Have you dealt with this reaction before?"

13. An 80-year-old patient was admitted to the hospital with a diagnosis of pneumonia. The patient is very lethargic and not communicating, and the patient's respirations are extremely labored. The nurse assesses that the patient is experiencing the general adaptation stage of:
    1. Alarm
    2. Resistance
    3. Exhaustion
    4. Reflex response

14. A patient has gone to the employee support center with complaints of fatigue and general uneasiness. The patient believes that the symptoms may be related to the increased amount of work that is expected in the job. The nurse initially recommends that the patient should attempt to reduce or control the stress by:
    1. Leaving the job immediately
    2. Enrolling in a self-awareness course
    3. Seeking the assistance of a psychiatrist
    4. Employing relaxation techniques, such as deep breathing

15. According to general adaptation syndrome (GAS), a nurse expects which of the following signs as part of an alarm reaction?
    1. Pupil dilation
    2. Decreased blood glucose levels
    3. Decreased heart rate
    4. Stabilized hormone levels

16. A nurse identifies that a patient is under stress. To determine the patient's perception of the stress, the nurse should ask:
    1. "Are you sure you are not taking drugs or alcohol?"
    2. "What does the situation mean to you?"
    3. "How did you handle this in the past?"
    4. "Why aren't you seeing a counselor?"

17. Which of the following patient observations does a nurse associate with the ego-defense mechanism of conversion?
    1. Assuming more job responsibilities
    2. Having difficulty sleeping
    3. Acting out inappropriately
    4. Refusing to talk about a problem

18. A patient has been having a hard time at home. He goes outside and begins to yell about the car and starts kicking the tires. This is an example of which of the following ego-defense mechanisms?
    1. Displacement
    2. Compensation
    3. Identification
    4. Denial

19. A nurse wants to assess whether a patient is using maladaptive coping strategies. The patient should be asked specifically about his or her:
    1. Dietary intake
    2. Social activities
    3. Cigarette smoking
    4. Exercise plan

STUDY GROUP QUESTIONS

- What is stress?
- What theories are associated with stress and the stress response?
- How does the general adaptation syndrome (GAS) work?
- How do nursing theorists explain stress and the stress response?
- What factors influence the response to stress?
- What assessment data may indicate the presence of a stress reaction?
- How does stress relate to illness?
- What are coping/defense mechanisms and how may they be used by individuals to deal with stress?
- What is the role of a nurse in reducing or eliminating stress for patients in health promotion, acute care, and restorative care settings?
- What is involved in crisis intervention?
- What are possible relaxation/stress reduction techniques?

Answers available through your instructor.

Loss and Grief 25

CASE STUDY

1. A woman's husband committed suicide and she is devastated by the event. In anticipation of potential difficulties, a nurse should be alert to the possibility of a complicated bereavement.
   a. What assessment data may indicate that the woman is experiencing a complicated period of bereavement?
   b. Identify a possible nursing diagnosis, goals, and nursing interventions for an individual who is experiencing a complicated bereavement.

CHAPTER REVIEW

Complete the following:

1. Grief resolution may be affected by:

2. Unexpected unemployment may be perceived as a loss.
   True _____ False _____

3. Provide an intervention that a nurse should implement for a family dealing with a patient's diagnosis of a terminal illness.

4. Which of the following interventions are appropriate for a terminally ill patient with constipation? Select all that apply.
   a. Maintenance of complete bed rest _____
   b. Increased intake of coffee _____
   c. Consumption of fresh vegetables _____
   d. Consumption of whole grain products _____
   e. Reducing fluid intake _____
   f. Obtaining an order for stool softeners _____

5. Identify at least two nursing measures that may be implemented to facilitate the mourning process.

6. Patients in the terminal stage of their lives may experience a sense of abandonment. What actions should a nurse implement to prevent or reduce this occurrence?

7. After a patient's death, there is federal and state legislation regarding policies and procedures for:

8. Formulate a question that a nurse could ask a patient regarding:
   a. The nature of a loss

   b. His/her cultural beliefs about loss

9. A patient has been in hospice care at home. A family member is taking care of the patient and is concerned about the patient's impending death, particularly what will happen to the patient. The nurse informs the family member that the signs of impending death include:

Select the best answer for each of the following questions:

10. A nurse is working with a patient who has been diagnosed with a terminal disease. The patient, who is moving into Kübler-Ross's denial stage of grieving, may respond:
    1. "I understand what the diagnosis means, and I know that I may die."
    2. "I would like to be able to make it to my son's wedding in June."
    3. "I think that the diagnostic tests are wrong, and they should be re-done."
    4. "I don't think that I can stand to have any more treatments. I just want to feel better."

11. While working with young children in a day care center, a nurse responds to instances that occur in their lives. Toddlers at the center generally experience loss and grief associated with:
    1. Anticipation of loss
    2. Separation from parents
    3. Changes in physical abilities
    4. Development of their identities

12. In a senior citizen center, a nurse is talking with a group of older adults. The recurrent theme associated with loss for this age-group is a:
    1. Confusion of fact and fantasy
    2. Perceived threat to their identity
    3. Change in status, role, and lifestyle
    4. Determination to reexamine life goals

13. A nurse who has recently graduated from nursing school is employed by an oncology unit. There are a number of patients who will not improve and will need assistance with dying. The nurse prepares for this experience by:
    1. Completing a detailed course on legal aspects of end of life issues
    2. Controlling his or her emotions about dying patients

CHAPTER 25 • Loss and Grief

3. Experiencing the death of a close family member
4. Identifying his or her own feelings about death and dying

14. A patient has had a long illness and is now approaching the end stages of his life. To assist this patient to meet his need for self-worth and support during this time, the nurse:
    1. Arranges for a grief counselor to visit
    2. Leaves the patient alone to deal with his life issues
    3. Asks the patient's family to take over his care
    4. Plans to visit the patient regularly throughout the day

15. The spouse of a patient who has just died is having more frequent episodes of headaches and generalized joint pain. The initial nursing intervention for this individual is to:
    1. Complete a thorough pain assessment
    2. Encourage more frequent use of analgesics
    3. Sit with the patient and encourage discussion of feelings
    4. Refer the patient immediately to a psychologist or grief counselor

16. A patient is experiencing a very serious illness that may not be curable. The nurse promotes hope for this patient in the affiliative dimension when:
    1. Reinforcing realistic goal setting
    2. Encouraging the development of supportive relationships
    3. Offering information about the illness and its treatment
    4. Demonstrating an understanding of the patient's strengths

17. A patient in the long-term care facility is to receive palliative care measures only during the end stages of a terminal illness. The nurse anticipates that this will include:
    1. Pain relief measures
    2. Emergency surgery
    3. Pulmonary resuscitation
    4. Transfer to intensive care if necessary

18. A patient arrives for outpatient chemotherapy. During this visit the patient tells the nurse that she is experiencing periods of nausea. The nurse promotes patient comfort by providing:
    1. Milk
    2. Coffee
    3. Ginger ale
    4. Orange juice

19. The loss of a known environment is associated with:
    1. Being hospitalized for several days
    2. The death of a pet
    3. Amputation of the right leg
    4. A recent burglary in the home

20. Of the following, a situational loss occurs when a:
    1. Parent requires physical assistance
    2. Family friend dies
    3. Child goes to college
    4. Job demotion and pay reduction occur

21. An individual in Bowlby's second phase of mourning, yearning, and searching may be expected to:
    1. Be unable to believe the loss
    2. Endlessly examine how the loss occurred
    3. Acquire new skills and build new relationships
    4. Experience emotional outbursts and sobbing

22. A nurse recognizes exaggerated grief in the person who:
    1. Has an active period of mourning that does not decrease and continues over time
    2. Postpones or holds back grieving and responds much later to the event
    3. Cannot function and is overwhelmed, with resulting substance abuse or phobias
    4. Is not aware that behaviors are interfering with daily activities, such as sleeping and eating

23. A nurse manager observes a new staff nurse performing care of the body after death. Which one of the following interventions requires correction and further instruction?
    1. The patient's remaining personal items are discarded.
    2. The family is allowed time alone with the deceased.
    3. Dentures are left in the patient's mouth.
    4. The patient's eyes are closed.

STUDY GROUP QUESTIONS

- What are loss and grief?
- What are the different types of loss and possible reactions to these losses?
- What are the differences and similarities between the theories of grief and loss?
- What is anticipatory grief?
- How may the grieving process be influenced by special circumstances?
- How are hope, spirituality, and self-concept related to loss and grieving?
- What behaviors are associated with loss and grieving?
- What resources are available for patient, family, and nurse that assist in the grieving process?
- What principles facilitate mourning?
- How may a nurse apply critical thinking and nursing processes to the patient/family experiencing loss and grieving?
- How are religious and cultural beliefs associated with loss, grief, death, and dying?
- How may a nurse intervene to assist a patient/family with loss and the grieving process?
- What is involved in care of the body after death?

Answers available through your instructor.

Exercise and Activity 26

CASE STUDY

1. A nurse is assigned to work with an 80-year-old woman residing in a nursing home. There is conflicting information in the chart about her ability to move around independently. The nurse is concerned about meeting her needs for proper body mechanics as well as her safety.
    a. What important assessment information is needed to plan meeting the patient's needs?
    b. If the patient is unable to ambulate independently, what nursing interventions should be planned?

CHAPTER REVIEW

Match the description/definition in Column A with the correct term in Column B.

Column A
____ 1. Awareness of the position of the body and its parts
____ 2. Resistance that moving body meets from the surface on which it moves
____ 3. Manner or style of walking
____ 4. Lying face up
____ 5. Lying face down
____ 6. Movement of the foot where the toes point upward
____ 7. Maintenance of optimal body position
____ 8. Body alignment during walking, turning, lifting, or carrying
____ 9. Mobility of the joint

Column B
a. Body mechanics
b. Prone
c. Range of motion
d. Posture
e. Dorsiflexion
f. Supine
g. Friction
h. Gait
i. Proprioception

Complete the following:

10. The three components to assess for a patient's mobility are:

11. Which of the following are correct principles of body mechanics? Select all that apply.
    a. Maintain a narrow base of support. ____
    b. Face the direction of movement. ____
    c. Maintain a higher center of gravity. ____
    d. Divide balanced activity between the arms and legs. ____
    e. Increase friction between the object and surface. ____
    f. Alternate periods of rest and activity. ____

12. The best way to determine a patient's level of pain is to observe for redness or swelling of the joints.
    True ____ False ____

13. Before ambulating a patient who has been in bed, the nurse should prepare the patient by:

14. Identify at least two pathological influences on alignment, exercise or activity.

15. Range of motion can be determined by observing the patient's gait and ability to perform activities of daily living.
    True ____ False ____

16. An example of a physiological factor that may influence activity tolerance is:

17. Identify a nursing diagnosis associated with a change in a patient's ability to maintain physical activity.

Copyright © 2011, 2007, 2003 by Mosby, Inc., an affiliate of Elsevier Inc. All rights reserved.

CHAPTER 26 • Exercise and Activity

18. For a patient who has severe arthritis and is unable to perform activities of daily living because of discomfort on movement, the priority is to:

19. A patient with a respiratory condition should be positioned in:

20. Complete the following about transferring patients.
    a. The general "rule of thumb" for transfers is:

    b. A nurse's priority during patient transfers is:

21. Identify the following patient positions:

    a. _____

    b. _____

    c. _____

22. Which of the following are expected findings for assessment of a patient while standing? Select all that apply.
    a. Head is erect and midline. _____
    b. Body parts are asymmetrical. _____
    c. The spine has a lateral curve. _____
    d. The abdomen protrudes. _____
    e. The knees are in a straight line between the hips and ankles. _____
    f. The feet are pointed at an angle and close together. _____
    g. The arms hang comfortably at the sides. _____

23. Which of the following indicate correct care or technique for a patient who is using crutches? Select all that apply.
    a. The patient leans on the axillae to support his or her weight. _____
    b. The rubber tips are cracked and worn. _____
    c. Crutches are placed 1 foot to the front and side of the feet. _____
    d. The patient has a non–weight-bearing left leg and is using a three-point gait. _____
    e. The unaffected leg is advanced first when the patient goes up the stairs. _____

24. Patients who are on prolonged bed rest need to be repositioned at least every _____ hours.

25. When transferring patients who are able to assist from the bed to a chair, the chair should be positioned:

26. Logrolling a patient in bed requires at least _____ caregivers to perform.

27. A nurse observes a patient and notes that there is limited range of motion in a few areas. This could be the result of:

Select the best answer for each of the following questions:

28. A patient is able to bear weight on one foot. The crutch walking gait that the nurse teaches this patient is the:
    1. Two-point gait
    2. Swing-through gait
    3. Three-point alternating gait
    4. Four-point alternating gait

29. A nurse is working with a patient who is able only to minimally assist the nurse in moving from the bed to the chair. The nurse needs to help the patient stand. The correct technique for lifting the patient to stand and pivot to the chair is to:
    1. Keep the legs straight
    2. Maintain a wide base with the feet
    3. Keep the stomach muscles loose
    4. Support the patient away from the body

30. A nurse is assisting a patient who has been prescribed total bed rest to perform range-of-motion exercises. The nurse performs the exercises by:
    1. Hyperextending the joints
    2. Working from proximal to distal joints
    3. Flexing the joints beyond where slight resistance is felt
    4. Providing support for joints distal to the joint being exercised

31. A patient has experienced an injury to his lower extremity. The orthopedist has prescribed the use of crutches and a four-point gait. The nurse instructs the patient using this gait to:
    1. Move the right foot forward first
    2. Move both crutches forward together
    3. Move the right foot and the left crutch together
    4. Move the right foot and the right crutch together

Copyright © 2011, 2007, 2003 by Mosby, Inc., an affiliate of Elsevier Inc. All rights reserved.

32. The patient had a cerebrovascular accident (CVA/stroke) with resultant left hemiparesis. The nurse is instructing the patient on the use of a cane for support during ambulation. The nurse instructs the patient to:
    1. Use the cane on the right side
    2. Use the cane on the left side
    3. Move the left foot forward first
    4. Move the right foot forward first

33. A patient is admitted to the rehabilitation facility for physical therapy after an automobile accident. To conduct an assessment of the patient's body alignment, the nurse should begin by:
    1. Observing the patient's gait
    2. Putting the patient at ease
    3. Determining the level of activity tolerance
    4. Evaluating the full extent of joint range of motion

34. An average-size female patient who resides in the extended care facility requires assistance to ambulate down the hall. The nurse has noticed that the patient has some weakness on her right side. The nurse assists this patient to ambulate by:
    1. Standing at her left side and holding the patient's arm
    2. Walking in front of her and having her hold onto her waist
    3. Standing behind her and encircling one arm around the patient's waist
    4. Standing at her right side and using a gait belt

35. A patient has a cast on the right foot and is being discharged home. Crutches will be used for ambulation, and the patient has stairs to manage to enter the house and to get to the bedroom and bathroom. The nurse observes the patient using the correct technique in using the crutches on the stairs when the patient:
    1. Advances the crutches first to ascend the stairs
    2. Uses one crutch for support while going up and down
    3. Uses the banister or wall for support when descending the stairs
    4. Advances the affected leg after moving the crutches when descending the stairs

36. A patient is getting up to ambulate for the first time since a surgical procedure. While ambulating in the hallway, the patient complains of severe dizziness. The nurse should first:
    1. Call for help
    2. Lower the patient gently to the floor
    3. Lean the patient against the wall until the episode passes
    4. Support the patient and move quickly back to the room

37. One of the expected benefits of exercise is:
    1. Decreased diaphragmatic excursion
    2. Decreased cardiac output
    3. Increased fatigue
    4. Decreased resting heart rate

38. A nurse selects which of the following for maintaining dorsiflexion of a patient?
    1. Pillows
    2. Foot boots
    3. Bed boards
    4. Trochanter rolls

39. A nurse recognizes that the position that is contraindicated for a patient who is at risk for aspiration is:
    1. Fowler's
    2. Lateral
    3. Sims'
    4. Supine

40. A patient had total hip replacement surgery and requires careful postoperative positioning to maintain the legs in abduction. The nurse will obtain a:
    1. Foot boot
    2. Trapeze bar
    3. Bed board
    4. Wedge pillow

STUDY GROUP QUESTIONS

- What are body mechanics?
- How is body movement regulated by the musculoskeletal and nervous systems?
- What general changes occur in the body's appearance and function throughout growth and development?
- How can body mechanics be influenced by pathological conditions?
- What patient assessment data should be obtained regarding body mechanics?
- What is activity tolerance?
- How can proper body mechanics be promoted for patients in different health care settings?
- What safety measures should be implemented before patient transfers and ambulation?
- What are the proper procedures for range-of-motion exercises, transfers, positioning, and ambulation?
- How should a patient be instructed to use assistive devices, such as canes, walkers, and crutches?

STUDY CHART

Create a study chart to describe how to *Safely Use Assistive Devices for Ambulation* that identifies the nursing actions and patient instruction required to reduce possible hazards for the following devices: gait belt, cane, walker, crutches.

Answers available through your instructor.

CHAPTER 26 • Exercise and Activity

Name _____ Date _____ Instructor's Name _____

Performance Checklist Skill 26-1: Moving and Positioning Patients in Bed

	S	U	NP	Comments

Assessment

1. Assess patient's body alignment and comfort level while patient is lying down.
2. Assess for risk factors that may contribute to complications of immobility.
3. Assess patient's physical ability to help with moving and positioning.
4. Assess health care provider's orders. Clarify whether patient's condition contraindicates any positions.
5. Assess for tubes, incisions, and equipment.
6. Assess ability and motivation of patient, family members, and primary caregiver to participate in moving and positioning patient in bed in anticipation of discharge to home.

Planning

1. Collect appropriate equipment. Get extra help as needed.
2. Perform hand hygiene.
3. Correctly identify patient and explain procedure.
4. Raise bed to comfortable working height.
5. Position patient flat in bed, if tolerated.
6. Keep patient aligned.

Implementation

1. Position patient in bed.
   A. **Assist Patient in Moving Toward Head of Bed (Two Nurses)**
      (1) Remove pillow from under head and shoulders, and place pillow at head of bed.
      (2) Face head of bed.
      (3) Each nurse should have one arm under patient's shoulders and one arm under patient's thighs.
      (4) Alternative position: position one nurse at patient's upper body. Nurse's arm nearest head of bed should be under patient's head and opposite shoulder; other arm should be under patient's closest arm and shoulder. Position other nurse at patient's lower torso. The nurse's arms should be under patient's lower back and torso.
      (5) Place feet apart, with foot nearest head of bed behind other foot (forward-backward stance).
      (6) Before moving patient, ask patient to flex knees with feet flat on bed.
      (7) Instruct patient to flex neck, tilting chin toward chest.
      (8) Have patient assist moving by pushing with feet on bed surface.
      (9) Flex knees and hips, bringing forearms closer to level of bed.

	S	U	NP	Comments

 (10) Instruct patient on count of three to push with heels and elevate trunk while breathing out, thus moving toward head of bed. ____ ____ ____ _____

 (11) On count of three, rock and shift weight from front to back leg. At the same time, patient pushes with heels and elevates trunk. ____ ____ ____ _____

B. Move Immobile Patient Toward Head of Bed With Drawsheet (Two Nurses)

 (1) Place drawsheet under patient by turning side to side. Extend sheet from shoulders to thighs. Return patient to supine position. ____ ____ ____ _____

 (2) Position one nurse at each side of patient's hips. ____ ____ ____ _____

 (3) Grasp drawsheet firmly near the patient. ____ ____ ____ _____

 (4) Place feet apart with forward-backward stance. Flex knees and hips. Shift weight from front to back leg, and move patient and drawsheet to desired position in bed. ____ ____ ____ _____

 (5) Realign patient in correct body alignment. ____ ____ ____ _____

C. Position Patient in Supported Fowler's Position

 (1) Elevate head of bed 45 to 60 degrees. ____ ____ ____ _____

 (2) Rest head against mattress or on small pillow. ____ ____ ____ _____

 (3) Use pillows to support arms and hands if patient does not have voluntary control or use of hands and arms. ____ ____ ____ _____

 (4) Position pillow at lower back. ____ ____ ____ _____

 (5) Place small pillow or roll under thigh. ____ ____ ____ _____

 (6) Place small pillow or roll under ankles. ____ ____ ____ _____

D. Position Hemiplegic Patient in Supported Fowler's Position

 (1) Elevate head of bed 45 to 60 degrees. ____ ____ ____ _____

 (2) Position patient in sitting position as straight as possible. ____ ____ ____ _____

 (3) Position head on small pillow with chin slightly forward. ____ ____ ____ _____

 (4) Flex knees and hips by using pillow or folded blanket under knees. ____ ____ ____ _____

 (5) Support feet in dorsiflexion with firm pillow or footboard. ____ ____ ____ _____

E. Position Patient in Supine Position

 (1) Be sure patient is comfortable on back with head of bed flat. ____ ____ ____ _____

 (2) Place small rolled towel under lumbar area of back. ____ ____ ____ _____

 (3) Place pillow under upper shoulders, neck, or head. ____ ____ ____ _____

 (4) Place trochanter rolls or sandbags parallel to lateral surface of patient's thighs. ____ ____ ____ _____

 (5) Place small pillow or roll under ankle to elevate heels. ____ ____ ____ _____

144 CHAPTER 26 • Exercise and Activity

		S	U	NP	Comments
(6)	Place footboard or firm pillows against bottom of patient's feet.	___	___	___	_____
(7)	Place pillows under pronated forearms, keeping upper arms parallel to patient's body.	___	___	___	_____
(8)	Place hand rolls in patient's hands.	___	___	___	_____

F. Position Hemiplegic Patient in Supine Position
  (1) Place head of bed flat.
  (2) Place folded towel or small pillow under shoulder or affected side.
  (3) Keep affected arm away from body with elbow extended and palm up. (Alternative is to place arm out to side, with elbow bent and hand toward head of bed.)
  (4) Place folded towel under hip of involved side.
  (5) Flex affected knee 30 degrees by supporting it on pillow or folded blanket.
  (6) Support feet with soft pillows at right angle to leg.

G. Position Patient in Prone Position
  (1) With patient supine, roll patient over arm positioned close to body, with elbow straight and hand under hip. Position on abdomen in center of bed.
  (2) Turn patient's head to one side and support head with small pillow.
  (3) Place small pillow under patient's abdomen below level of diaphragm.
  (4) Support arms in flexed position level at shoulders.
  (5) Support lower legs with pillow to elevate toes.

H. Position Hemiplegic Patient in Prone Position
  (1) With patient lying supine, move patient toward unaffected side.
  (2) Roll patient onto affected side.
  (3) Place pillow on patient's abdomen.
  (4) Roll patient onto abdomen by positioning involved arm close to patient's body, with elbow straight and hand under hip. Roll patient carefully over arm.
  (5) Turn head toward involved side.
  (6) Position involved arm out to side, with elbow bent, hand toward head of bed, and fingers extended (if possible).
  (7) Flex knees slightly by placing pillow under legs from knees to ankles.
  (8) Keep feet at right angle to legs by using pillow high enough to keep toes off mattress.

I. Position Patient in Lateral (Side-Lying) Position
  (1) Lower head of bed completely or as low as patient can tolerate.

Copyright © 2011, 2007, 2003 by Mosby, Inc., an affiliate of Elsevier Inc. All rights reserved.

	S	U	NP	Comments

    (2) Position patient to side of bed. Use mechanical lift if needed. ____ ____ ____ _____
    (3) Prepare to turn patient onto side. Flex patient's knee that will not be next to mattress. Place one hand on patient's hip and one hand on patient's shoulder. ____ ____ ____ _____
    (4) Roll patient onto side toward you.
    (5) Place pillow under patient's head and neck.
    (6) Bring shoulder blade forward.
    (7) Position both arms in slightly flexed position. Upper arm is supported by pillow level with shoulder.
    (8) Place tuck-back pillow behind patient's back. (Make by folding pillow lengthwise. Smooth area is slightly tucked under patient's back.)
    (9) Place pillow under semiflexed upper leg level at hip from groin to foot.
    (10) Place sandbag parallel to plantar surface of dependent foot.

J. Position Patient in Sims' (Semiprone) Position
    (1) Lower head of bed completely.
    (2) Be sure patient is comfortable in supine position.
    (3) Position patient to one side of bed, then roll over one arm positioned close to body. Roll patient to lateral position, lying partially on abdomen. Position dependent arm out from body.
    (4) Place small pillow under patient's head.
    (5) Place pillow under flexed upper arm, supporting arm level with shoulder.
    (6) Place pillow under flexed upper legs, supporting leg level with hip.
    (7) Place sandbags parallel to plantar surface of foot.

K. Logrolling the Patient (Three Nurses)
    (1) Place small pillow between patient's knees.
    (2) Cross patient's arms on chest.
    (3) Position two nurses on side of bed to which the patient will be turned. Position third nurse on the other side of bed.
    (4) Fanfold or roll the drawsheet.
    (5) Move the patient as one unit in a smooth, continuous motion on the count of three.
    (6) Nurse on the opposite side of the bed places pillows along the length of the patient.
    (7) Gently lean the patient as a unit back toward the pillows for support.

2. Perform hand hygiene.

	S	U	NP	Comments

Evaluation
1. Evaluate patient's body alignment, position, and comfort.
2. Measure range of motion.
3. Observe skin for areas of erythema or breakdown.
4. Record each position change, including frequency, amount of assistance needed, and patient's response and tolerance.
5. Record and report any signs of redness in areas such as over bony prominences.

CHAPTER 26 • Exercise and Activity   147

Name_____   Date_____   Instructor's Name_____

Performance Checklist Skill 26-2: Using Safe and Effective Transfer Techniques

	S	U	NP	Comments

Assessment
1. Assess patient's physiologic capacity to transfer.
2. Assess patient's sensory status.
3. Assess patient's cognitive status.
4. Assess patient's level of motivation.
5. Assess previous mode of transfer (if applicable).
6. Assess patient's specific risk for falling or being injured when transferred.
7. Assess special transfer equipment needed for home setting. Assess home environment for hazards.

Planning
1. Gather appropriate equipment.
2. Determine number of people needed to assist with transfer.
3. Perform hand hygiene. Verify that bed's brakes are locked.
4. Explain procedure to patient.

Implementation
1. Transfer patient.
   A. **Assist Cooperative Patient to Sitting Position Bed in Bed**
      (1) Raise bed to waist level. Place patient in supine position.
      (2) Face head of bed at a 45-degree angle, and remove pillows.
      (3) Position feet apart with foot closest to bed in front of other foot.
      (4) Place hand nearer to patient under shoulders, supporting patient's head and cervical vertebrae.
      (5) Place other hand on bed surface.
      (6) Raise patient to sitting position by shifting weight from front to back leg.
      (7) Push against bed using arm that is placed on bed surface.
   B. **Assist Cooperative Patient Who Can Partially Bear Weight to Sitting Position on Side of Bed**
      (1) With bed flat and at waist level, turn patient to side, facing you on side of bed on which patient will be sitting.
      (2) Raise head of bed 30 degrees.
      (3) Stand opposite patient's hips. Turn diagonally so you face the patient and far corner of the foot of bed.
      (4) Place feet apart with foot closer to bed in front of other foot.
      (5) Place arm nearer head of bed under patient's shoulders, supporting head and neck.
      (6) Place other arm over patient's thighs.

Copyright © 2011, 2007, 2003 by Mosby, Inc., an affiliate of Elsevier Inc. All rights reserved.

	S	U	NP	Comments

(7) Move patient's lower legs and feet over side of bed. Pivot toward rear leg, allowing patient's upper legs to swing downward.

(8) At same time, shift weight to rear leg and elevate patient.

(9) Remain in front until patient regains balance, and continue to provide physical support to weak or cognitively impaired patient.

C. **Transferring Cooperative Patient Who Is Partially Weight Bearing From Bed to Chair**

(1) Assist patient to sitting position on side of bed. Have chair in position at 45-degree angle to bed on patient's strong side.

(2) Apply transfer belt or other transfer aids.

(3) Ensure that patient has stable nonskid shoes. Place weight-bearing or strong leg forward, with weak foot back.

(4) Spread your feet apart.

(5) Flex hips and knees, aligning knees with patient's knees.

(6) Grasp transfer belt from underneath along patient's sides.

(7) Rock patient up to standing position on count of three while straightening hips and legs and keeping knees slightly flexed. Unless contraindicated, patient may be instructed to use hands to push up if applicable.

(8) Maintain stability of patient's weak or paralyzed leg with knee.

(9) Pivot on foot farther from chair.

(10) Instruct patient to use armrests on chair for support and ease into chair.

(11) Flex hips and knees while lowering patient into chair.

(12) Assess patient for proper alignment for sitting position. Provide support for paralyzed extremities. Lapboard or sling will support flaccid arm. Stabilize leg with bath blanket or pillow.

(13) Praise patient's progress, effort, or performance.

D. **Use Mechanical Lift and Full Body Sling to Transfer Uncooperative Patient Who Can Bear Partial Weight or Patient Who Cannot Bear Weight and is Either Uncooperative or Does Not Have Upper Body Strength to Move From From Bed to Chair**

(1) Position lift properly at bedside.

(2) Position chair near bed, and allow adequate space to maneuver lift.

(3) Raise bed to high position with mattress flat. Lower side rail.

(4) Keep bed side rail up on side opposite to you.

(5) Roll patient away from you.

	S	U	NP	Comments

(6) Place sling under patient. Place lower edge under patient's knees (wide edge), and upper edge fits under patient's shoulders (narrow piece).

(7) Roll patient to opposite side towards you and pull body sling through.

(8) Roll patient supine onto canvas seat.

(9) Remove patient's glasses, if appropriate.

(10) If using a transportable Hoyer lift, place lift's horseshoe bar under side of bed (on side with chair).

(11) Lower horizontal bar to sling following manufacturer's directions. Some lifts require valve to be locked.

(12) Attach hooks on strap to holes in sling. Short straps hook to top holes of sling; longer straps hook to bottom of sling.

(13) Elevate head of bed.

(14) Fold patient's arms over chest.

(15) Use lift to raise patient.

(16) Use steering handle to pull lift from bed and maneuver to chair.

(17) Move lift to chair.

(18) Position patient and lower slowly into chair.

(19) Remove straps and hydraulic lift.

(20) Check patient's sitting alignment and correct if necessary.

2. Perform hand hygiene.

E. **Transfer Patient From Bed to Stretcher (Bed at Stretcher Level)**

(1) Place bed flat, and position at same level as stretcher. Ensure bed brakes are locked. Cross patient's arms on chest.

(2) Lower side rails. Two caregivers stand on the side where the stretcher will be while third caregiver stands on the other side.

(3) Two caregivers help patient roll onto side toward them (use of drawsheet is optional) with a smooth, continuous motion.

(4) Place slide board under drawsheet or follow manufacturer's guidelines (see illustrations). Gently roll patient back onto the slide board.

(5) Roll stretcher alongside the bed. Lock wheels of stretcher once it is in place. Instruct the patient not to move.

(6) All three caregivers place feet widely apart with one slightly in front of the other, and grasp the friction-reducing device.

(7) On the count of three, the two caregivers pull the drawsheet or patient from the bed onto the stretcher while the third person holds the slide board in place. Using the friction-reducing device, shift weight from front foot to back foot. Position patient in center of stretcher.

CHAPTER 26 • Exercise and Activity

	S	U	NP	Comments
(8) Put up side rail of stretcher on side where caregivers are, then roll stretcher away from bed and put side rail up on that side. Cover patient with sheet or blanket.	___	___	___	_____
(9) Perform hand hygiene.	___	___	___	_____
(10) Evaluate patient's body alignment.	___	___	___	_____

Evaluation

1. Evaluate vital signs. Ask if patient feels fatigued.
2. Observe for correct body alignment and presence of pressure points on skin.
3. Ask if patient experienced pain.
4. Record each transfer and position change and patient's response.
5. Report patient progress and any unusual occurrence to nurse in charge.

Safety 27

CASE STUDIES

1. You will be accompanying the visiting nurse to the home of a family with two young children who are ages 2 and 4 years.
   a. What general assessment information should be obtained regarding home safety during the visit?
   b. What specific safety observations should be made because there are two young children residing in the home?
2. A patient with diabetes mellitus is living at home and needs to take daily insulin injections.
   a. What are some of the precautions that this patient should take to avoid pathogen transmission and for safety?
3. You are currently working in a long-term care facility. There are a number of patients who are recognized as being at risk for falls. A restraint-free environment is desired.
   a. What specific interventions may be implemented to prevent falls and provide for patient safety without the use of restraints?

CHAPTER REVIEW

Complete the following:

1. Identify an example of a problem that may be encountered if a basic human need of a safe environment is not met.

2. Identify an example of a possible physical hazard that may be found in the home.

3. Older adults are predisposed to accidents as a result of:

4. For each of the following, identify a nursing intervention that may be implemented to prevent injury and promote patient safety.
   a. Falls:
   b. Patient-inherent accidents:
   c. Procedure-related risks:
   d. Equipment-related risks:

5. List the eight conditions identified as preventable in the Deficit Reduction Act (2005).

6. Immunity that occurs as a result of injection of weakened or dead organisms and modified toxins is called:

7. For each of the following age-groups, identify an example of a potential hazard.

   a. Infant, toddler, preschooler:
   b. School age child:
   c. Adolescent:
   d. Adult:
   e. Older adult:

8. During an assessment, a nurse determines that a patient with a high risk for injury is an individual experiencing:

9. For each of the following potential bioterrorist methods, identify a possible agent that may be used.
   a. Biological:
   b. Chemical:
   c. Radiological:

10. There is a greater risk for poisoning as a result of finding multiple medications in the home of an older adult.
    True _____ False _____

11. An example of safety instruction for a school age child would be:

12. The primary goal when using restraints (safety reminder devices) is to:

13. When using restraints, nursing homes are required to:

CHAPTER 27 • Safety

14. Side rails may be used at any time to keep a patient in bed.
    True _____ False _____
15. An older adult patient who often forgets to take medication or does not remember if it was taken may benefit from a(n):

16. Identify an example of a medication safety strategy that is used in a health care agency.

17. For the following areas, identify a specific environmental adjustment that should be made to promote safety.
    a. Tactile deficit:

    b. Visual deficit:

18. Identify an example of an intervention that may be implemented as an alternative to patient restraint.

19. An example of a nursing diagnosis associated with patient safety concerns is:

Select the best answer for each of the following questions:

20. To prevent sudden infant death syndrome (SIDS), a nurse instructs parents to:
    1. Use proper infant car seats
    2. Remove poisonous substances from the home
    3. Have the child immunized as recommended
    4. Place the infant on the back or side to sleep
21. An older adult patient is being discharged home. The patient will be taking furosemide (Lasix) on a daily basis. A specific consideration for this patient is:
    1. Exposure to the sun
    2. Food consumption when taking take the medication
    3. The location of the bathroom
    4. Financial considerations for long-term care
22. While walking through a hallway in the extended care facility, a nurse notices smoke coming from a wastebasket in a patient's room. Upon closer investigation, the nurse identifies that there is a fire that is starting to flare up. The nurse should first:
    1. Extinguish the fire
    2. Remove the patient from the room
    3. Contain the fire by closing the door to the room
    4. Turn off all of the surrounding electrical equipment
23. A patient is newly admitted to the hospital and appears to be disoriented. There is a concern for the patient's immediate safety. The nurse is considering the use of restraints to prevent an injury. The nurse recognizes that the use of restraints in a hospital requires:
    1. A physician's order
    2. The patient's consent
    3. A family member's consent
    4. Agreement among the nursing staff
24. A nurse is completing admission histories for newly admitted patients to the unit. The nurse is aware that the patient with the greatest risk of injury:
    1. Is 84 years of age
    2. Uses corrective lenses
    3. Has a history of falls
    4. Has arthritis in the lower extremities
25. A child has ingested a poisonous substance. The parent is instructed by the nurse to:
    1. Take the child to the hospital immediately
    2. Call the poison control center
    3. Take the child to the pediatrician
    4. Administer 30 mL of emetic
26. Using the Morse Fall Scale, a nurse identifies what score for the patient with no history of falls, the presence of a secondary diagnosis, use of a walker for ambulation with a weak gait, and awareness of his own limitations.
    1. 25
    2. 30
    3. 40
    4. 55
27. A restraint that may be used to prevent an adult patient from pulling on and removing tubes or an IV is a(n):
    1. Vest restraint
    2. Jacket restraint
    3. Extremity restraint
    4. Mummy restraint
28. An older adult patient in the extended care facility has been wandering outside of the room during the late evening hours. The patient has a history of falls. The nurse intervenes initially by:
    1. Placing an abdominal restraint on the patient during the night
    2. Keeping both the light and the television on in the patient's room all night
    3. Reassigning the patient to a room close to the nursing station
    4. Having the family members check on the patient during the night
29. A parent with three children has gone to the outpatient clinic. The children range in age from 2½ to 15 years old. A nurse is discussing safety issues with the parent. The nurse evaluates that further teaching is required if the parent states:
    1. "I have spoken to my teenager about safe sex practices."
    2. "I make sure that my child wears a helmet when he rides his bicycle."

3. "My 8-year-old is taking swimming classes at the local community center."
4. "Now my 2½-year-old can finally sit in the front seat of the car with me."

30. A viral disease that is spread through contaminated food or water is:
    1. Shigella
    2. *E. coli*
    3. Listeria
    4. Hepatitis A

STUDY GROUP QUESTIONS

- What are the basic human needs regarding safety?
- What are some physical hazards and how can they be reduced or eliminated?
- What developmental changes and abilities predispose individuals to accidents or injury?
- What additional risk factors may affect an individual's level of safety?
- What risks exist in a health care agency, and how can they be prevented?
- What safety measures and patient teaching should be implemented in different health care settings?
- What are the procedures for the correct use of side rails and restraints?
- How can a nurse avoid the use of patient restraints?
- What assessment information should be obtained regarding patient/family safety?
- How can a nurse assist patients and families in reducing or eliminating safety hazards?

Answers available through your instructor.

Name _____ Date _____ Instructor's Name _____

Performance Checklist Skill 27-1: Applying Physical Restraints

	S	U	NP	Comments

Assessment
1. Assess if the patient needs a restraint.
2. Assess patient's behavior, such as confusion, disorientation, agitation, restlessness, combativeness, or inability to follow directions.
3. Review agency policies regarding restraints. Check physician's order for purpose and type of restraint, location and duration of restraint. Determine if signed consent for use of restraint is needed.

Planning
1. Review manufacturer's instructions for restraint application before entering patient's room.
2. Perform hand hygiene and collect equipment.
3. Approach patient in a calm, confident manner and explain what you plan to do. Correctly identify patient using two identifiers according to agency policy.
4. Introduce self to patient and family and assess their feelings about restraint use. Explain that restraint is temporary and designed to protect patient from injury.
5. Inspect area where restraint is to be placed. Assess condition of skin underlying area on which restraint is to be applied.

Implementation
1. Provide privacy. Position and drape patient as needed.
2. Adjust bed to proper height and lower side rail on side of patient contact.
3. Be sure patient is comfortable and in correct anatomical position.
4. Pad skin and bony prominences, if necessary, that will be under the restraint.
5. Apply proper-size selected restraint:
   Always refer to manufacturer's directions.
   a. **Belt restraint:** Have patient in a sitting position. Apply over clothes, gown, or pajamas. Remove wrinkles or creases from front and back of restraint while placing it around patient's waist. Bring ties through slots in belt. Help patient lie down if in bed. Avoid applying belt too tightly.
   b. **Extremity (ankle or wrist) restraint:** This restraint is designed to immobilize one or all extremities. Wrap limb restraint around wrist or ankle with soft part toward skin and secured snugly in place by Velcro straps.
   c. **Mitten restraint:** Thumb-less mitten device that restrains patient's hands. Place hand in mitten, being sure Velcro strap is around the wrist and not the forearm.
6. Attach restraint straps to portion of bed frame that moves when head of bed is raised or lowered. **Do not attach to side rails.**
7. Secure restraints with a quick-release tie. Do not tie in a knot.

Copyright © 2011, 2007, 2003 by Mosby, Inc., an affiliate of Elsevier Inc. All rights reserved.

	S	U	NP	Comments

8. Insert two fingers under secured restraint.
9. Assess proper placement of restraint, skin integrity, pulses, temperature, color, and sensation of the restrained body part.
10. Remove restraints **at least every 2 hours** or more frequently as determined by agency policy (JCAHO, 2007). If patient is violent or noncompliant, remove one restraint at a time and/or have additional staff assistance while removing restraints.
11. Secure call light or intercom system within reach.
12. Leave bed or chair with wheels locked. Make sure bed is in the lowest position.
13. Perform hand hygiene.

Evaluation

1. Inspect patient every 15 minutes for any injury, including all hazards of immobility, while restraints are in use.
2. Observe IV lines, urinary catheters, and drainage tubes to determine that they are positioned correctly.
3. The physician, health care provider, or registered nurse needs to evaluate the patient within 1 or 4 hours after initiation of restraint, depending on agency policy, to reevaluate need for continued restraints.
4. Reassess patient's need for continued use of restraints at least every 24 hours.
5. Provide appropriate sensory stimulation and reorients patient as needed.
6. Document patient's response and expected or unexpected outcomes after restraint is applied.

CHAPTER 27 • Safety

Name _____ Date _____ Instructor's Name_____

Procedural Guidelines 27-1: Intervening in Accidental Poisoning

	S	U	NP	Comments
1. Assess for signs or symptoms of accidental ingestion of harmful substances; symptoms may include nausea, vomiting, foaming at the mouth, drooling, difficulty breathing, sweating, lethargy.	___	___	___	_____
2. Terminate the toxic exposure by emptying the mouth of pills, plant parts, or other material.	___	___	___	_____
3. If poisoning is due to skin or eye contact, irrigate the skin or eye with copious amounts of tap water for 15 to 20 minutes. In the case of an inhalation exposure, safely remove the victim from the potentially dangerous environment.	___	___	___	_____
4. Identify the type and amount of substance ingested to help determine the correct type and amount of antidote needed.	___	___	___	_____
5. **If the victim is conscious and alert, call the local poison control center or the national toll-free poison control center number (1-800-222-1222) before attempting any intervention.**	___	___	___	_____
6. If the victim has collapsed or stopped breathing, call 9-1-1 for emergency transportation to the hospital. Initiate CPR if indicated. Ambulance personnel will be able to provide emergency measures if needed.	___	___	___	_____
7. Position victim with head turned to side to reduce risk of aspiration.	___	___	___	_____
8. Never induce vomiting if the victim has ingested poisonous substances such as lye, household cleaners, hair care products, grease or petroleum products, furniture polish, paint thinner, or kerosene.	___	___	___	_____
9. Never induce vomiting in an unconscious or convulsing victim.	___	___	___	_____

Hygiene 28

CASE STUDIES

1. Your clinical experience is scheduled to be on a medical unit. It will be your responsibility to provide instruction to a patient who has just been diagnosed with diabetes mellitus.
    a. What specific information on hygienic care will be included for the patient's teaching session?
2. An older adult patient residing in an extended care facility requires assistance with hygienic care.
    a. What developmental changes are considered when assisting this patient to meet hygienic needs?

CHAPTER REVIEW

Match the description/definition in Column A with the correct term in Column B.

Column A

_____ 1. Inflammation of the skin characterized by abrupt onset with erythema, pruritus, pain, and scaly oozing lesions
_____ 2. Thickened portion of the epidermis, usually flat and painless, on the undersurface of the foot or hand
_____ 3. Inflammation of the tissue surrounding the nail
_____ 4. Scraping or rubbing away of the epidermis, resulting in localized bleeding
_____ 5. Keratosis caused by friction and pressure from shoes, mainly on toes
_____ 6. Fungating lesion that appears on the sole of the foot
_____ 7. Loss of hair

Column B

a. Abrasion
b. Callus
c. Plantar wart
d. Paronychia
e. Contact dermatitis
f. Corn
g. Alopecia

Complete the following:

8. Which of the following techniques are appropriate for diabetic foot care? Select all that apply.
    a. Soaking the feet _____
    b. Rubbing the feet vigorously to dry them _____
    c. Walking barefoot to toughen the feet _____
    d. Applying bland powder if the feet perspire _____
    e. Applying lanolin for dryness _____
    f. Wearing clean, white cotton socks _____
    g. Using a heating pad to warm the feet _____
    h. Applying a mild antiseptic to small cuts _____
    i. Avoiding elastic stockings _____
9. A nurse-initiated treatment for a skin rash is:

10. When cleansing a patient's eyes, the nurse should use:

11. The patient's eyeglasses should be kept:

12. Ear irrigation is contraindicated in the presence of:

13. Asepsis is maintained during linen changes by the nurse when:

14. Provide an example of how the nurse prepares a comfortable environment for the patient in the health care facility:

15. The best type of light to use to assess a patient's skin is:

16. Identify physiological conditions that may place a patient at risk for impaired skin integrity.

17. How does the use of a commercial "bag bath" differ from a regular patient bed bath?

18. Identify a safety measure that is implemented when providing a tub bath for a patient.

Copyright © 2011, 2007, 2003 by Mosby, Inc., an affiliate of Elsevier Inc. All rights reserved.

19. How may patients' cultural background influence their hygienic care practices?

20. A nurse notes that a young adult patient has acne of the face and back. What care should be provided?

21. Identify at least three guidelines for patient bathing and skin care.

22. What patients may require special oral hygiene?

23. Place the steps of the bed bath in the correct order:
    a. Back _____
    b. Arms _____
    c. Face _____
    d. Abdomen _____
    e. Legs _____
    f. Perineal area _____
    g. Chest _____

Select the best answer for each of the following questions:

24. A nurse is caring for an older adult patient in an extended care facility. The patient wears dentures, and the nurse delegated their care to the nursing assistant. The nurse instructs the assistant that the patient's dentures should be:
    1. Cleaned in hot water
    2. Left in place during the night
    3. Brushed with a soft toothbrush
    4. Wrapped in a soft towel when not worn

25. A nurse determines, after completing an assessment, that an expected outcome for a patient with impaired skin integrity will be that the:
    1. Skin remains dry
    2. Skin has increased erythema
    3. Skin tingles in areas of pressure
    4. Skin demonstrates increased diaphoresis

26. A patient has been hospitalized following a traumatic injury. The nurse is now able to provide hair care for the patient. The nurse includes:
    1. Using hot water to rinse the scalp
    2. Cutting away matted or tangled hair
    3. Using nails to massage the patient's scalp
    4. Applying peroxide to dissolve blood in the hair and then rinsing with saline

27. While completing a patient's bath, a nurse notices a red, raised skin rash on the patient's chest. The next step for the nurse to take is to:
    1. Moisturize the skin with lotion
    2. Wash the area again with hot water and soap
    3. Discuss proper hygienic care with the patient
    4. Assess for any other areas of inflammation

28. A nurse is planning patient assignment with a nursing assistant. In delegating the morning care for a patient, the nurse expects the assistant to:
    1. Cut the patient's nails with scissors
    2. Use soap to wash the patient's eyes
    3. Wash the patient's legs with long strokes from the ankle to the knee
    4. Place the unconscious patient in high-Fowler's position to provide oral hygiene

29. A patient is receiving chemotherapy and is experiencing stomatitis. To promote comfort for this patient, a nurse recommends that the patient use:
    1. A firm toothbrush
    2. Normal saline rinses
    3. A commercial mouthwash
    4. An alcohol and water mixture

30. For a patient with dry skin, a nurse should:
    1. Apply moisturizing lotion
    2. Use hot water for bathing
    3. Obtain a dehumidifier
    4. Wash the skin frequently

31. When integrating cultural considerations into hygienic care, a nurse recognizes that Hindu or Muslim patients:
    1. Consider the top part of the body cleaner
    2. Do not desire gender-congruent care
    3. Use the left hand for bathing
    4. Have no specific hygienic care practices

32. Use of an electric razor is specifically indicated for a patient who is being treated with:
    1. Diuretics
    2. Antibiotics
    3. Anticoagulants
    4. Narcotic analgesics

33. When making an occupied bed, the first step for a nurse is to:
    1. Cover the patient with a bath blanket
    2. Position the patient on the far side of the bed
    3. Explain the procedure to the patient
    4. Adjust the height of the bed to waist level

STUDY GROUP QUESTIONS

- What hygienic care measures are necessary for the integumentary system?
- What factors may influence a patient's hygienic care practices?
- How do growth and development influence hygienic care needs?
- What are the patient teaching needs for hygienic care across the life span?

- What assessments of the integumentary system are necessary to determine integumentary alterations and hygienic care needs?
- What are the correct procedures for providing hygienic care and a comfortable environment for patients?
- How does a patient's self-care ability influence the provision of hygienic care?
- How is physical assessment integrated into the provision of hygienic care?
- What actions should be taken if a patient refuses hygienic care?

Answers available through your instructor.

Name _____ Date _____ Instructor's Name _____

Performance Checklist Skill 28-1: Bathing and Perineal Care

	S	U	NP	Comments

Assessment

1. Assess patient's tolerance for bathing including activity tolerance, comfort level, cognitive ability, musculoskeletal function, and respiratory status.
2. Assess patient's visual status, ability to sit without support, hand grasp, ROM of extremities.
3. Assess for presence of equipment.
4. Assess patient's bathing preferences.
5. Ask if patient has noticed any problems related to condition of skin and genitalia.
6. Assess condition of patient's skin.
7. Identify risks for skin impairment.
8. Assess patient's knowledge of skin hygiene in terms of its importance, preventive measures to take, and common problems.

Planning

1. Check physician's or health care provider's therapeutic bath order for type of solution, length of time for bath, and body part to be treated.
2. Review orders for specific precautions concerning patient's movement or positioning.
3. Explain procedure and ask patient for suggestions on how to prepare supplies. If partial bath, ask how much of bath patient wishes to complete.
4. Adjust room temperature and ventilation, close room doors and windows, and draw room divider curtain.
5. Prepare equipment and supplies.

Implementation

1. **Complete or Partial Bed Bath**
   A. Offer patient bedpan or urinal. Provide towel and washcloth.
   B. Perform hand hygiene. Apply clean gloves. Note if patient has latex allergy.
   C. Place hospital bed at comfortable working height. Lower side rail closest to you, and assist patient in assuming comfortable supine position, maintaining body alignment. Bring patient toward side closest to you.
   D. Place bath blanket over patient, and then loosen and remove top covers without exposing patient. Place soiled linen in laundry bag being careful not to allow linen to touch uniform. If possible, have patient hold top of bath blanket.
   E. Remove patient's gown or pajamas. If an extremity is injured or has reduced mobility, begin removal from *unaffected* side. If patient has IV access, remove gown from arm *without* IV first. Then remove gown from arm with IV. Remove IV from pole, and slide IV tubing and bag through the arm of patient's gown. Rehang IV container and check flow rate. If IV pump is in use, turn pump off, clamp tubing, remove tubing from pump, and proceed as above. Reinsert tubing into pump, unclamp tubing, and turn pump on at correct rate. Observe flow rate and regulate if necessary. *Do not disconnect tubing.*
   F. Pull side rail up. Fill washbasin two-thirds full with warm water. Check water temperature, and have patient place fingers in water to test temperature tolerance. Place plastic container of bath lotion in bathwater to warm if desired.

CHAPTER 28 • Hygiene   161

	S	U	NP	Comments

G. Lower side rail, remove pillow, and raise head of bed 30 to 45 degrees if allowed. Place bath towel under patient's head. Place second bath towel over patient's chest.

H. Wash face.
   (1) Ask if patient is wearing contact lenses. If so, perform correct eye care.
   (2) Fold washcloth around fingers of your hand to form a mitt. Immerse mitt in water and wring thoroughly.
   (3) Wash patient's eyes with plain warm water. Use different section of mitt for each eye. Move mitt from inner to outer canthus. Soak any crusts on eyelid for 2 to 3 minutes with damp cloth before attempting removal. Dry around eyes gently and thoroughly.
   (4) Ask if patient prefers to use soap on face. Wash, rinse, and dry forehead, cheeks, nose, neck, and ears. (Men may wish to shave at this point or after bath.)
   (5) Provide eye care for an unconscious patient.

I. Wash trunk and upper extremities.
   (1) Remove bath blanket from patient's arm closest to you. Place bath towel lengthwise under arm. Bathe with minimal soap and water using long, firm strokes from distal to proximal (fingers to axilla).
   (2) Raise and support arm above head (if possible) to wash, rinse, and dry axilla thoroughly. Apply deodorant or powder to underarms if desired or needed.
   (3) Move to other side of bed and repeat steps (1) and (2) with other arm.
   (4) Cover patient's chest with bath towel and fold bath blanket down to umbilicus. Bathe chest using long, firm strokes. Take special care with skin under female's breasts, lifting breast upward, if necessary, using back of your hand. Rinse and dry well.

J. Wash hands and nails.
   (1) Fold bath towel in half and lay it on bed beside patient. Place basin on towel. Immerse patient's hand in water. Allow hand to soak for 2 to 3 minutes before washing hand and fingernails. Remove basin and dry hand well. Repeat for other hand.

K. Check temperature of bathwater and change if necessary.

L. Wash the abdomen.
   (1) Place bath towel lengthwise over chest and abdomen. (Two towels may be needed.) Fold bath blanket down to just above pubic region. Bathe, rinse, and dry abdomen with special attention to umbilicus and skinfolds of abdomen and groin. Keep abdomen covered between washing and rinsing. Dry well.
   (2) Apply clean gown or pajama top.

M. Wash the lower extremities.
   (1) Cover chest and abdomen with top of bath blanket. Cover legs with bottom of blanket. Expose near leg by folding blanket toward midline. Be sure to drape perineum with blanket.
   (2) Place bath towel under leg, supporting leg at knee and ankle. If appropriate, place patient's foot in the bath basin to soak while washing and rinsing. (Bend patient's leg at knee, and while grasping patient's heel, elevate leg from mattress slightly and place bath basin on towel.) If patient is unable to support leg, cleansing can simply be done by washing feet thoroughly with washcloth.

Copyright © 2011, 2007, 2003 by Mosby, Inc., an affiliate of Elsevier Inc. All rights reserved.

CHAPTER 28 • Hygiene

		S	U	NP	Comments

- (3) Wash leg using long, firm strokes from ankle to knee, then knee to thigh. Do not rub or massage the back of the calf. Dry well. Wash between the toes of foot. Cleanse foot, making sure to bathe between toes. Clean and clip nails as needed. Dry toes and feet completely. Remove and discard towel.
- (4) Raise side rail, move to opposite side of bed, lower side rail, and repeat steps (2) and (3) for other leg and foot.

N. Raise side rail for patient's safety, remove contaminated gloves, and change bathwater.

O. Provide perineal hygiene.
- (1) If patient is able to maneuver and handle washcloth, allow to cleanse perineum on own.
- (2) Female patient
  - (a) Apply new pair of disposable gloves. Lower side rail. Assist patient in assuming dorsal recumbent position. Note restrictions or limitations in patient's positioning. Be sure waterproof pad is positioned under patient's buttocks. Drape patient with bath blanket placed in the shape of a diamond. Lift lower edge of bath blanket to expose perineum.
  - (b) Fold lower corner of bath blanket up between patient's legs onto abdomen. Wash and dry patient's upper thighs.
  - (c) Wash labia majora. Use nondominant hand to gently retract labia from thigh: with dominant hand, wash carefully in skinfolds. Wipe in direction from perineum to rectum. Repeat on opposite side using separate section of washcloth. Rinse and dry area thoroughly.
  - (d) Gently separate labia with nondominant hand to expose urethral meatus and vaginal orifice. With dominant hand, wash downward from pubic area toward rectum in one smooth stroke the middle and both sides of the perineum. Use separate section of cloth for each stroke. Cleanse thoroughly around labia minora, clitoris, and vaginal orifice. Avoid placing tension on indwelling catheter if present, and clean area around it thoroughly.
  - (e) Provide catheter care as needed.
  - (f) Rinse area thoroughly. If patient uses bedpan, pour warm water over perineal area. Dry thoroughly, using front to back method.
  - (g) Fold lower corner of bath blanket back between patient's legs and over perineum. Ask patient to lower legs and assume comfortable position.
- (3) Male patient
  - (a) Lower side rail. Assist patient to supine position. Note any restriction in mobility.
  - (b) Fold lower half of bath blanket up to expose upper thighs. Wash and dry thighs.
  - (c) Cover thighs with bath towels. Raise bath blanket up to expose genitalia. Gently raise penis and place bath towel underneath. Gently grasp shaft of penis. If patient is uncircumcised, retract foreskin. If patient has an erection, defer procedure until later.
  - (d) Wash tip of penis at urethral meatus first. Using circular motion, cleanse from meatus outward. Discard washcloth and repeat with a clean cloth until penis is clean. Rinse and dry gently.

	S	U	NP	Comments

      (e) Return foreskin to its natural position. This is extremely important in patients with decreased sensation in their lower extremities.

      (f) Gently cleanse shaft of penis and scrotum by having patient abduct legs. Pay special attention to underlying surface of penis. Lift scrotum carefully, and wash underlying skinfolds. Rinse and dry thoroughly.

      (g) Avoid placing tension on indwelling catheter if present.

  P. Dispose of bathwater and dispose of gloves.

  Q. Wash back.

    (1) Reapply clean pair of gloves. Lower side rail. Assist patient in assuming prone or side-lying position (as applicable). Place towel lengthwise along patient's side, and keep patient covered with bath blanket.

    (2) If fecal material is present, enclose in a fold of underpad or toilet tissue, and remove with disposable wipes.

    (3) Keep patient draped by sliding bath blanket over shoulders and thighs during bathing. Wash, rinse, and dry back from neck to buttocks using long, firm strokes. Pay special attention to folds of buttocks and anus.

    (4) Cleanse buttocks and anus, washing front to back. Cleanse, rinse, and dry area thoroughly. If needed, place a clean absorbent pad under patient's buttocks. Remove contaminated gloves.

    (5) Give a back rub if appropriate for patient.

  R. Apply additional body lotion or oil as desired.

  S. Remove soiled linen and place in dirty linen bag. Clean and replace bathing equipment. Wash hands.

  T. Assist patient in dressing. Comb patient's hair. Women may want to apply makeup.

  U. Make patient's bed.

  V. Check the function and position of external devices.

  W. Place bed in lowest position.

2. **Commercial Bag Bath or Cleansing Pack**
   A. The cleansing pack contains 8 to 10 premoistened towels for cleansing. Warm the package contents in a microwave following package directions.
   B. Use a single towel for each general body part cleansed. Follow the same order of cleansing as the total or partial bed bath.
   C. Allow the skin to air-dry for 30 seconds. It is permissible to lightly cover patient with a bath towel to prevent chilling.
   NOTE: If there is excessive soiling (e.g., in the perineal region), use an extra bag bath or conventional washcloths, soap, water, and towels.

3. **Tub Bath or Shower**
   A. Consider patient's condition, and review orders for precautions concerning patient's movement or positioning.
   B. Schedule use of shower or tub.
   C. Check tub or shower for cleanliness. Use cleaning techniques outlined in agency policy. Place rubber mat on tub or shower bottom. Place disposable bath mat or towel on floor in front of tub or shower.
   D. Collect all hygienic aids, toiletry items, and linens requested by patient. Place within easy reach of tub or shower.
   E. Assist patient to bathroom if necessary. Have patient wear robe and slippers to bathroom.
   F. Demonstrate how to use call signal for assistance.
   G. Place "occupied" sign on bathroom door.

	S	U	NP	Comments

H. Fill bath tub halfway with warm water. Check temperature of bath water; then have patient test water and adjust temperature if water is too warm. Explain which faucet controls hot water. If patient is taking shower, turn shower on and adjust water temperature before patient enters shower stall. Use shower seat or tub chair if needed.

I. Instruct patient to use safety bars when getting in and out of tub or shower. Caution patient against use of bath oil in tub water.

J. Instruct patient not to remain in tub longer than 10 to 15 minutes. Check patient every 5 minutes.

K. Return to bathroom when patient signals, and knock before entering.

L. For patient who is unsteady, drain tub of water before patient attempts to get out of it. Place bath towel over patient's shoulders. Assist patient in getting out of tub as needed and assist with drying.

M. Assist patient as needed with getting dressed in a clean gown or pajamas, slippers, and robe. (In home setting, patient may put on regular clothing.)

N. Assist patient to room and comfortable position in bed or chair.

O. Clean tub or shower according to agency policy. Remove soiled linen and place in dirty linen bag. Discard disposable equipment in proper receptacle. Place "unoccupied" sign on bathroom door. Return supplies to storage area.

P. Perform hand hygiene.

Evaluation

1. Observe skin, paying particular attention to areas previously soiled or reddened or showing early signs of breakdown.
2. Observe range of motion during bath.
3. Ask patient to rate level of comfort.
4. Record bath on flow sheet. Note level of assistance required.
5. Record condition of skin and any significant findings.
6. Report evidence of alterations in skin integrity to nurse in charge or physician.

CHAPTER 28 • Hygiene

Name _____ Date _____ Instructor's Name _____

Performance Checklist Skill 28-2: Providing Oral Hygiene

	S	U	NP	Comments

Assessment
1. Perform hand hygiene, and apply clean gloves. ___ ___ ___ _____
2. Inspect integrity of lips, teeth, buccal mucosa, gums, palate, and tongue. ___ ___ ___ _____
3. Identify presence of common oral problems. ___ ___ ___ _____
4. Remove gloves, and perform hand hygiene. ___ ___ ___ _____
5. Assess patient's risk for aspiration, impaired swallowing, or reduced gag reflex. ___ ___ ___ _____
6. Assess risk for oral hygiene problems. ___ ___ ___ _____
7. Determine patient's oral hygiene practices and willingness to perform oral hygiene. ___ ___ ___ _____
8. Assess patient's ability to grasp and manipulate toothbrush. ___ ___ ___ _____

Planning
1. Explain procedure to patient. ___ ___ ___ _____
2. Place paper towels on over-bed table, and arrange other equipment within easy reach. ___ ___ ___ _____

Implementation
1. Raise bed to comfortable working position. Raise head of bed (if allowed) and lower side rail. Move patient, or help patient move closer. Side-lying position can be used. ___ ___ ___ _____
2. Place towel over patient's chest. ___ ___ ___ _____
3. Apply clean gloves. ___ ___ ___ _____
4. Apply enough toothpaste to cover length of bristles. Holding brush over emesis basin, pour small amount of water over toothpaste. ___ ___ ___ _____
5. Encourage patient to assist with brushing. Hold toothbrush bristles at 45-degree angle to gum line. Be sure tips of bristles rest against and penetrate under gum line. Brush inner and outer surfaces of upper and lower teeth by brushing from gum to crown of each tooth. Clean biting surfaces of teeth by holding top of bristles parallel with teeth and brushing gently back and forth. Brush sides of teeth by moving bristles back and forth. ___ ___ ___ _____
6. Have patient hold brush at 45-degree angle and lightly brush over surface and sides of tongue. Avoid initiating gag reflex. ___ ___ ___ _____
7. Allow patient to rinse mouth thoroughly by taking several sips of water, swishing water across all tooth surfaces, and spitting into emesis basin. ___ ___ ___ _____
8. Have patient rinse mouth with antiseptic mouth rinse for 30 seconds. Then have patient spit rinse into emesis basin. ___ ___ ___ _____
9. Assist in wiping patient's mouth. ___ ___ ___ _____
10. Allow patient to floss. ___ ___ ___ _____
11. Allow patient to rinse mouth thoroughly with cool water and spit into emesis basin. Assist in wiping patient's mouth. ___ ___ ___ _____
12. Assist patient to comfortable position, remove emesis basin and bedside table, raise side rail, and lower bed to original position. ___ ___ ___ _____
13. Wipe off over-bed table, discard soiled linen and paper towels in appropriate containers, remove soiled gloves, and return equipment to proper place. ___ ___ ___ _____
14. Perform hand hygiene. ___ ___ ___ _____

Copyright © 2011, 2007, 2003 by Mosby, Inc., an affiliate of Elsevier Inc. All rights reserved.

CHAPTER 28 • Hygiene

	S	U	NP	Comments

Evaluation
1. Ask patient if any area of oral cavity feels uncomfortable or irritated. _____ _____ _____ _____
2. Apply gloves, and inspect condition of oral cavity. _____ _____ _____ _____
3. Ask patient to describe proper hygiene techniques. _____ _____ _____ _____
4. Observe patient brushing. _____ _____ _____ _____
5. Record procedure, noting condition of oral cavity. _____ _____ _____ _____
6. Report bleeding or presence of lesions to nurse in charge or physician. _____ _____ _____ _____

Name _____ Date _____ Instructor's Name _____

Performance Checklist Skill 28-3: Performing Mouth Care for an Unconscious or Debilitated Patient

	S	U	NP	Comments

Assessment
1. Perform hand hygiene. Apply clean gloves.
2. Assess patient's risk for oral hygiene problems.
3. Test for presence of gag reflex by placing tongue blade on back half of tongue.
4. Inspect condition of oral cavity.
5. Remove gloves. Perform hand hygiene.

Planning
1. Explain procedure to patient.
2. Collect equipment.
3. Unless contraindicated lower side rail and position patient on side (Sims' position) with head turned well toward dependent side and head of bed lowered. Raise side rail.

Implementation
1. Apply disposable gloves.
2. Place paper towels on over-bed table, and arrange equipment. If needed, turn on suction machine, and connect tubing to suction catheter.
3. Pull curtain around bed, or close room door.
4. Raise bed to its highest horizontal level; lower side rail.
5. Position patient close to side of bed; turn patient's head toward mattress.
6. Place towel under patient's head and emesis basin under chin.
7. Remove dentures or partial plates if present.
8. Place towel under patient's head and emesis basin under chin.
9. If patient is unconscious, uncooperative, or has difficulty keeping mouth open, insert an oral airway. Insert upside down, then turn the airway sideways and then over tongue to keep teeth apart. Insert when patient is relaxed, if possible. Do not use force.
10. Clean mouth with brush moistened with dental cleansing agent, such as commercial diluted hydrogen peroxide and sodium bicarbonate solution or chlorhexidine, if prescribed. Clean chewing and inner tooth surfaces first. Clean outer tooth surfaces. Brush roof of mouth, gums, and inside cheeks. Gently brush tongue but avoid stimulating gag reflex (if present). Moisten brush with water to rinse. (Bulb syringe also may be used to rinse.) Repeat rinse several times.
11. For patients without teeth, use a toothette moistened in water or normal saline to clean oral cavity.
12. Suction oral secretions as they accumulate.
13. Apply thin layer of water-soluble jelly to lips.
14. Inform patient that procedure is completed.
15. Raise side rails as appropriate or ordered. Remove gloves, and dispose in proper receptacle.
16. Lower side rails. Reposition patient comfortably, raise side rail, and return bed to original position.
17. Apply clean gloves to clean equipment and return to its proper place. Place soiled linen in proper receptacle.
18. Remove gloves and discard.
19. Perform hand hygiene.

	S	U	NP	Comments

Evaluation
1. Apply gloves, and inspect oral cavity.
2. Ask debilitated patient if mouth feels clean.
3. Evaluate patient's respirations, and auscultate lung sounds on an ongoing basis.
4. Record procedure, including pertinent observations.
5. Report any unusual findings to nurse in charge or physician.

Name _____ Date _____ Instructor's Name _____

Performance Checklist Skill 28-4: Making an Occupied Bed

	S	U	NP	Comments

Assessment
1. Assess potential for patient incontinence or for excess drainage on bed linen.
2. Check chart for orders or specific precautions concerning movement and positioning.

Planning
1. Explain procedure to patient, noting that the patient will be asked to turn on side and roll over linen.

Implementation
1. Perform hand hygiene, and apply gloves (gloves are worn only if linen is soiled or there is risk for contact with body secretions).
2. Assemble equipment, and arrange on bedside chair or table. Remove unnecessary equipment such as a dietary tray or items used for hygiene.
3. Draw room curtain around bed or close door.
4. Adjust bed height to comfortable working position. Lower any raised side rail on one side of bed. Remove call light.
5. Loosen top linen at foot of bed.
6. Remove bedspread and blanket separately. If spread and blanket are soiled, place them in linen bag. Keep soiled linen away from uniform.
7. If you reuse blanket and spread, fold them by bringing the top and bottom edges together. Fold farthest side over onto nearer bottom edge. Bring top and bottom edges together again. Place folded linen over back of chair.
8. Cover patient with bath blanket placed over top sheet. If patient is unable to help, tuck top of bath blanket under shoulder. Grasp top edge of sheet under bath blanket, and remove sheet. Discard sheet in linen bag.
9. With assistance slide mattress toward head of bed.
10. Position patient on the far side of the bed, turned onto side and facing away from you. Be sure side rail in front of patient is up. Adjust pillow under patient's head.
11. Loosen bottom linens, moving from head to foot. With seam side down (facing the mattress), fanfold bottom sheet and drawsheet toward patient—first drawsheet, then bottom sheet. Tuck edges of linen just under buttocks, back, and shoulders. Do not fanfold mattress pad if it is to be reused.
12. Wipe off any moisture on exposed mattress with towel and use appropriate disinfectant.
13. Apply clean linen to exposed half of bed:
    A. Place clean mattress pad on bed by folding it lengthwise with center crease in middle of bed. Fanfold top layer over mattress. (If pad is reused, simply smooth out any wrinkles.)
    B. Unfold bottom sheet lengthwise so that center crease is situated lengthwise along center of bed. Fanfold sheet's top layer toward center of bed alongside the patient. Smooth bottom layer of sheet over mattress, and bring edge over closest side of mattress. Pull fitted sheet smoothly over mattress ends. Allow edge of flat unfitted sheet to hang about 25 cm (10 inches) over mattress edge. Lower hem of bottom flat sheet should lie seam-down and even with bottom edge of mattress.

Copyright © 2011, 2007, 2003 by Mosby, Inc., an affiliate of Elsevier Inc. All rights reserved.

CHAPTER 28 • Hygiene

		S	U	NP	Comments

14. Miter bottom flat sheet at head of bed:
    A. Face head of bed diagonally. Place hand away from head of bed under top corner of mattress, near mattress edge, and lift.
    B. With other hand, tuck top edge of bottom sheet smoothly under mattress so that side edges of sheet above and below mattress meet if brought together.
    C. Face side of bed and pick up top edge of sheet at approximately 45 cm (18 inches) from top of mattress.
    D. Lift sheet, and lay it on top of mattress to form a neat triangular fold, with lower base of triangle even with mattress side edge.
    E. Tuck lower edge of sheet, which is hanging free below the mattress, under mattress. Tuck with palms down, without pulling triangular fold.
    F. Hold portion of sheet covering side of mattress in place with one hand. With the other hand, pick up top of triangular linen fold and bring it down over side of mattress. Tuck this portion under mattress.
15. Tuck remaining portion of sheet under mattress, moving toward foot of bed. Keep linen smooth.
16. *(Optional)* Open clean drawsheet so that it unfolds in half. Lay centerfold along middle of bed lengthwise, and position sheet so that it will be under the patient's buttocks and torso. Fanfold top layer toward patient, with edge along patient's back. Smooth bottom layer out over mattress, and tuck excess edge under mattress (keep palms down).
17. Place waterproof pad over drawsheet, with centerfold against patient's side. Fanfold top layer toward patient.
18. Have patient roll slowly toward you, over the layers of linen. Raise side rail on working side, and go to other side.
19. Lower side rail. Assist patient in positioning on other side, over folds of linen. Loosen edges of soiled linen from under mattress.
20. Remove soiled linen by folding it into a bundle or square, with soiled side turned in. Discard in linen bag. If necessary, wipe mattress with antiseptic solution, and dry mattress surface before applying new linen.
21. Pull clean, fanfolded linen smoothly over edge of mattress from head to foot of bed.
22. Assist patient in rolling back into supine position. Reposition pillow.
23. Pull fitted sheet smoothly over mattress ends. Miter top corner of bottom sheet (see step 11). When tucking corner, be sure that sheet is smooth and free of wrinkles.
24. Facing side of bed, grasp remaining edge of bottom flat sheet. Lean back, keep back straight, and pull while tucking excess linen under mattress. Proceed from head to foot of bed. (Avoid lifting mattress during tucking to ensure fit.)
25. Smooth fanfolded drawsheet out over bottom sheet. Grasp edge of sheet with palms down, lean back, and tuck sheet under mattress. Tuck from middle to top and then to bottom.
26. Place top sheet over patient with center fold lengthwise down middle of bed. Open sheet from head to foot, and unfold over patient.
27. Ask patient to hold clean top sheet, or tuck sheet around patient's shoulders. Remove bath blanket and discard in linen bag.

Copyright © 2011, 2007, 2003 by Mosby, Inc., an affiliate of Elsevier Inc. All rights reserved.

		S	U	NP	Comments

28. Place blanket on bed, unfolding it so that crease runs lengthwise along middle of bed. Unfold blanket to cover patient. Make sure top edge is parallel with edge of top sheet and 15 to 20 cm (6 to 8 inches) from top sheet's edge.
29. Place spread over bed according to step 28. Be sure that top edge of spread extends about 2.5 cm (1 inch) above blanket's edge. Tuck top edge of spread over and under top edge of blanket.
30. Make cuff by turning edge of top sheet down over top edge of blanket and spread.
31. Standing on one side at foot of bed, lift mattress corner slightly with one hand and tuck linens under mattress. Top sheet and blanket are tucked under together. Be sure that linens are loose enough to allow movement of patient's feet. Making a horizontal toe pleat is an option.
32. Make modified mitered corner with top sheet, blanket, and spread:
    A. Pick up side edge of top sheet, blanket, and spread approximately 45 cm (18 inches) from foot of mattress. Lift linen to form triangular fold, and lay it on bed.
    B. Tuck lower edge of sheet, which is hanging free below mattress, under mattress. Do not pull triangular fold.
    C. Pick up triangular fold, and bring it down over mattress while holding linen in place along side of mattress. Do not tuck tip of triangle.
33. Raise side rail. Make other side of bed; spread sheet, blanket, and bedspread out evenly. Fold top edge of spread over blanket and make cuff with top sheet (see step 30); make modified mitered corner at foot of bed (see step 32).
34. Change pillowcase:
    A. Have patient raise head. While supporting neck with one hand, remove pillow. Allow patient to lower head.
    B. Remove soiled case by grasping pillow at open end with one hand and pulling case back over pillow with the other hand. Discard case in linen bag.
    C. Grasp clean pillowcase at center of closed end. Gather case, turning it inside out over the hand holding it. With the same hand, pick up middle of one end of the pillow. Pull pillowcase down over pillow with the other hand.
    D. Be sure pillow corners fit evenly into corners of pillowcase. Place pillow under patient's head.
35. Place call light within patient's reach, and return bed to comfortable position.
36. Open room curtains, and rearrange furniture. Place personal items within easy reach on over-bed table or bedside stand. Return bed to a comfortable height.
37. Discard dirty linen in hamper or chute and wash hands.
38. Ask if patient feels comfortable.

Evaluation
1. Inspect skin for areas of irritation.
2. Observe patient for signs of fatigue, dyspnea, pain, or discomfort.

Name _____ Date _____ Instructor's Name _____

Procedural Guidelines 28-1: Performing Nail and Foot Care

	S	U	NP	Comments
1. Obtain health care provider's order for cutting nails if agency policy requires.	___	___	___	_____
2. Explain procedure to patient, including fact that proper soaking requires several minutes.	___	___	___	_____
3. Perform hand hygiene. Arrange equipment on over-bed table.	___	___	___	_____
4. Pull curtain around bed, or close room door.	___	___	___	_____
5. Assist ambulatory patient with sitting in bedside chair. Help bed-bound patient to supine position with head of bed elevated. Place disposable bath mat on floor under patient's feet or place towel on mattress.	___	___	___	_____
6. Fill washbasin with warm water. Test water temperature.	___	___	___	_____
7. Place basin on bath mat or towel, and help patient place feet in basin. Place call light within patient's reach.	___	___	___	_____
8. Adjust over-bed table to low position, and place it over patient's lap. (Patient sits in chair or lies in bed.)	___	___	___	_____
9. Fill emesis basin with warm water, and place basin on paper towels on over-bed table.	___	___	___	_____
10. Instruct patient to place fingers in emesis basin and place arms in comfortable position.	___	___	___	_____
11. When patient has diabetes or peripheral vascular disease, allow patient's feet and fingernails to soak for 10 to 20 minutes. Rewarm water in basin after 10 minutes.	___	___	___	_____
12. Clean gently under fingernails with orange stick while fingers are immersed. Remove emesis basin and dry fingers thoroughly.	___	___	___	_____
13. With nail clippers, clip fingernails straight across and even with tops of fingers. Shape nails with emery board or file. If patient has circulatory problems, do not cut nail; file the nail only.	___	___	___	_____
14. Push cuticle back gently with orange stick.	___	___	___	_____
15. Move over-bed table away from patient.	___	___	___	_____
16. Put on clean gloves and scrub callused areas of feet with washcloth.	___	___	___	_____
17. Clean gently under nails with orange stick. Remove feet from basin, and dry thoroughly.	___	___	___	_____
18. Clean and trim toenails using procedures stated previously for fingernails. Do not file corners of toenails.	___	___	___	_____
19. Apply lotion to feet and hands, and assist patient back to bed and into comfortable position.	___	___	___	_____
20. Remove gloves, discarding in trash. Perform hand hygiene.	___	___	___	_____
21. Return supplies to appropriate location and place soiled linen in bag or hamper	___	___	___	_____
22. Perform hand hygiene.	___	___	___	_____
23. Record care given.	___	___	___	_____
24. Report any breaks in skin, reddened or tender areas, or any discomfort.	___	___	___	_____

Name _____ Date _____ Instructor's Name _____

Procedural Guidelines 28-2: Cleaning Dentures

	S	U	NP	Comments
1. Perform hand hygiene.	___	___	___	_____
2. Assess patient for fit of dentures and any gum soreness or irritation.	___	___	___	_____
3. Ask patient about preferences for denture care.	___	___	___	_____
4. Clean dentures for patient during routine mouth care. Dentures need to be cleansed as often as natural teeth.	___	___	___	_____
5. Fill emesis basin with tepid water. If using sink, place washcloth in bottom of sink, and fill sink with approximately 1 inch of water.	___	___	___	_____
6. Remove dentures: If patient is unable to do this independently, don gloves, grasp upper plate at front with thumb and index finger wrapped in gauze, and pull downward. Gently lift lower denture from jaw, and rotate one side downward to remove from patient's mouth. Place dentures in emesis basin or sink.	___	___	___	_____
7. Apply dentifrice or toothpaste to denture, and brush surfaces of dentures. Hold dentures close to water. Hold brush horizontally, and use back and forth motion to cleanse biting surfaces. Use short strokes from top of denture to biting surfaces of teeth to clean outer tooth surface. Hold brush vertically, and use short strokes to clean inner tooth surfaces. Hold brush horizontally, and use back-and-forth motion to clean undersurface of dentures.	___	___	___	_____
8. Rinse dentures thoroughly in tepid water.	___	___	___	_____
9. Return dentures to patient, or store in tepid water in denture cup.	___	___	___	_____

Copyright © 2011, 2007, 2003 by Mosby, Inc., an affiliate of Elsevier Inc. All rights reserved.

Name _____ Date _____ Instructor's Name _____

Procedural Guidelines 28-3: Shampooing Hair of Bed-Bound Patient

	S	U	NP	Comments
1. Before washing patient's hair, determine that there are no contraindications to this procedure. Certain medical conditions, such as head and neck injuries, spinal cord injuries, and arthritis, place the patient at risk for injury during shampooing because of positioning and manipulation of patient's head and neck.	___	___	___	_____
2. Perform hand hygiene. Apply clean gloves if open lesions present.	___	___	___	_____
3. Inspect the hair and scalp before initiating the procedure. This determines the presence of any conditions that require the use of special shampoos or treatments.	___	___	___	_____
4. Place waterproof pad under patient's shoulders, neck, and head. Position patient supine, with head and shoulders at top edge of bed. Place trough under patient's head and washbasin at end of trough spout. Be sure trough spout or tubing extends beyond edge of mattress.	___	___	___	_____
5. Place rolled towel under patient's neck and bath towel over patient's shoulders.	___	___	___	_____
6. Brush and comb patient's hair.	___	___	___	_____
7. Obtain warm water.	___	___	___	_____
8. Ask patient to hold face towel or washcloth over eyes.	___	___	___	_____
9. Slowly pour water from water pitcher over hair until it is completely wet. If hair contains matted blood, put on gloves, apply peroxide to dissolve clots, and then rinse hair with saline. Apply small amount of shampoo.	___	___	___	_____
10. Work up lather with both hands. Start at hairline, and work toward back of neck. Lift head slightly with one hand to wash back of head. Shampoo sides of head. Massage scalp by applying pressure with fingertips.	___	___	___	_____
11. Rinse hair with water. Make sure water drains into basin. Repeat rinsing until hair is free of soap.	___	___	___	_____
12. Apply conditioner or cream rinse if requested, and rinse hair thoroughly.	___	___	___	_____
13. Wrap patient's head in bath towel. Dry patient's face with cloth used to protect eyes. Dry off any moisture along neck or shoulders.	___	___	___	_____
14. Dry patient's hair and scalp. Use second towel if first becomes saturated.	___	___	___	_____
15. Comb hair to remove tangles and dry with dryer if desired.	___	___	___	_____
16. Apply oil preparation or conditioning product to hair, if desired by patient.	___	___	___	_____
17. Assist patient to comfortable position and complete styling of hair.	___	___	___	_____

CHAPTER 28 • Hygiene   175

Name _____   Date _____   Instructor's Name _____

Procedural Guidelines 28-4: Making an Unoccupied Bed

	S	U	NP	Comments

1. Perform hand hygiene.
2. Determine if patient has been incontinent. Gloves will be necessary if any body fluids are present on linen.
3. Assess activity orders or restrictions in mobility to determine if patient can get out of bed for procedure. Assist to bedside chair or recliner.
4. Lower side rails on both sides of bed and raise bed to comfortable working position.
5. Remove soiled linen and place in laundry bag. Avoid shaking or fanning linen.
6. Reposition mattress and wipe off any moisture using a washcloth moistened in antiseptic solution. Dry thoroughly.
7. Apply all bottom linen on one side of bed before moving to opposite side. Apply bottom sheet, flat or fitted.
8. Be sure to place fitted sheet smoothly over mattress. To apply a flat unfitted sheet, allow about 25 cm (10 inches) to hang over mattress edge. Lower hem of sheet lies seam-down, even with bottom edge of mattress. Pull remaining top portion of sheet over top edge of mattress.
9. While standing at head of bed, miter top corner of bottom flat sheet.
10. Tuck remaining portion of unfitted sheet under mattress.
11. *Optional:* Apply drawsheet, laying center fold along middle of bed lengthwise. Smooth drawsheet over mattress and tuck excess edge under mattress, keeping palms down.
12. Move to opposite side of bed and spread bottom sheet smoothly over edge of mattress from head to foot of bed.
13. Apply fitted sheet smoothly over each mattress corner. For an unfitted sheet, miter top corner of bottom sheet (see step 8), making sure corner is stretched tight.
14. Grasp remaining edge of unfitted bottom sheet and tuck tightly under mattress while moving from head to foot of bed. Smooth folded drawsheet over bottom sheet and tuck under mattress, first at middle, then at top, and then at bottom.
15. If needed, apply waterproof pad over bottom sheet or drawsheet.
16. Place top sheet over bed with vertical center fold lengthwise down middle of bed. Open sheet out from head to foot, being sure top edge of sheet is even with top edge of mattress.
17. Make horizontal toe pleat: stand at foot of bed and fanfold top sheet 5 to 10 cm (2 to 4 inches) across bed. Pull sheet up from bottom to make fold approximately 15 cm (6 inches) from bottom edge of mattress.
18. Tuck in remaining portion of sheet under foot of mattress. Then place blanket over bed with top edge parallel to top edge of sheet and 15 to 20 cm (6 to 8 inches) down from edge of sheet. (*Optional:* Apply additional spread over bed.)
19. Make cuff by turning edge of top sheet down over top edge of blanket and spread.
20. Standing on one side at foot of bed, lift mattress corner slightly with one hand, and with other hand tuck top sheet, blanket, and spread under mattress. Be sure toe pleats are not pulled out.
21. Make modified mitered corner with top sheet, blanket, and spread. After making triangular fold, do not tuck tip of triangle.

Copyright © 2011, 2007, 2003 by Mosby, Inc., an affiliate of Elsevier Inc. All rights reserved.

S	U	NP	Comments

22. Go to other side of bed. Spread sheet, blanket, and spread out evenly. Make cuff with top sheet and blanket. Make modified corner at foot of bed. _____ _____ _____ _____
23. Apply clean pillowcase. _____ _____ _____ _____
24. Place call light within patient's reach on bed rail or pillow and return bed to height allowing for patient transfer. Assist patient to bed. _____ _____ _____ _____
25. Arrange patient's room. Remove and discard supplies. Perform hand hygiene. _____ _____ _____ _____

Oxygenation

29

CASE STUDY

1. You are the nurse in an outpatient clinic where a 32-year-old woman has gone for ongoing medical treatment. She tells you that she had asthma since she was a young child. While speaking with the patient, you notice that she is exhibiting mild wheezing and a productive cough. She appears slightly pale.
   a. What additional assessment questions should be asked of this patient?
   b. Identify a possible nursing diagnosis for this patient.
   c. What nurse-initiated actions may be taken at this time?
   d. Identify general information that should be included in patient teaching for promoting oxygenation.

CHAPTER REVIEW

Match the description/definition in Column A with the correct term in Column B.

Column A

_____ 1. Collapse of alveoli, preventing exchange of oxygen
_____ 2. Tachypnea pattern of breathing associated with metabolic acidosis
_____ 3. Need to sit upright to breathe easier
_____ 4. Collection of air in the pleural space
_____ 5. Bloody sputum
_____ 6. Inadequate tissue oxygenation at the cellular level
_____ 7. Amount of blood in the ventricles at the end of diastole
_____ 8. Collection of blood in the pleural space
_____ 9. Resistance of ejection of blood from the left ventricle
_____ 10. Difficulty breathing, sensation of breathlessness

Column B

a. Hypoxia
b. Pneumothorax
c. Atelectasis
d. Kussmaul respiration
e. Orthopnea
f. Hemothorax
g. Preload
h. Afterload
i. Hemoptysis
j. Dyspnea

Complete the following:

11. The average resting heart rate for an adult is _____ beats per minute.

12. Chest movement is affected by the what conditions?

13. Identify whether the following signs and symptoms are associated with left ventricular or right ventricular heart failure:
    a. Distended neck veins _____
    b. Ankle edema _____
    c. Pulmonary congestion _____
    d. Increased arterial blood pressure _____

14. Which of the following may cause hyperventilation? Select all that apply.
    a. Anxiety _____
    b. Fever _____
    c. Severe atelectasis _____
    d. Head injury _____
    e. Excessive administration of oxygen _____

15. Provide an example of a physiological alteration or problem that may result in each of the following:
    a. Decreased oxygen carrying capacity

    b. Decreased inspired oxygen concentration

    c. Hypovolemia

    d. Increased metabolic rate

16. A premature infant has a deficiency of _____ and is at risk for hyaline membrane disease.

17. An example of a modifiable risk factor for cardiopulmonary disease is:

18. Which of the following pathophysiological changes in the heart and lungs occur with aging? Select all that apply.
    a. Thinning of the ventricular wall of the heart _____
    b. SA node becoming fibrotic from calcification _____
    c. Increased elastin in the arterial vessel walls _____
    d. Increased chest wall compliance and elastic recoil _____
    e. Decreased alveolar surface area _____
    f. Increased responsiveness of central and peripheral chemoreceptors _____
    g. Decreased number of cilia _____
    h. Increased respiratory drive _____

19. A patient awakes in a panic and feels as though she is suffocating. This is noted by the nurse as:

20. A musical, high-pitched lung sound that may be heard on inspiration or expiration is:

21. Identify the following two cardiac rhythms:
    a.

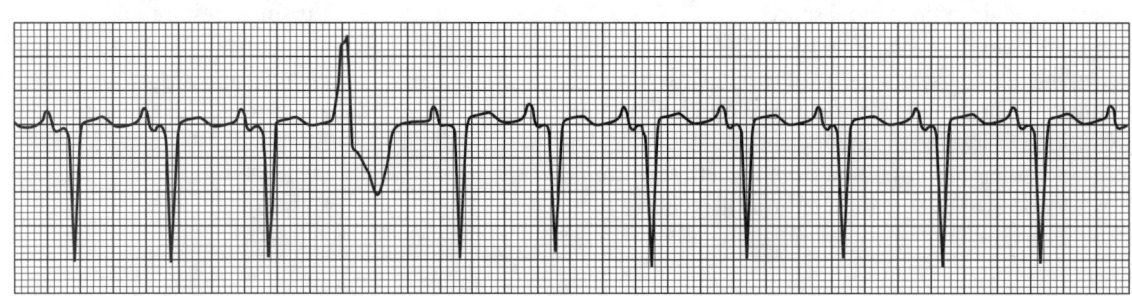

    b.

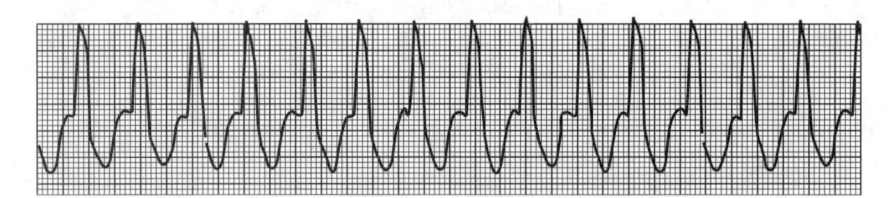

22. Briefly define the following abnormal chest wall movements:
    a. Retraction

    b. Paradoxical breathing

23. Which type of asepsis is used for tracheal suctioning?

24. Continuous bubbling in the chest tube water-seal chamber indicates:

25. Identify an example of a nursing intervention for promotion of each of the following:
    a. Dyspnea management

    b. Patent airway

    c. Lung expansion

    d. Mobilization of secretions

CHAPTER 29 • Oxygenation

26. Identify the following types of oxygen delivery systems and the flow rate for each:
    a.

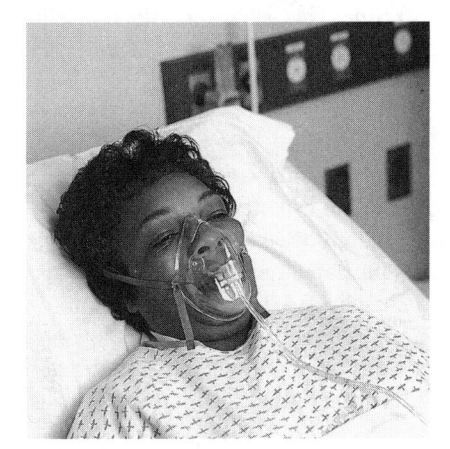

    b.

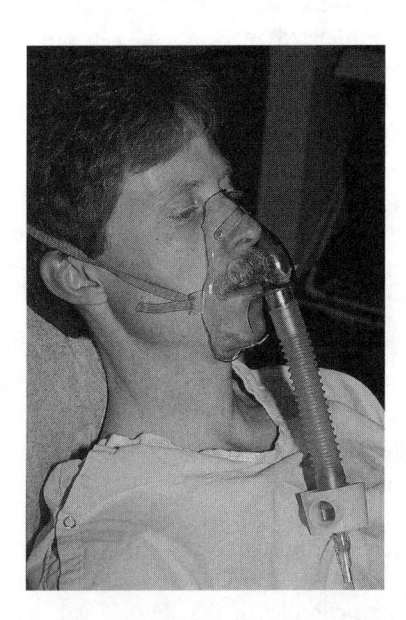

27. Identify the following for tuberculin (Mantoux) testing:
    a. A skin test is administered on a patient's:

    b. The test is read after _____ hours.
    c. A reddened, flat area is a(n) _____ reaction.
28. For chest percussion, vibration, and postural drainage:
    a. Chest percussion is contraindicated for a patient with:

    b. Vibration is used only during:

    c. The position for a 2-year-old for postural drainage is:

29. For continuous positive airway pressure (CPAP):
    a. CPAP is used for:

    b. The usual pressure setting is:

    c. A disadvantage of CPAP is:

30. An indication for home oxygen therapy is an SaO_2 value of:

31. The ABCs of CPR are:
    A
    B
    C
32. Defibrillation is recommended within _____ (time) for an out-of-hospital sudden cardiac arrest and within _____ (time) for an inpatient.
33. a. The prevalence of atrial fibrillation increases with age and is the leading contributing factor for stroke in the older adult.
    True _____ False _____
    b. Care of chest tubes can be delegated to a nursing assistant.
    True _____ False _____
34. Identify an example of a safety measure that should be implemented when a patient is using home oxygen therapy.

35. For the nursing diagnosis *Ineffective airway clearance related to the presence of tracheobronchial secretions*, identify a patient outcome and a nursing intervention to assist the patient to meet the outcome.

36. Which of the following are appropriate interventions for patient suctioning? Select all that apply.
    a. Performing pharyngeal suctioning before tracheal suctioning _____
    b. Avoiding routine use of normal saline instillations when suctioning _____
    c. Applying suction for 30 seconds at a time _____
    d. Suctioning during the insertion and removal of the tube _____
    e. Allowing 1 to 2 minutes between suction passes _____
    f. Providing regular suctioning every 1 to 2 hours around the clock _____
37. Cardiac output is the result of the stroke volume × _____.
38. What are the signs and symptoms that are associated with decreased oxygenation?

CHAPTER 29 • Oxygenation

39. Identify a possible nursing diagnosis for a patient with anemia.

40. Provide examples of dietary risks that may influence cardiopulmonary status and oxygenation.

41. The most effective positioning for a patient with cardiopulmonary disease is:

42. A method to encourage voluntary deep breathing for a postoperative patient is the use of an:

43. Identify at least two environmental or occupational hazards that may affect an individual's cardiopulmonary functioning:

44. Cardiac dysrhythmias may be caused by:

Select the best answer for each of the following questions:

45. Individuals have gone to the health fair to receive their free influenza vaccine. The nurse briefly discusses the medical backgrounds of the patients. The influenza vaccine will be withheld from the:
    1. HIV-positive man
    2. Older adult woman
    3. Man with chronic arthritis
    4. Woman with a hypersensitivity to eggs

46. A patient has a chest tube in place to drain bloody secretions from the chest cavity. When caring for a patient with a chest tube, a nurse should:
    1. Keep the drainage device above chest level
    2. Clamp the chest tube when the patient is ambulating
    3. Have the patient cough if the tubing becomes disconnected
    4. Leave trapped fluid in the tubing and estimate the amount

47. A nurse is making a home visit to a patient who has emphysema (chronic obstructive pulmonary disease [COPD]). Specific instruction to control exhalation pressure for this patient with an increased residual volume of air should include:
    1. Coughing
    2. Deep breathing
    3. Pursed-lip breathing
    4. Diaphragmatic breathing

48. A patient has been admitted to a medical center with a respiratory condition and dyspnea. A number of medications are prescribed for the patient. For a patient with this difficulty, the nurse should question the order for:
    1. Steroids
    2. Mucolytics
    3. Bronchodilators
    4. Narcotic analgesics

49. After a patient assessment, the nurse suspects hypoxemia. This is based on the nurse finding that the patient is experiencing:
    1. Restlessness
    2. Bradypnea
    3. Bradycardia
    4. Hypotension

50. A patient has experienced some respiratory difficulty and is placed on oxygen via nasal cannula. A nurse assists the patient with this form of oxygen delivery by:
    1. Changing the tubing every 4 hours
    2. Assessing the nares for breakdown
    3. Inspecting the back of the mouth q8h
    4. Securing the cannula to the nose with nonallergic tape

51. A patient is being seen in an outpatient medical clinic. A nurse has reviewed the patient's chart and finds that there is a history of a cardiopulmonary abnormality. This is supported by the nurse's assessment of the patient having:
    1. Scleral jaundice
    2. Reddened conjunctivae
    3. Symmetrical chest movement
    4. Splinter hemorrhages in the nails

52. A 65-year-old patient is seen in a physician's office for a routine annual checkup. As part of the physical examination, an ECG is performed. The ECG reveals a normal P wave, P-R interval, and QRS complex and a heart rate of 58 beats per minute. The nurse evaluates this finding as:
    1. Sinus tachycardia
    2. Sinus bradycardia
    3. Sinus dysrhythmia
    4. Supraventricular bradycardia

53. A patient is admitted to a medical center with a diagnosis of left ventricular congestive heart failure. A nurse is completing the physical assessment and is anticipating finding that the patient has:
    1. Liver enlargement
    2. Peripheral edema
    3. Pulmonary congestion
    4. Jugular neck vein distention

54. A patient has just returned to the unit after abdominal surgery. A nurse is planning care for this patient and is considering interventions to promote pulmonary function and prevent complications. The nurse:
    1. Teaches the patient leg exercises to perform
    2. Asks the physician to order nebulizer treatments
    3. Demonstrates the use of a flow-oriented incentive spirometer
    4. Informs the patient that his secretions will need to be suctioned

55. A nurse manager is evaluating the care that is provided by a new staff nurse during the orientation period. One of the patients requires nasotracheal suctioning,

and the nurse manager determines that the appropriate technique is used when the new staff nurse:
1. Places the patient in the supine position
2. Prepares for a clean or nonsterile procedure
3. Suctions the oropharyngeal area first, then moves to the nasotracheal area
4. Applies intermittent suction for 10 seconds while the suction catheter is being removed

56. Chest tubes have been inserted into a patient after thoracic surgery. In working with this patient, a nurse should:
1. Coil and secure excess tubing next to the patient
2. Clamp off the chest tubes except during respiratory assessments
3. Milk or strip the tubing every 15 to 30 minutes to maintain drainage
4. Remove the tubing from the connection to check for adequate suction

57. A patient is being discharged home with an order for oxygen prn. In preparing to teach the patient and family, a priority for the nurse is to provide information on the:
1. Use of the oxygen delivery equipment
2. Physiology of the respiratory system
3. Use of PaO_2 levels to determine oxygen demand
4. Length of time that the oxygen is to be used by the patient

58. In discriminating types of chest pain that a patient may experience, a nurse recognizes that pain associated with inflammation of the pericardial sac is noted by the patient experiencing:
1. Knifelike pain to the upper chest
2. Constant, substernal pain
3. Pain with inspiration
4. Pain aggravated by coughing

59. A nurse is checking a patient who has a chest tube in place and finds that there is constant bubbling in the water-seal chamber. The nurse should:
1. Tighten loose connections
2. Leave the chest tube clamped
3. Raise the tubing above the level of the insertion site
4. Prepare the patient for the removal of the tube

60. For a patient who is receiving noninvasive ventilation and states that he feels claustrophobic, the nurse should:
1. Discontinue the treatment
2. Lower the pressure settings
3. Notify the health care provider immediately
4. Demonstrate use of the quick-release straps

61. The patient is admitted with a diagnosis of COPD. The appropriate oxygen delivery method for this patient is a:
1. Simple face mask with 5 to 8 L/min (50%) O_2
2. Venuri mask with 8 L/min (35%–40%) O_2
3. Nasal cannula with 1 to 2 L/min (28%) O_2
4. Partial nonrebreather mask with 6 to 10 L/min (80%) O_2

62. A nurse is completing a physical assessment of a patient with a history of a cardiopulmonary abnormality. A finding associated with hyperlipidemia is the patient having:
1. Cyanosis
2. Xanthelasma
3. Petechiae
4. Ecchymosis

STUDY GROUP QUESTIONS

- How do the anatomy and physiology of the cardiovascular and respiratory systems promote oxygenation?
- What physiological factors affect oxygenation?
- How do growth and development influence oxygenation?
- How do behavioral and environmental factors influence oxygenation?
- What are some common alterations in cardiovascular and pulmonary functioning?
- How are the critical thinking and nursing processes applied to patients having difficulty with oxygenation?
- What assessment information should be obtained to determine the patient's oxygenation status?
- What findings are usually seen in a patient who has inadequate oxygenation?
- How can the nurse promote oxygenation for patients in the health promotion, acute care, and restorative care settings?
- What specific measures and procedures should be implemented by the nurse to manage dyspnea, maintain a patent airway, mobilize secretions, and expand the lungs?
- What should be included in patient/family teaching for promotion and maintenance of oxygenation?
- What safety measures should be implemented for the use of oxygen in the home?

Answers available through your instructor.

CHAPTER 29 • Oxygenation

Name _____ Date _____ Instructor's Name _____

Performance Checklist Skill 29-1: Suctioning

	S	U	NP	Comments

Assessment
1. Assess signs and symptoms of upper and lower airway obstruction requiring nasal or oral tracheal suctioning.
2. Determine the presence of hypoxemia.
3. Assess for risk factors for upper or lower airway obstruction.
4. Determine additional factors that normally influence upper or lower airway function.
5. Assess factors that influence character of secretions.
6. Identify contraindications to nasotracheal suctioning.
7. Examine sputum microbiology data.
8. Obtain patient's vital signs and oxygen saturation via pulse oximetry. Continuously monitor pulse oximetry during suctioning.
9. Assess patient's understanding of procedure.

Planning
1. Explain to patient how procedure will help clear airway and relieve breathing problems. Explain that temporary coughing, sneezing, gagging, or shortness of breath is normal during the procedure. Encourage patient to cough out secretions. Practice coughing, if able. Splint surgical incisions, if necessary.
2. Assist patient with assuming position comfortable for nurse and patient (usually semi-Fowler's or sitting upright with head hyperextended, unless contraindicated).
3. Place towel across patient's chest, if needed.

Implementation
1. Perform hand hygiene, and apply mask, goggles, or face shield if splashing is likely.
2. Connect one end of connecting tubing to suction machine, and place other end in convenient location near patient. Turn suction device on, and set vacuum regulator to appropriate negative pressure 120 to 150 mm Hg.
3. If indicated, increase supplemental oxygen therapy to 100% or as ordered by physician or health care provider. Encourage patient to breathe deeply.
4. Prepare suction catheter.
   A. One-time-use catheter
      (1) Open suction kit or catheter using aseptic technique. If sterile drape is available, place it across patient's chest or on the over-bed table. Do not allow the suction catheter to touch any nonsterile surfaces.
      (2) Unwrap or open sterile basin, and place on bedside table. Be careful not to touch inside of basin. Fill basin with about 100 mL of sterile normal saline solution or water.
      (3) Open lubricant. Squeeze small amount onto open sterile catheter package without touching package. NOTE: Lubricant is not necessary for artificial airway suctioning.
   B. Closed (in-line) suction catheter
5. Turn on suction device, and set regulator to appropriate pressure.
6. Apply a pair of clean gloves for oropharyngeal suction. Apply sterile glove to each hand, or clean glove to nondominant hand and sterile glove to dominant hand for all other suction techniques.

Copyright © 2011, 2007, 2003 by Mosby, Inc., an affiliate of Elsevier Inc. All rights reserved.

	S	U	NP	Comments

7. Pick up suction catheter with dominant hand without touching nonsterile surfaces. Pick up connecting tubing with nondominant hand. Secure catheter to tubing.
8. Check that the equipment is functioning properly by suctioning small amount of normal saline solution from basin.
9. Suction airway.
   A. **Oropharyngeal suctioning**
      (1) Remove oxygen mask if present. Insert Yankauer catheter along gum line to pharynx. With suction applied, move catheter around mouth until you clear the secretions. Encourage patient to cough. Replace oxygen mask, as appropriate.
      (2) Rinse catheter with water in basin until catheter and connecting tube are cleared of secretions.
      (3) Place catheter or Yankauer in a clean, dry area for reuse with suction turned off. If patient able to suction self, place within patient's reach with suction on.
   B. **Nasopharyngeal and nasotracheal suctioning**
      (1) Lightly coat distal 6 to 8 cm (2 to 3 inches) of catheter tip with water-soluble lubricant.
      (2) Remove oxygen delivery device, if applicable, with nondominant hand. Without applying suction and using dominant thumb and forefinger, gently but quickly insert catheter into naris during inhalation. Following the natural course of the naris, slightly slant the catheter downward or through mouth. Do not force through naris.
         (a) *Nasopharyngeal suctioning:* In adults, insert catheter about 16 cm (6 inches); in older children, 8 to 12 cm (3 to 5 inches); in infants and young children, 4 to 8 cm (2 to 3 inches). Rule of thumb is to insert catheter distance from tip of nose (or mouth) to base of earlobe.
         (b) *Nasotracheal suctioning:* In adults, insert catheter about 20 cm (8 inches); in older children, 14 to 20 cm (5.5 to 8 inches); and in young children and infants, 8 to 14 cm (3 to 5.5 inches).
            1) *Positioning:* In some instances turning patient's head to right helps nurse suction left mainstem bronchus; turning head to left helps nurse suction right mainstem bronchus. If resistance felt after insertion of catheter maximum recommended distance, catheter has probably hit carina. Pull catheter back 1 to 2 cm before applying suction.
      (3) With catheter tip in position, apply intermittent suction for up to 10 seconds by placing and releasing nondominant thumb over vent of catheter and slowly withdrawing catheter while rotating it back and forth between dominant thumb and forefinger. Encourage patient to cough. Replace oxygen device, if applicable.
      (4) Rinse catheter and connecting tubing with normal saline or water until cleared.
      (5) Assess for need to repeat suctioning procedure. Observe for alterations in cardiopulmonary status. When possible, allow adequate time (1 to 2 minutes) between suction passes for ventilation and oxygenation. Assist patient to deep breathe and cough.

	S	U	NP	Comments

  C. **Artificial airway suctioning**
   (1) Hyperinflate and/or hyperoxygenate patient before suctioning, using manual resuscitation bag valve-mask connected to oxygen source or sigh mechanism on mechanical ventilator.
   (2) If patient is receiving mechanical ventilation, open swivel adapter, or if necessary remove oxygen or humidity delivery device with nondominant hand.
   (3) Without applying suction, gently but quickly insert catheter using dominant thumb and forefinger into artificial airway (it is best to try to insert catheter into the artificial airway while patient is inhaling) until you meet resistance or until patient coughs; then pull back 1 cm (½ inch).
   (4) Apply intermittent suction by placing and releasing nondominant thumb over vent of catheter; slowly withdraw catheter while rotating it back and forth between dominant thumb and forefinger. Encourage patient to cough. Observe patient for any respiratory distress.
   (5) If patient is receiving mechanical ventilation, close swivel adapter, or replace oxygen delivery device.
   (6) Encourage patient to deep breathe, if able. Some patients respond well to several manual breaths from the mechanical ventilator or bag-valve-mask.
   (7) Rinse catheter and connecting tubing with normal saline until clear. Use continuous suction.
   (8) Assess patient's cardiopulmonary status for secretion clearance. Repeat steps (1) through (7) once or twice more to clear secretions. Allow at least 1 full minute between suction passes.
   (9) When you have cleared pharynx and trachea sufficiently of secretions, perform oropharyngeal suctioning to clear mouth of secretions. Do not suction nose again after suctioning mouth.
10. When you have completed suctioning, disconnect catheter from connecting tubing. Roll catheter around fingers of dominant hand. Pull glove off inside out so that catheter remains coiled in glove. Pull off other glove over first glove in same way to seal in contaminants. Discard in appropriate receptacle. Turn off suction device.
11. Remove towel, place in laundry or appropriate receptacle, and reposition patient.
12. If indicated, readjust oxygen to original level because patient's blood oxygen level should have returned to baseline.
13. Discard remainder of normal saline into appropriate receptacle. If basin is disposable, discard into appropriate receptacle. If basin is reusable, rinse it out and place it in soiled utility room.
14. Remove face shield, and discard into appropriate receptacle. Perform hand hygiene.
15. Place unopened suction kit on suction machine table or at head of bed.
16. Assist patient to a comfortable position, and provide oral hygiene as needed.

Evaluation
1. Compare patient's respiratory assessment before and after suctioning.
2. Observe airway secretions.

	S	U	NP	Comments

3. Ask patient if breathing is easier and if there is less congestion.
4. Record the amount, consistency, color, and odor of secretions.
5. Record the patient's response to the suction procedure.
6. Record and report the presuctioning and postsuctioning cardiopulmonary status.

Name _____ Date _____ Instructor's Name _____

Performance Checklist Skill 29-2: Care of Patients With Chest Tubes

	S	U	NP	Comments

Assessment
1. Perform hand hygiene.
2. Assess pulmonary status.
3. Obtain vital signs, oxygen saturation level, and level of cognition.
4. Ask patient to rate level of comfort.
5. Observe:
   A. Chest tube dressing.
   B. Tubing for kinks, dependent loops, or clots.
   C. Chest drainage system, which should be upright and below level of tube insertion.

Planning
1. Provide two shodded hemostats for each chest tube, attached to top of patient's bed with adhesive tape. Chest tubes are only clamped under specific circumstances per physician order or nursing policy and procedure.
2. Position the patient.
   A. Semi-Fowler's position to evacuate air (pneumothorax).
   B. High-Fowler's position to drain fluid (hemothorax).

Implementation
1. Be sure tube connection between chest and drainage tubes is intact and taped.
   A. Make sure water-seal vent is not occluded.
   B. Make sure suction-control chamber vent is not occluded when using suction.
2. Coil excess tubing on mattress next to patient. Secure with rubber band, tape, or plastic clamp.
3. Adjust tubing to hang in straight line from top of mattress to drainage chamber.
4. If chest tube is draining fluid, indicate time that you began drainage on drainage bottle's adhesive tape or on write-on surface of disposable commercial system.
5. Strip or milk chest tube only if indicated.
6. Perform hand hygiene.

Evaluation
1. Monitor vital signs and pulse oximetry.
2. Observe:
   A. Chest tube dressing.
   B. Tubing, which should be free of kinks and dependent loops.
   C. The chest drainage system, which should be upright and below level of tube insertion. Note presence of clots or debris in tubing.
   D. Water seal for fluctuations with patient's inspirations and expirations.
      (1) Waterless system: diagnostic indicator for fluctuations with patient's inspirations and expirations.
      (2) Water-seal system: bubbling in the water-seal chamber.

	S	U	NP	Comments

    E. Waterless system: bubbling is diagnostic indicator.

    F. Type and amount of fluid drainage. Note color and amount of drainage, patient's vital signs, and skin color.

    G. Waterless system: the suction control (float ball) indicates the amount of suction the patient's intrapleural space is receiving.

3. Ask patient to rate comfort level.

4. Record patency of chest tubes, presence of drainage, presence of fluctuations, patient's vital signs, chest dressing status, type of suction, and level of comfort.

Name _____ Date _____ Instructor's Name _____

Performance Checklist Skill 29-3: Care of the Patient With Noninvasive Ventilation

	S	U	NP	Comments

Assessment
1. Assess patient's respiratory status and observe for signs and symptoms associated with hypoxia.
2. Observe patient's ability to clear and remove airway secretions.
3. If available, note patient's most recent arterial blood gas (ABG) results or arterial oxygen saturation.
4. Obtain vital signs before initiation of therapy.
5. Review patient's medical record for medical order for CPAP/BiPAP and appropriate settings.

Planning
1. Explain to patient and family the purpose and reasons for CPAP/BiPAP.

Implementation
1. Perform hand hygiene; apply gloves and goggles. Apply barrier gown if secretions are projectile.
2. Determine correct mask size. Use supplied masking charts to determine correct size.
3. Connect CPAP/BiPAP device delivery tubing to pressure generator.
4. Connect patient to pulse oximetry.
5. Set CPAP/BiPAP initial settings:
   CPAP: 4 to 8 cm H_2O
   BiPAP:
   Inspiratory usually set at 8 cm H_2O
   Expiratory usually set at 4 cm H_2O
6. Perform frequent skin assessment to determine the presence of pressure, skin irritation, or skin breakdown.
7. Dispose of supplies as appropriate and perform hand hygiene.

Evaluation
1. Evaluate patient's response to noninvasive ventilation. Observe for decreased anxiety; improved LOC and cognitive abilities; decreased fatigue; absence of dizziness; decreased pulse rate, regular rhythm; decreased respiratory rate and work of breathing; return to normal blood pressure; improved color.
2. Monitor pulse oximetry.
3. Observe skin integrity over the bridge of patient's nose.
4. Monitor patient's and family's ability to manipulate device and face mask.
5. Record respiratory assessment findings; CPAP/BiPAP settings; SpO_2; patient's response to noninvasive ventilation.
6. Report any sudden change in patient's respiratory status or decreasing pulse oximetry.

Name _____ Date _____ Instructor's Name _____

Procedural Guidelines 29-1: Closed (In-Line) Suctioning

	S	U	NP	Comments
1. Perform respiratory assessment.	___	___	___	_____
2. Explain the procedure to the patient and the importance of coughing during the suctioning procedure.	___	___	___	_____
3. Assist patient with assuming a position of comfort for both patient and nurse, usually semi-Fowler's or high-Fowler's position. Place towel across the patient's chest.	___	___	___	_____
4. Perform hand hygiene and attach suction.				
A. If catheter is not already in place, open suction catheter package using aseptic technique, attach closed suction catheter to ventilator circuit by removing swivel adapter and placing closed suction catheter apparatus on ET or tracheostomy tube, and connect Y on mechanical ventilator circuit to closed suction catheter with flex tubing.	___	___	___	_____
B. Connect one end of connecting tubing to suction machine, and connect other to the end of a closed system or in-line suction catheter, if not already done. Turn suction device on, and set vacuum regulator to appropriate negative pressure (see manufacturer's directions). Many closed system suction catheters require slightly higher suction; consult manufacturer's guidelines.	___	___	___	_____
5. Hyperinflate and/or hyperoxygenate patient with bag-valve-mask or manual breathing mechanism on mechanical ventilator according to institution protocol and clinical status (usually 100% oxygen).	___	___	___	_____
6. Unlock suction control mechanism if required by manufacturer. Open saline port and attach saline syringe or vial.	___	___	___	_____
7. Pick up suction catheter enclosed in plastic sleeve with dominant hand.	___	___	___	_____
8. Insert catheter; use a repeating maneuver of pushing catheter and sliding (or pulling) plastic sleeve back between thumb and forefinger until you feel resistance or patient coughs.	___	___	___	_____
9. Encourage patient to cough, and apply suction by squeezing on suction control mechanism while withdrawing catheter. It is difficult to apply intermittent pulses of suction and nearly impossible to rotate the catheter compared with a standard catheter. Be sure to withdraw catheter completely into plastic sheath so it does not obstruct airflow.	___	___	___	_____
10. Reassess cardiopulmonary status, including pulse oximetry, to determine need for subsequent suctioning or presence of complications. Repeat steps 5 through 9 one to two more times to clear secretions. Allow adequate time (at least 1 full minute) between suction passes for ventilation and reoxygenation.	___	___	___	_____
11. When airway is clear, withdraw catheter completely into sheath. Be sure that colored indicator line on catheter is visible in the sheath. Squeeze vial or push syringe while applying suction to rinse inner lumen of catheter. Use at least 5 to 10 mL of saline to rinse the catheter. Lock suction mechanism, if applicable, and turn off suction.	___	___	___	_____

	S	U	NP	Comments
12. If patient requires oral or nasal suctioning, perform Skill 28-1 with separate standard suction catheter.	___	___	___	_____
13. Reposition patient.	___	___	___	_____
14. Remove gloves and discard them, and perform hand hygiene.	___	___	___	_____
15. Compare patient's cardiopulmonary assessments before and after suctioning and observe airway secretions.	___	___	___	_____

Sleep 30

CASE STUDY

1. A middle-aged adult patient has gone to a physician's office to obtain a prescription for a "sleeping pill" because she has been having difficulty either falling or staying asleep. You are completing the initial nursing assessment and discover that the patient is recently divorced and trying to juggle extensive work and child care responsibilities.
   a. Identify a possible nursing diagnosis and outcome for this patient.
   b. Indicate nursing interventions and teaching areas for this patient.

CHAPTER REVIEW

Match the description/definition in Column A with the correct term in Column B.

Column A
_____ 1. Cessation of breathing for periods of time during sleep
_____ 2. A decrease in the amount, quality, and consistency of sleep
_____ 3. Awaking at night to urinate
_____ 4. Sudden muscle weakness during intense emotions
_____ 5. Difficulty falling or staying asleep
_____ 6. 24-hour day/night cycle
_____ 7. Disorder that produces abnormal behavior or emotions
_____ 8. Excessive sleepiness during the day

Column B
a. Cataplexy
b. Sleep deprivation
c. Circadian rhythm
d. Parasomnia
e. Narcolepsy
f. Sleep apnea
g. Insomnia
h. Nocturia

Complete the following:

9. An example of a factor that may affect sleep is:

10. Which of the following are appropriate nursing interventions to assist the older adult patient to achieve adequate sleep? Select all that apply.
    a. Altering the daily sleep and wake times _____
    b. Encouraging the patient to stay in bed even if not feeling sleepy _____
    c. Limiting patient's caffeine intake in the late afternoon or evening _____
    d. Lowering the head of the bed as flat as possible _____
    e. Encouraging increased fluid intake 2 to 4 hours before sleep _____
    f. Avoiding use of sedatives and hypnotics, if possible _____
    g. Encouraging daytime naps of 1 to 2 hours _____
    h. Provide social activities and exercise _____

11. Identify a way in which a nurse can promote a restful environment.

12. It is expected that during sleep the heart rate will decrease by 10 beats per minute from the daytime average rate.
    True _____ False _____

13. Very few older adults experience sleep problems.
    True _____ False _____

14. Normal sleep cycles usually last _____ (time) and are followed by _____ sleep.

15. Identify at least two nursing interventions that may be implemented related to a patient's sleep:
    a. Comfort measures

    b. Safety measures

16. A nurse tells a patient to include what information in a sleep log?

17. What are the best types of bedtime snacks for promoting sleep?

18. A nurse recommends to the parents of a newborn that the best way to position the child for sleep is on his/her:

19. Which of the following medications may be prescribed for a patient with narcolepsy? Select all that apply.
    a. Diazepam _____
    b. Modafinil _____
    c. Theophylline _____
    d. Sodium oxybate _____
    e. Zolpidem _____
20. Identify at least one patient outcome related to sleep.

Select the best answer for each of the following questions:

21. Individuals experience changes in their sleep patterns as they progress through the life cycle. A nurse assesses that a patient is experiencing bedtime fears, restlessness during the night, and nightmares. These behaviors are associated with:
    1. Infants
    2. Toddlers
    3. Preschoolers
    4. School-age children
22. A nurse is making rounds during the night to check on patients. When she enters one of the rooms at 3:00 AM, she finds that the patient is sitting up in a chair. The patient tells the nurse that she is not able to sleep. The nurse should first:
    1. Obtain an order for a hypnotic
    2. Assist the patient back to bed
    3. Provide a glass of warm milk and a back rub
    4. Ask about activities that have previously helped her sleep
23. A nurse is working on a pediatric unit at the local hospital. A 4-year-old boy is admitted to the unit. To assist this child to sleep, the nurse:
    1. Reads to him
    2. Teaches him relaxation activities
    3. Allows him to watch TV until he is tired
    4. Has him get ready for bed very quickly, without advance notice
24. A patient is found to be awakening frequently during the night. There are a number of medications prescribed for this patient. The nurse determines that the medication that may be creating this patient's particular sleep disturbance is the:
    1. Narcotic
    2. Beta blocker
    3. Antidepressant
    4. Antihistamine
25. A nurse suspects that a patient may be experiencing sleep deprivation. This suspicion is validated by the nurse's finding that the patient has:
    1. Increased reflex response
    2. Blurred vision
    3. Cardiac arrhythmia
    4. Increased response time
26. A nurse is working in a sleep clinic that is part of the local hospital. In preparing to work with patients with different sleep needs, the nurse understands that:
    1. Bedtime rituals are most important for adolescents.
    2. Regular use of sleeping medications is appropriate.
    3. Warm milk before bedtime may help a patient sleep.
    4. Individuals are most easily aroused from sleep during stages 3 and 4.
27. A nurse is visiting a patient in his home. While completing a patient history and home assessment, the nurse finds that there are many prescription medications kept in the bathroom cabinet. In determining possible areas that may influence the patient's sleep patterns, the nurse looks for a classification of medication that may suppress the patient's rapid eye movement (REM) sleep. The nurse looks in the cabinet for a:
    1. Diuretic
    2. Stimulant
    3. Beta blocker
    4. Nasal decongestant
28. A newborn is taken to a pediatrician's office for the first physical exam. The parents ask the nurse when they can expect the baby to sleep through the night. The nurse responds that, although there may be individual differences, infants usually develop a nighttime pattern of sleep by the age of:
    1. 6 weeks
    2. 3 months
    3. 6 months
    4. 10 months
29. A nurse is working with older adults in the senior center. A group is discussing problems with sleep. The nurse recognizes that older adults:
    1. Take less time to fall asleep
    2. Are more difficult to arouse from sleep
    3. Have a significant decline in stage 4 sleep
    4. Require more sleep than a middle-aged adult
30. A patient with congestive heart failure is being discharged from the hospital to her home. The patient will be taking a diuretic daily. The nurse recognizes that, with this drug, the patient may experience:
    1. Nocturia
    2. Nightmares
    3. Reduced REM sleep
    4. Increased daytime sleepiness
31. During a home visit, a nurse discovers that the patient has been having difficulty sleeping. To assist the patient to achieve sufficient sleep, an appropriate question the nurse might ask is the following:
    1. "Do you keep your bedroom completely dark at night?"
    2. "Do you nap enough during the day?"

3. "Why don't you eat something right before you go to bed?"
4. "What kinds of things do you do right before bedtime?"

32. A patient has gone to the sleep clinic to determine what may be creating his sleeping problems. In addition, his partner is having sleep pattern interruptions. If this patient is experiencing sleep apnea, the nurse may expect the partner to identify that the patient:
    1. Snores excessively
    2. Talks in his sleep
    3. Is very restless
    4. Walks in his sleep

33. A nurse anticipates that the patient who is in non–rapid eye movement (NREM) stage 1 sleep is:
    1. Easily aroused
    2. Completely relaxed
    3. Having vivid, full-color dreams
    4. Experiencing significantly reduced vital signs

34. A nurse is working with a patient who has a history of respiratory disease. This patient is expected to demonstrate:
    1. Longer time falling asleep
    2. Decreased NREM sleep
    3. Increased awakenings in the early morning
    4. Need for extra pillows for comfort

35. To help promote sleep for a patient, a nurse recommends:
    1. Exercise about 2 hours before bedtime
    2. Intake of a large meal about 3 hours before bedtime
    3. Drinking alcoholic beverages at bedtime
    4. Napping frequently during the afternoon

36. An expected treatment for sleep apnea is:
    1. Biofeedback
    2. Full body massage
    3. Administration of hypnotics
    4. Continuous positive airway pressure (CPAP)

37. As sleep aids, medications that are considered relatively safe to use are:
    1. Nonbenzodiazepines
    2. Barbiturates
    3. Psychotropics
    4. Antihistamines

38. An expected observation of a patient in REM sleep is:
    1. Possible enuresis
    2. Sleepwalking
    3. Loss of skeletal muscle tone
    4. Easy arousal from external noise

39. A parent asks the nurse what the appropriate amount of sleep is for her 11-year-old child. The nurse responds correctly by informing the parent that children in this age-group should average:
    1. 14 hours per night
    2. 12 hours per night
    3. 10 hours per night
    4. 7 hours per night

STUDY GROUP QUESTIONS

- What is sleep?
- What are the physiological processes involved in sleep?
- How is sleep regulated by the body?
- What are the functions of sleep?
- What purpose do dreams serve?
- What are the normal requirements and patterns of sleep across the life span?
- What factors may influence sleep?
- What are some common sleep disorders and nursing interventions?
- What information should be included in a sleep history?
- How are the critical thinking and nursing processes applied with patients experiencing insufficient sleep or rest?
- What measures may be implemented by the nurse to promote sleep for patients/families?
- What information should be included in patient/family teaching for the promotion of rest and sleep?

STUDY CHART

Create a study chart to describe the *Sleep Patterns Across the Life Span* that identifies the sleep patterns and needs for infants, toddlers, preschoolers, school-age children, adolescents, adults, and older adults.

Answers available through your instructor.

31 Pain Management

CASE STUDY

1. A patient is going to be using a PCA pump with a morphine infusion after surgery.
    a. What assessments need to be made before and while the patient uses the pump?
    b. What information is needed in the teaching plan for this patient?

CHAPTER REVIEW

Match the description/definition in Column A with the correct term in Column B.

Column A

_____ 1. Local anesthesia, with minimal sedation, given between the vertebrae
_____ 2. Unpleasant, subjective sensory and emotional experience
_____ 3. Partial or complete disappearance of symptoms
_____ 4. Extends from the point of injury to another body area
_____ 5. Rapid onset, lasts briefly
_____ 6. Localized, sharp sensation resulting from stimulation of the skin
_____ 7. Increase in the severity of symptoms
_____ 8. Classification of medication used for pain relief
_____ 9. Prolonged, varying in intensity
_____ 10. Diffuse, radiating, and varying in intensity from dull to sharp

Column B

a. Pain
b. Analgesic
c. Exacerbation
d. Remission
e. Acute pain
f. Chronic pain
g. Superficial pain
h. Visceral pain
i. Radiating pain
j. Epidural infusion

Complete the following:

11. The first structure in the brain to process pain impulses is the:

12. The gate control theory of pain suggests that pain can be reduced through the use of:

13. Which of the following are physiological responses to acute pain as a result of sympathetic stimulation? Select all that apply.
    a. Decreased respiratory rate _____
    b. Increased heart rate _____
    c. Peripheral vasodilation _____
    d. Increased blood glucose level _____
    e. Diaphoresis _____
    f. Pupil constriction _____
    g. Pallor _____
    h. Decreased blood pressure _____

14. Provide an example of a lifestyle response to chronic pain.

15. Identify two responses that an infant or child would have to pain.

16. The single most reliable indicator of pain is the:

17. Using the PQRSTU assessment guide, identify nursing interventions for the following.
    a. Quality

    b. Region

    c. Timing

18. Identify how a nurse may assess the level of pain for the following patients.
    a. Toddler

    b. Person for whom English is a second language

19. To determine the location of a patient's pain, a nurse should ask the patient to:

20. A pain rating of _____ on a scale of 0 to 10 is an emergency and requires immediate action.

21. For a patient who experiences discomfort upon ambulation or during a dressing change, a nurse should plan to:

22. An example of how a nurse may individualize a patient's treatment for pain is:

23. Which of the following are correct statements regarding transcutaneous electrical nerve stimulation (TENS)? Select all that apply.
    a. It is an invasive procedure. _____
    b. It requires a health care provider's order. _____
    c. Skin preparation is required before electrode placement. _____
    d. Electrodes are applied directly onto dry skin. _____
    e. Controls are adjusted until the patient feels a buzzing sensation. _____
    f. Electrodes remain in the same area for the next treatment. _____

24. Which of the following medications are indicated for the treatment of mild to moderate pain? Select all that apply.
    a. Ibuprofen (Motrin) _____
    b. Morphine _____
    c. Codeine _____
    d. Tramadol (Ultram) _____
    e. Fentanyl _____
    f. Acetaminophen (Tylenol) _____
    g. Propoxyphene (Darvon) _____

25. Identify two examples of nonpharmacological interventions that may be implemented to relieve pain.

26. An example of an adjuvant medication that may be used in conjunction with an analgesic to manage a patient's pain is:

27. The usual dosage of on-demand morphine in the PCA is:

28. Complete the following about analgesics.
    a. A priority nursing intervention specifically for the patient with an epidural analgesic infusion is:
    b. A priority nursing assessment for all patients before and while receiving analgesics is:

29. Identify an intervention that a nurse should implement to adapt or alter the environment to promote a patient's comfort:

30. Identify examples of patients who may be unable to effectively communicate their pain experience.

31. The ABCDE approach to pain assessment and management is:
    A
    B
    C
    D
    E

32. Concomitant symptoms associated with pain include:

Select the best answer for each of the following questions:

33. Identify whether the following statements are true or false.
    a. Nurses can allow their own misconceptions about or interpretations of the pain experience to affect their willingness to intervene for their patient.
       True _____ False _____
    b. The degree and quality of pain are related to the patient's definition of pain.
       True _____ False _____
    c. When patients are experiencing pain, they will not hesitate to inform you.
       True _____ False _____
    d. Fatigue decreases a patient's perception of pain.
       True _____ False _____
    e. A nurse should provide descriptive words for a patient to assist in assessing the quality of the pain.
       True _____ False _____
    f. Pain assessment can be delegated to assistive personnel.
       True _____ False _____
    g. Large doses of opioids for the terminally ill patient will hasten the onset of death.
       True _____ False _____
    h. Health care providers will initially order higher doses than needed for patients with cancer pain.
       True _____ False _____
    i. The Joint Commission (TJC) has a standard that requires health care workers to assess all patients for pain.
       True _____ False _____

j. Pain is a normal part of aging.
      True _____ False _____
   k. Nurses should anticipate that higher doses of oral opioids will be ordered after patients are converted from the IV form.
      True _____ False _____
34. A patient is experiencing pain that is not being managed by analgesics given by the oral or intramuscular routes. Epidural analgesia is initiated. The nurse is alert for a complication of this treatment and observes the patient for:
   1. Diarrhea
   2. Hypertension
   3. Urinary retention
   4. An increased respiratory rate
35. A patient had a laparoscopic procedure this morning and is requesting a pain medication. The nurse assesses the patient's vital signs and decides to withhold the medication based on the finding of:
   1. Pulse rate = 90 beats per minute
   2. Respirations = 10 per minute
   3. Blood pressure = 130/80 mm Hg
   4. Temperature = 99°F, rectally
36. A nurse is working with an older adult population in the extended care facility. Many of the patients experience discomfort associated with arthritis and have analgesics prescribed. In administering an analgesic medication to an older adult patient, the nurse should:
   1. Give the medication when the pain increases in severity
   2. Combine opioids for a greater effect
   3. Use the IM route whenever possible
   4. Give the medication before activities or procedures
37. One of the patients that a nurse is working with on an outpatient basis at the local clinic has rheumatoid arthritis. The patient has no known allergies to any medications, so the nurse anticipates that the physician will prescribe:
   1. Amitriptyline
   2. Butorphanol
   3. Indomethacin
   4. Morphine
38. An adolescent has been carried to the sidelines of the soccer field after experiencing a twisted ankle. The level of pain is identified as low to moderate. The nurse observes that the patient has:
   1. Pupil constriction
   2. Diaphoresis
   3. A decreased heart rate
   4. A decreased respiratory rate
39. A nurse on the pediatric unit is finding that it is sometimes difficult to determine the presence and severity of pain in very young patients. The nurse recognizes that toddlers may be experiencing pain when they have:
   1. An increased appetite
   2. A relaxed posture
   3. An increased degree of cooperation
   4. Disturbances in their sleep patterns
40. A patient on the oncology unit is experiencing severe pain associated with his cancer. Although analgesics have been prescribed and administered, the patient is having "breakthrough pain." The nurse anticipates that his treatment will include:
   1. The use of a placebo
   2. Experimental medications
   3. An increase in the opioid dose
   4. Administration of medications every hour
41. A patient is experiencing pain that is being treated with a fentanyl transdermal patch. The nurse advises this patient to:
   1. Avoid exposure to the sun
   2. Change the patch site every 2 hours
   3. Apply a heating pad over the site
   4. Expect immediate pain relief when the patch is applied
42. A patient is experiencing severe pain and has been placed on a morphine drip. During the patient's assessment, the nurse finds that the patient's respiratory rate is 6 breaths per minute. The nurse anticipates that the patient will receive:
   1. Naloxone
   2. Morphine
   3. Incentive spirometry
   4. No additional treatment for this expected response
43. An assessment tool that allows for total freedom in identification of pain severity is the:
   1. Brief Pain Inventory (BPI)
   2. Visual Analog Scale (VAS)
   3. Verbal Descriptor Scale (VDS)
   4. Critical Care Pain Observation Tool (CCPOT)
44. A nurse is working for an oncology unit in the medical center. All of the patients experience pain that requires management. The nurse should visit first with the patient who is also exhibiting signs of:
   1. Anxiety
   2. Fatigue
   3. Distraction
   4. Depression
45. For a patient with a consistent level of discomfort, the most effective pain relief is achieved with administration of analgesics:
   1. PRN
   2. Every 3 to 4 hours
   3. Every 12 hours
   4. Around the clock
46. A nurse anticipates that the patient with visceral pain will describe the pain as:
   1. Sharp
   2. Cramping
   3. Burning
   4. Shooting

47. Which of the following orders would the nurse question for the patient who has an epidural infusion for pain relief?
    1. Use of pulse oximetry
    2. Tubing changes every 24 hours
    3. An order for a sedative
    4. Use of fentanyl in the infusion
48. A patient will be using an ambulatory infusion pump at home for analgesia. Additional teaching is required if the patient is observed:
    1. Wearing the pump in the shower
    2. Flushing the catheter with saline
    3. Clamping the catheter after the infusion
    4. Using stool softeners
49. Because of the possible cardiovascular and neurological effects, which of the following analgesic orders for an older adult patient should be questioned?
    1. Acetaminophen
    2. Aspirin
    3. Ibuprofen
    4. Propoxyphene

STUDY GROUP QUESTIONS

- How may a nurse use a holistic approach to assist a patient in achieving comfort?
- What is pain?
- What are the physiological components of the pain experience?
- How may a patient respond, physiologically and behaviorally, to a pain experience?
- What factors influence the pain experience?
- How are acute and chronic pain different?
- How should a nurse assess a patient's pain?
- How may a patient characterize pain?
- What nonpharmacological measures may be used to relieve pain?
- What interventions may a nurse implement to promote comfort and relieve pain?
- What pharmacological measures are available for pain relief?
- How is a back rub/massage performed to achieve an optimum effect?
- What actions should a nurse take if comfort or pain relief measures are not effective?
- What information should be included in patient/family teaching for pain control or relief?

STUDY CHART

Create a study chart to describe the *Factors Influencing Pain and Comfort* that identifies how age, sex, culture, meaning of pain, and previous experience of a patient alter the pain experience.

Answers available through your instructor.

CHAPTER 31 • Pain Management

Name_____   Date_____   Instructor's Name_____

Procedural Guidelines 31-1: Massage

	S	U	NP	Comments

1. Based on patient assessment, decide on performing massage on one or more body parts. Assess if patient has had neck or spinal trauma.
2. Perform hand hygiene.
3. Help patient to assume comfortable lying or sitting position.
4. Dim room lights and/or turn on soft music.
5. Use warm body lotion as lubricant.
6. Massage each body part at least 10 minutes.
   A. *Hands:* Make contact with the patient's skin, first with one hand and then the other. Using both hands, slowly open the patient's palm, gliding your fingers over the palmar surface. While supporting the hand, use both thumbs to apply friction to the palm and use them in a circular motion to stretch the palm outward. Massage each finger outward and then separately, using a corkscrew-like motion from base of finger to the tip. With thumb and finger, knead each small muscle in the patient's fingers. Glide hands smoothly from fingertips to wrists. Repeat for other hand.
   B. *Arms:* Use a gliding stroke to massage from the patient's wrist to forearm. With thumb and forefinger of both hands, knead muscles from forearm to shoulder. Continue kneading biceps, deltoid, and triceps muscles. Finish with gliding strokes from the wrist to the shoulder.
   C. *Neck:* Support the neck at the hairline with one hand, and, starting at the base of the neck, massage upward with a gliding stroke. Knead muscles on one side. Switch hands to support neck and knead other side. Stretch the neck slightly, with one hand at the top and the other at the bottom.
   D. *Back:* Begin at sacral area and massage in circular motion while moving upward from buttocks to shoulders. Use a firm, smooth stroke over the scapula. Continue in one smooth stroke to upper arms and laterally along sides of back down to iliac crests. Use long, gliding strokes along muscles of spine. Knead any muscles that feel tense or tight.
7. At end of massage, have patient relax, taking slow, deep breaths.

Nutrition 32

CASE STUDIES

1. You are working with a patient who is being discharged from the acute care unit after a heart attack (myocardial infarction). The patient's primary care provider has prescribed medical nutrition therapy, with a diet that is low in sodium and saturated fat. The patient comes from a family where food plays an important role in traditional culture practices.
   a. What do you need to know about the patient and the family to assist in dietary planning?
   b. How can you assist this patient to meet the prescribed dietary requirements?
2. A pregnant woman is at the medical office for a prenatal checkup. What nutritional recommendations should be provided to this patient?
3. You are working in a home care agency and have a large older adult patient population. In planning care, what nutritional considerations should be taken into account for these patients?
4. As an occupational health nurse, you are concerned with positive health behaviors for the employees. You have noticed that some of the workers are overweight. What should you include in a teaching plan to promote nutritional health for the employees?

CHAPTER REVIEW

Match the description/definition in Column A with the correct term in Column B.

Column A

_____ 1. Increase in blood glucose level
_____ 2. Breakdown of food products into smaller particles
_____ 3. Production of more complex chemical substances through the synthesis of nutrients
_____ 4. All biochemical and physiological processes by which the body maintains itself
_____ 5. Organic substances in food that are present in small amounts and act as coenzymes in biochemical reactions
_____ 6. Inorganic elements that act as catalysts in biochemical reactions
_____ 7. Substances necessary for body functioning
_____ 8. Breakdown of complex body substances into simpler substances
_____ 9. Decrease in blood glucose level
_____ 10. Measurement of size and makeup of body at specific sites

Column B

a. Anabolism
b. Hypoglycemia
c. Digestion
d. Anthropometry
e. Catabolism
f. Nutrients
g. Minerals
h. Metabolism
i. Hyperglycemia
j. Vitamins

Complete the following:

11. Identify an example of a nutrition objective from Healthy People 2010.

12. A vitamin that is synthesized by the body is:

13. Identify whether the following represent carbohydrates, proteins, or fats.
    a. Starches _____
    b. Meats _____
    c. Linoleic acid _____
    d. Fiber _____
    e. 9 kcal/g of energy _____
    f. Amino acids _____
    g. Fruits _____

14. What information can you provide to an individual at a health fair who is interested in general nutritional guidelines?

15. Provide an example of an alternative dietary pattern.

16. For each area of nutritional assessment, identify specific elements to pursue with the patient.
    a. Food and nutrient intake

Copyright © 2011, 2007, 2003 by Mosby, Inc., an affiliate of Elsevier Inc. All rights reserved.

b. Physical examination

c. Anthropometric measurements

17. Which of the following are indicators of malnutrition? Select all that apply.
    a. Listlessness _____
    b. Straight arms and legs _____
    c. Some fat under the skin _____
    d. Paresthesia _____
    e. Loss of ankle reflexes _____
    f. Rapid heart rate _____
    g. No palpable masses _____
    h. Apathy _____
    i. Dry, scaly skin _____
    j. Reddish-pink mucous membranes _____
    k. Spongy gums with marginal redness _____
    l. Surface papillae present on the tongue _____
    m. Pale conjunctivae _____
    n. Corneal xerosis _____
    o. Firm, pink nails _____
    p. Calf tenderness and tingling _____

18. A nurse calculates a patient's body mass index (BMI) by dividing the weight in kilograms by the height in square meters. If the patient weighs 180 pounds and is 6 feet tall, what is the BMI?

19. A neurogenic cause of dysphagia is:

    A myogenic cause is:

20. A common sign or symptom of food-borne illnesses is:

21. A nurse on an acute care unit wishes to promote a patient's appetite. Identify at least two interventions that should be implemented by the nurse.

22. Identify the interventions that a nurse should implement for the patient who is experiencing dysphagia.

23. An advantage of enteral nutrition over parenteral nutrition is that enteral nutrition:

24. Regarding complications of tube feedings:
    a. The most serious complication of tube feedings is:

    b. To avoid this complication, the nurse should:

25. The method of choice for long-term enteral feeding is:

26. The pH of the gastric aspirate for a patient who has been fasting is:

27. A parenteral nutrition formula that is hyperosmolar (greater than 10% dextrose) should be administered through a(n) _____ venous line.

28. A patient will be receiving parenteral nutrition (PN). Identify the following:
    a. The main reason for use of PN:

    b. A major nursing goal for the patient receiving PN:

    c. A nursing intervention to assist the patient in the prevention of metabolic complications related to PN therapy:

    d. Guidelines and precautions for lipid infusions:

29. Identify a dietary measure that should be implemented for a patient without teeth or with ill-fitting dentures.

30. Identify a nursing diagnosis and goal for a patient who is underweight.

31. Indicate whether the following statements are true or false.
    a. Infants require more protein than adults.
       True _____ False _____
    b. Childhood obesity has doubled in the last 20 years.
       True _____ False _____
    c. Unsaturated fatty acids have a minimal effect on blood cholesterol.
       True _____ False _____

32. Identify an example of an antioxidant vitamin.

33. What interventions should be implemented for a patient who is receiving enteral feedings? Select all that apply.
    a. Keep the head of the bed elevated to 30 to 45 degrees _____
    b. Withhold the feeding if the residual is 50 to 100 mL. _____
    c. Tube placement is confirmed by monitoring the pH of aspirate. _____
    d. Gastric residual volume is measured daily. _____
    e. Continuous feedings are administered through an infusion pump. _____
    f. Tubing should be flushed with 200 mL of water before and after each feeding. _____

Select the best answer for each of the following questions:

34. A nurse is working with a patient who requires an increase in complete proteins in the diet. The nurse recommends:
    1. Milk
    2. Cereals
    3. Legumes
    4. Vegetables

35. A nurse is talking with a community resident who has gone to the health fair. The resident tells the nurse that he takes a lot of extra vitamins every day. Because of the greater potential for toxicity, the resident is advised not to exceed the dietary guidelines for:
    1. Vitamin A
    2. Vitamin B_1
    3. Vitamin B_{12}
    4. Folic acid

36. A nurse is working with a patient who is a lactovegetarian. The food that is selected as appropriate for this dietary pattern is:
    1. Fish
    2. Milk
    3. Eggs
    4. Poultry

37. A patient states that he does not eat fish anymore. An appropriate follow-up question by the nurse is which of the following?
    1. "Why don't you like fish?"
    2. "What caused you to lose interest in fish?"
    3. "Fish makes you feel ill in some way?"
    4. "Aren't you aware that fish is a valuable source of nutrients?"

38. A nurse is preparing to insert a nasogastric tube for enteral feedings. The nurse recognizes that this intervention is used when the patient:
    1. Has a gag reflex
    2. Is not able to chew foods
    3. Is slow to eliminate food
    4. Is not able to ingest foods

39. A nurse is preparing the enteral feeding for a patient who has a nasogastric tube in place. The most effective method that the nurse can use to check for placement of a nasogastric tube is to:
    1. Perform a pH analysis of aspirated secretions
    2. Measure the visible tubing exiting from the nose
    3. Inject air into the tube and auscultate over the stomach
    4. Place the end of the tube into water and observe for bubbling

40. A female patient who has gone to a family planning center is taking an oral contraceptive. This patient should increase vitamin B_6 and niacin intake. The nurse recommends that the patient consume more:
    1. Tomatoes
    2. Whole grains
    3. Citrus fruits
    4. Green, leafy vegetables

41. A patient has heard on television that zinc is an important element in the body's immune response. The patient asks the nurse what foods contain zinc. Because of its zinc content, the nurse recommends:
    1. Fish
    2. Liver
    3. Whole grains
    4. Green, leafy vegetables

42. A nurse is assigned to make home visits to a number of patients. Of the patients that the nurse visits, the patient with the greatest risk of a nutritional deficiency is the patient with:
    1. Decreased metabolic requirements
    2. An alteration in dietary schedule
    3. A body weight that is 5% over the ideal weight
    4. A weight loss of 3% within the past 6 months

43. After surgery, a patient is having her dietary intake advanced. After a period of NPO, the patient is placed on a clear liquid diet. What food does the nurse request for the patient?
    1. Milk
    2. Soup
    3. Custard
    4. Popsicles

44. While completing an assessment during a home visit, a nurse discovers that the patient has a history of congestive heart failure and is taking digoxin 0.25 mg daily. Being aware that medications may influence the patient's dietary patterns, the nurse is alert to the patient experiencing:
    1. Anorexia
    2. Gastric distress
    3. An alteration in taste
    4. An alteration in smell

45. A patient on the unit has an enteral tube in place for feedings. When the nurse enters the room, the patient says that he is experiencing cramps and nausea. The nurse should:
    1. Cool the formula
    2. Remove the tube
    3. Use a more concentrated formula
    4. Decrease the administration rate

46. Which of the following statements made by the parent of an infant indicates the need for additional teaching?
    1. "I'll wait to give the baby regular cow's milk until he is a year old."
    2. "I'll start with cereal as the first solid food that I give to the baby after about 4 months."
    3. "I'll add a little honey to the baby's bottle to help him digest the formula."
    4. "When he can have them, I'll wait a few days in between giving the baby any new foods."

47. A nurse instructs a patient who is a vegan to specifically include which supplement in the diet?
    1. Vitamin A
    2. Vitamin C
    3. Vitamin B_{12}
    4. Niacin

CHAPTER 32 • Nutrition

48. The individual with the highest percentage of water in the body is a(n):
    1. Infant
    2. Obese patient
    3. Lean patient
    4. Older adult
49. A patient with a gastrostomy has an excessive residual volume. The nurse should:
    1. Request an order for a chest x-ray
    2. Alter the type of feeding being given
    3. Request an order for an antidiarrheal agent
    4. Maintain the patient in high-Fowler's position
50. A nurse is monitoring a patient's laboratory reports. Which of the following, if decreased, is indicative of anemia?
    1. BUN level
    2. Creatinine level
    3. Albumin level
    4. Hemoglobin level
51. A nurse is instructing the family of a patient who is on an National Dysphagia Diet Task Force (NDDTF) dysphagia puree diet to include:
    1. Mashed potatoes
    2. Moistened breads
    3. Well-cooked noodles
    4. Soft fruits
52. A nurse recognizes that a patient on a low cholesterol diet requires additional teaching if he indicates that he eats which of the following?
    1. Oatmeal
    2. Pastries
    3. Dried fruits
    4. Green peppers
53. A realistic weight loss goal for the patient who is overweight is:
    1. 1 pound per week
    2. 3 pounds per week
    3. 5 pounds per week
    4. 7 pounds per week
54. To prevent the presence of *E. coli* in food, a nurse specifically instructs a patient and family to:
    1. Carefully can foods at home
    2. Boil shellfish completely
    3. Cook ground beef well
    4. Keep dairy products refrigerated
55. A nurse is visiting a patient in the home and notes that additional teaching is required if the patient is observed:
    1. Cooking poultry to 180° F
    2. Thawing frozen foods at room temperature
    3. Discarding all foods that may be spoiled
    4. Cleaning the inside of the refrigerator with bleach
56. Tube feedings are ordered for a patient with a nasogastric tube. Unless the agency specifies otherwise, the nurse should:
    1. Dilute the feedings with water
    2. Infuse the feedings over the course of 1 to 2 hours
    3. Begin with 150 to 250 mL at a time
    4. Increase feedings by 100 to 150 mL per feeding every 8 hours

STUDY GROUP QUESTIONS

- What are the basic principles of nutrition?
- What body processes are involved in the intake, use, and elimination of foods?
- What are the six major nutrients, their purposes, and food sources?
- What are the current recommendations for daily nutritional intake?
- How do nutritional needs change across the life span?
- How does culture/ethnicity influence dietary intake?
- What are some common alternative food patterns?
- How should a nurse assess a patient's nutritional status?
- What patients are at a greater risk for nutritional deficiencies?
- What nursing diagnoses may be appropriate for patients with nutritional alterations?
- How does a nurse assist patients to meet nutritional needs in the health promotion, acute care, and restorative care settings?
- What special diets may be prescribed for individuals?
- What are the nursing procedures for implementation of enteral and parenteral nutrition?
- What guidelines and precautions should be considered by a nurse in assisting a patient with enteral or parenteral nutrition?
- What general information should be included for patients/families for promotion or restoration of an adequate nutritional intake?

STUDY CHART

Create a study chart to describe the Six Nutrients that identifies the uses of each in the body and their food sources: carbohydrates, proteins, lipids, vitamins, minerals, and water.

Answers available through your instructor.

CHAPTER 32 • Nutrition 203

Name _____ Date _____ Instructor's Name _____

Performance Checklist Skill 32-1: Aspiration Precautions

	S	U	NP	Comments

Assessment
1. Perform nutritional screening.
2. Assess patients who are at increased risk of aspiration for signs and symptoms of dysphagia.
3. Observe patient during mealtimes for signs of dysphagia, and allow patient to attempt to feed self. Note at end of meal if patient fatigues.
4. Ask patient about any difficulties with chewing or swallowing various textures of food.
5. Report signs and symptoms of dysphagia to the physician or health care provider.
6. Place identification on patient's chart or Kardex form indicating that dysphagia is present.

Planning
1. Instruct patient about what you are going to do and why.
2. Explain to patient why you are observing him or her while he or she eats.
3. Provide a 30-minute rest period before feeding time.

Implementation
1. Perform hand hygiene.
2. Provide thorough oral hygiene, including brushing of tongue, before meal.
3. Using penlight and tongue blade, gently inspect mouth for pockets of food.
4. Elevate head of patient's bed so that hips are flexed at a 90-degree angle or help patient to same position in a chair. Have patient assume a chin-tuck position.
5. Add thickener to thin liquids to create the consistency of mashed potatoes, or serve patient pureed foods.
6. Place ½ to 1 teaspoon of food on unaffected side of the mouth, allowing utensil to touch the mouth or tongue.
7. Place hand on throat to gently palpate swallowing event as it occurs. Swallowing twice is often necessary to clear the pharynx.
8. Observe patient consume various consistencies of foods and liquids.
9. Provide verbal coaching while feeding patient and positive reinforcement to patient.
10. Observe for coughing, choking, gagging, and drooling of food; suction airway as necessary.
11. Provide rest periods as necessary during meal.
12. Ask patient to remain sitting upright for at least 30 minutes after the meal.
13. Help patient to perform hand hygiene and mouth care.
14. Return patient's tray to appropriate place and perform hand hygiene.

Evaluation
1. Observe patient's ability to ingest foods of various textures and thicknesses.
2. Monitor patient's food and fluid intake.
3. Weigh patient weekly.
4. Observe patient's oral cavity after meal to detect pockets of food.
5. Record patient's tolerance of food textures, amount of assistance required, patient position during meal, absence or presence of dysphagia, and amount eaten.
6. Report any coughing, gagging, choking, or swallowing difficulties.

Copyright © 2011, 2007, 2003 by Mosby, Inc., an affiliate of Elsevier Inc. All rights reserved.

CHAPTER 32 • Nutrition

Name _____ Date _____ Instructor's Name _____

Performance Checklist Skill 32-2: Inserting a Nasogastric or Nasointestinal Feeding Tube

	S	U	NP	Comments

Assessment
1. Verify patient's identity and type of tube ordered with health care provider's order.
2. Verify patient's need for enteral tube feeding.
3. Assess patency of nares. Have patient close each nostril alternately and breathe. Examine each naris for patency and skin breakdown.
4. Assess patient's medical history for nasal problems and risk of aspiration.
5. Assess patient for gag reflex.
6. Assess patient's mental status.
7. Assess for bowel sounds.

Planning
1. Explain procedure to patient. Identify patient using at least two identifiers.
2. Explain to patient how to communicate during intubation by raising index finger to indicate gagging or discomfort.
3. Perform hand hygiene. Stand on same side of bed as naris for insertion. Position patient in sitting or high-Fowler's position. If patient is comatose, place in semi-Fowler's position with head propped forward with a pillow.
4. Place towel over patient chest. Keep facial tissues in reach.
5. Examine feeding tube for flaws: rough or sharp edges on distal end and closed or clogged outlet holes.
6. Determine length of tube you will insert, and mark with tape or indelible ink.
7. Prepare NG or NI tube for intubation.
    A. If the tube has a guide wire or stylet, inject 10 mL of water from 60-mL Luer-Lok or catheter-tip syringe into the tube.
    B. Make certain that you position guide wire securely against weighted tip and that both Luer-Lok connections fit snugly together.
8. Cut adhesive tape 10 cm (4 inches) long, or prepare tube fixation device.

Implementation
1. Put on clean gloves.
2. Dip tube with surface lubricant into glass of room temperature water or apply water-soluble lubricant.
3. Hand patient a glass of water with a straw or a glass with crushed ice (if able to swallow).
4. Gently insert tube through nostril to back of throat (posterior nasopharynx). May cause patient to gag. Aim back and down toward ear.
5. Check for position of tube in back of throat with penlight and tongue blade.
6. Have patient flex head toward chest after tube has passed through nasopharynx.
7. Emphasize need to mouth breathe and swallow during the procedure.
8. When you insert the tip of tube approximately 10 inches (in the adult), stop and listen for air exchange from the distal portion of the tube.
9. Encourage patient to swallow by giving small sips of water or ice chips. Advance tube as patient swallows. Rotate tube 180 degrees while inserting.
10. Advance tube each time patient swallows until it has advanced the desired length.

Copyright © 2011, 2007, 2003 by Mosby, Inc., an affiliate of Elsevier Inc. All rights reserved.

	S	U	NP	Comments

11. Check position of tube in back of throat with penlight and tongue blade.
12. Obtain gastric aspirate, and check placement of tube by measuring gastric pH.
13. After you obtain gastric aspirates, anchor tube to nose and avoid pressure on nares. Mark exit site with indelible ink. Use one of the following options for anchoring.
    A. **Apply tape**
        (1) Apply tincture of benzoin or other skin adhesive on tip of patient's nose and allow it to become "tacky."
        (2) Split one end of the adhesive tape strip lengthwise 5 cm (2 inches).
        (3) Wrap each of the 5-cm strips around tube as it exits nose.
    B. **Apply tube fixation device using shaped adhesive patch**
        (1) Apply wide end of patch to bridge of nose.
        (2) Slip connector around feeding tube as it exits nose.
14. Fasten end of NG tube to patient's gown using a piece of tape. Do not use safety pins.
15. Assist patient to a comfortable position.
16. Obtain x-ray film of chest/abdomen.
17. Change gloves, and administer oral hygiene. Cleanse tubing at nostril with washcloth dampened in soap and water.
18. Remove gloves, dispose of equipment, and perform hand hygiene.

Evaluation

1. Observe patient to determine response to NG or NI tube intubation. Have the patient speak. Check vital signs and oxygen saturation.
2. Confirm radiographic results.
3. Remove guide wire or stylet after radiographic confirmation.
4. Routinely assess location of external exit site marking on the tube as well as color and pH of fluid withdrawn from the NG or NI tube.
5. Record and report type and size of tube placed, location of distal tip of tube, patient's tolerance of procedure, pH value of gastric aspirate, and confirmation of tube position by x-ray films.

Name _____ Date _____ Instructor's Name _____

Performance Checklist Skill 32-3: Verifying Feeding Tube Placement

	S	U	NP	Comments

Assessment
1. Know the policy and procedures for frequency and method of checking tube placement in your facility.
2. Identify signs and symptoms of coughing, choking, or cyanosis.
3. Identify conditions that increase the risk for spontaneous tube dislocation from the intended position.
4. Observe the external portion of the tube for movement of the ink mark away from the mouth or nares.
5. Review patient's medication record to determine if patient is receiving a gastric acid inhibitor or a proton pump inhibitor.
6. Review patient's record for history of previous tube displacement.

Planning
1. Explain procedure to patient.

Implementation
1. Perform hand hygiene and apply gloves.
2. Measures to verify placement of tube should be conducted at the following times.
   A. For intermittently tube-fed patients, test placement immediately before each feeding and before administration of medications.
   B. For continuously tube-fed patients, test placement every 4 to 6 hours and before medication administration.
   C. Wait at least 1 hour after medication administration by tube or mouth.
3. Draw up 10 to 30 mL of air into a 60-mL syringe; then attach to end of feeding tube. Flush tube with 30 mL of air before attempting to aspirate fluid. Repositioning the patient from side to side is helpful. More than one bolus of air through the tube is necessary in some cases.
4. Draw back on syringe slowly and obtain 5 to 10 mL of gastric aspirate. Observe appearance of aspirate to help assess the position of the tube.
5. Gently mix aspirate in syringe and expel into medicine cup. Dip the pH strip into the fluid or apply a few drops of the fluid to the strip. Compare the color of the strip with the color on the chart provided by the manufacturer to determine pH.
6. If unable to aspirate fluid after repeated attempts, determine correct placement by verification of original x-ray examination of positioning, maintenance of tube in original taped position, absence of risk factors for tube dislocation, and no signs of the patient experiencing respiratory distress.
7. Irrigate tube.
8. Remove and dispose of gloves. Perform hand hygiene.

Evaluation
1. Observe patient for respiratory distress.
2. Verify that color, pH, and appearance of aspirate are consistent with the initial tube placement according to x-ray results.
3. Record and report pH and appearance of aspirate.

CHAPTER 32 • Nutrition

Name _____ Date _____ Instructor's Name _____

Performance Checklist Skill 32-4: Administering Enteral Nutrition via Nasoenteric, Gastrostomy, or Jejunostomy Tubes

	S	U	NP	Comments

Assessment
1. Assess patient's need for enteral tube feeding.
2. Assess for food allergies.
3. Auscultate for bowel sounds.
4. Obtain baseline weight and review laboratory values. Assess patient for fluid volume excess or deficit, electrolyte abnormalities, and metabolic abnormalities such as hyperglycemia.
5. Verify health care provider's order for formula, rate, route, and frequency.
6. For tubes placed through abdominal wall, assess stoma site for breakdown, irritation, or drainage.

Planning
1. Explain procedure to patient.
2. Perform hand hygiene.
3. Prepare feeding container to administer formula continuously.
   A. Verify patient's name, tube, and feeding with health care provider's order; use two patient identifiers to verify correct patient.
   B. Check expiration date on formula and integrity of container.
   C. Have tube feeding at room temperature.
   D. Connect tubing to container or prepare ready-to-hang container.
   E. Shake formula container well, and fill container with formula. Open stopcock on tubing, and fill tubing with formula to remove air. Hang formula on feeding pump pole.
4. For intermittent feeding, measure formula and have syringe ready. Be sure formula is at room temperature.
5. Place patient in high-Fowler's position or elevate head of bed at least 30 degrees.

Implementation
1. Perform hand hygiene. Apply gloves.
2. Determine tube placement.
3. Check for gastric residual.
   A. Draw up 10 to 30 mL of air and connect syringe to end of feeding tube. Flush tube with air. Pull back slowly, and aspirate the total amount of gastric contents that may be aspirated.
   B. Return aspirated contents to stomach unless the volume is greater than 200 mL. (Review agency policy.)
   C. Flush tube with 30 mL of water.
4. Initiate feeding.
   A. Syringe or intermittent feeding
      (1) Pinch proximal end of feeding tube.
      (2) Remove plunger from syringe and attach barrel of syringe to end of tube.
      (3) Fill syringe with measured amount of formula. Release tube, elevate syringe to no more than 18 inches (45 cm) above insertion site, and allow it to empty gradually by gravity. Repeat steps (1) to (3) until you have prescribed amount delivered to patient.
      (4) If using feeding bag, prime tubing and attach gavage tubing to end of feeding tube. Set rate by adjusting roller clamp on tubing or placing on a feeding pump. Allow bag to empty gradually over 30 to 60 minutes. Label bag with tube-feeding type, strength, and amount. Include date, time, and initials.
      (5) Maintain patient's head elevated 30 degrees for 30 minutes after tube feeding.

Copyright © 2011, 2007, 2003 by Mosby, Inc., an affiliate of Elsevier Inc. All rights reserved.

	S	U	NP	Comments

B. Continuous-drip method
  (1) Prime and hang feeding bag and tubing on IV pole.
  (2) Connect distal end of tubing to proximal end of feeding tube.
  (3) Connect tubing through infusion pump, and set rate (see manufacturer's directions).
5. Advance rate of concentration of tube feeding gradually.
6. Maintain head of bed elevated 30 degrees during continuous tube feeding.
7. After intermittent infusion or at end of infusion, irrigate feeding tube per hospital policy. Have registered dietitian recommend total free water requirement per day.
8. When you are not administering tube feedings, cap or clamp the proximal end of the feeding tube.
9. Rinse bag and tubing with warm water whenever feedings are interrupted. Use a new administration set every 24 hours.
10. For tubes placed through the abdominal wall, the exit site of the tube is usually left open to air. Clean insertion site per agency policy.

Evaluation
1. Measure residual volume per agency policy.
2. Monitor finger-stick blood glucose level (usually at least every 6 hours until maximum administration rate is reached and maintained for 24 hours).
3. Monitor intake and output every 8 hours.
4. Weigh patient daily until patient reaches and maintains maximum administration rate for 24 hours; then weigh patient 3 times per week.
5. Monitor laboratory values.
6. Observe patient's respiratory status.
7. Observe patient's level of comfort.
8. Auscultate bowel sounds.
9. For tubes placed through the abdominal wall, observe stoma site for integrity.
10. Record patient's response to tube feeding, patency of tube, and any side effects.
11. Record and report type and amount of feeding, status of feeding tube, amount of water administered, patient's tolerance, and adverse effects.

Urinary Elimination 33

CASE STUDIES

1. A patient is going to the medical center for an intravenous pyelogram (IVP).
   a. What nursing assessments and patient teaching should be completed before this test is performed?
   b. What are the nurse's responsibilities for the patient following an IVP?
2. You will be working with unlicensed assistive personnel in an extended care setting.
   a. What urinary care may be safely delegated by a nurse?
3. On an acute care unit, a patient is to have her catheter removed. The primary nurse tells you that all that is necessary is to "cut it, wait for the balloon to deflate, and pull it out."
   a. How will you proceed with this catheter removal?
4. A clean-voided or midstream urine specimen is required from a male patient. He is able to perform activities of daily living, including hygienic care.
   a. How will you teach this patient to obtain the specimen?
5. A patient had surgery and an incontinent urinary diversion was created.
   a. What are the special needs of this patient and the interventions that you will implement?

CHAPTER REVIEW

Match the description/definition in Column A with the correct term in Column B.

Column A	Column B
1. Accumulation of urine in the bladder because of inability to empty bladder completely	a. Urgency
2. Painful or difficult urination	b. Hematuria
3. Difficulty in initiating urination	c. Oliguria
4. Volume of urine remaining in the bladder after voiding	d. Retention
5. Feeling the need to void immediately	e. Nocturia
6. Voiding large amounts of urine	f. Frequency
7. Urination, particularly excessive, at night	g. Dysuria
8. Presence of blood in the urine	h. Residual urine
9. Voiding very often	i. Hesitancy
10. Diminished urinary output in relation to fluid intake	j. Polyuria

Complete the following:

11. An example of a noninvasive procedure that may be used to examine the urinary system is:

12. What are the indications for the use of intermittent and indwelling urinary catheterization?

13. What positions may be used for catheterization of a female patient?

14. The recommended daily fluid intake for dilution of urine, promotion of micturition, and flushing the urethra of microorganisms is:

    The minimum urinary output for an adult is _____ per hour.

15. Provide an example of how each of the following factors may influence urination.
    a. Sociocultural

    b. Fluid intake

c. Pathological conditions

d. Medications

16. a. The type of urinary incontinence that results from increased intra-abdominal pressure with leakage of a small amount of urine is called:

   b. The treatment for this type of incontinence includes:

17. Which of the following are the expected characteristics of a normal urine specimen? Select all that apply.
    a. pH 10 _____
    b. Protein 4 mg _____
    c. Presence of glucose _____
    d. Specific gravity 1.2 _____
    e. Amber color _____

18. What is a priority when managing a patient's condom catheter?

19. To maintain a patient's dignity and self-esteem when assisting with urinary elimination, the nurse makes sure to:

20. Manual compression of the bladder is called:

21. Which of the following statements are correct for urinary diversions? Select all that apply.
    a. A ureterostomy is a continent diversion. _____
    b. A transureterostomy connects the ureters and repositions one ureter through the abdominal wall. _____
    c. Continent diversions have pouches created to store urine. _____
    d. Patients with urinary diversions need special clothing and have activity restrictions. _____

22. For a patient on strict intake and output, urinary output is measured with:

23. Identify a method that a nurse may implement to stimulate a patient to void:

24. To assist a patient to start and stop the urine stream, a nurse instructs the patient that a way to strengthen the pelvic floor muscles is by performing:

25. Identify the distance of catheter insertion:
    a. Female adult patient:

    b. Male adult patient:

26. Which of the following are appropriate techniques for indwelling catheter care? Select all that apply.
    a. Keep the drainage bag below the level of the bladder. _____
    b. Provide perineal care daily. _____
    c. Cleanse in a direction toward the urinary meatus. _____
    d. Attach the drainage bag to the side rail of the bed. _____
    e. Open the connection at the drainage bag to obtain a urine specimen. _____
    f. Avoid having any dependent loops of tubing. _____
    g. Drain all urine in the bag before patient ambulation or exercise. _____
    h. For the immobile patient, empty the drainage bag every 24 hours. _____

27. To prevent nocturia, a nurse instructs a patient to:

28. Identify how the mobility status of an older adult may influence urination.

29. Which of the following are correct in regards to urodynamic testing? Select all that apply.
    a. Fasting is not required before the test. _____
    b. Patients stand during the procedure. _____
    c. Patients will be catheterized during the procedure. _____
    d. No discomfort is expected after the procedure. _____
    e. Fluids are restricted after the procedure. _____

30. How can urinary infection be prevented or reduced for a patient with an indwelling catheter?

31. Which of the following statements are correct regarding a cystoscopy? Select all that apply.
    a. The procedure may be performed under general anesthesia. _____
    b. Fluids are restricted before and during the procedure. _____
    c. Antibiotics are often administered intravenously. _____
    d. An informed consent is not required. _____
    e. Bowel preparation is performed the evening before the test. _____
    f. The patient is NPO if the test is performed with local anesthesia. _____
    g. Bed rest is usually indicated immediately after the test. _____

h. Bloody or cloudy urine may be observed after the test. _____
i. Fluid intake is encouraged after the test is completed. _____

Select the best answer for each of the following questions:

32. A patient on the medical unit is scheduled to have a 24-hour urine collection to diagnose a urinary disorder. The nurse should:
    1. Note the start time on the container
    2. Have the patient void while defecating
    3. Start with the first voiding sample from the patient
    4. Continue with the test if a specimen is flushed away
33. One of a nurse's assigned patients is experiencing urinary retention. The nurse anticipates a medication that may be ordered for this difficulty is:
    1. Propantheline
    2. Oxybutynin
    3. Bethanechol
    4. Phenylpropanolamine
34. Several patients in a long-term care unit have indwelling urinary catheters in place. A nurse is delegating catheter care to the nursing assistant. The nurse includes instruction in:
    1. Using lotion on the perineal area
    2. Disinfecting the first 2 to 3 inches of the catheter every 2 hours
    3. Ensuring that the drainage bag is secured to the side rail
    4. Cleansing about 4 inches along the length of the catheter, proximal to distal
35. A patient with recurrent urinary tract infections asks a nurse how they may be avoided. In addition to hygienic care, the nurse discusses with the patient that selected foods may help prevent infections, while other foods may not. The nurse recommends that the patient promote urinary acidity by avoiding:
    1. Eggs
    2. Prunes
    3. Orange juice
    4. Whole grain breads
36. Prevention of infection is a patient outcome that is identified for a patient with a urinary alteration and an indwelling catheter. The nurse assists the patient to attain this outcome by:
    1. Emptying the drainage bag daily
    2. Draining all urine after the patient ambulates
    3. Performing perineal care q8h and prn
    4. Opening the drainage system only at the connector points to obtain specimens
37. A patient being seen at a urologist's office suffers from urge incontinence. The nurse anticipates that treatment for this difficulty will include:
    1. Biofeedback
    2. Catheterization
    3. Cholinergic drug therapy
    4. Electrical stimulation
38. A nurse notes that there is an order on a patient's record for a sterile urine specimen. The patient has an indwelling urinary catheter. The nurse will proceed to obtain this specimen by:
    1. Withdrawing the urine from a urinometer
    2. Opening the drainage bag and removing urine
    3. Disconnecting the catheter from the drainage tubing
    4. Using a syringe to withdraw urine from the catheter port
39. A patient had a laparoscopic procedure in the morning and is having difficulty voiding later that day. Before initiating invasive measures, the nurse intervenes by:
    1. Administering a cholinergic agent
    2. Applying firm pressure over the perineal area
    3. Increasing the patient's daily fluid intake to 3000 mL
    4. Rinsing the perineal area with warm water
40. To determine the possibility of a renal problem, a patient is scheduled to have an intravenous pyelogram (IVP). Immediately after the procedure, a nurse will need to evaluate the patient's response and be alert to:
    1. An infection in the urinary bladder
    2. An allergic reaction to the contrast material
    3. Urinary suppression from injury to kidney tissues
    4. Incontinence from paralysis of the urinary sphincter
41. A unit manager is evaluating the care that has been given to a patient by a new nursing staff member. The manager determines that the staff member has implemented an appropriate technique for clean-voided urine specimen collection if:
    1. Fluids were restricted before the collection
    2. Sterile gloves were applied for the procedure
    3. The specimen was collected after the initial stream of urine had passed
    4. The specimen was placed in a clean container and then placed in the utility room
42. A patient at the urology clinic is diagnosed with reflex incontinence. This problem was identified by the patient's statement of experiencing:
    1. A constant dribbling of urine
    2. An urge to void and not enough time to reach the bathroom
    3. An uncontrollable loss of urine when coughing or sneezing
    4. No urge to void and being unaware of bladder fullness
43. A female patient has an order for urinary catheterization. A nursing student will be evaluated by the instructor on the insertion technique. The student is identified as implementing appropriate technique if:
    1. The catheter is advanced 7 to 8 inches
    2. The balloon is inflated before insertion to test its patency

3. The catheter is reinserted if it is accidentally placed in the vagina
4. Both hands are kept sterile throughout the procedure

44. A patient is diagnosed with prostate enlargement. The nurse is alert to a specific indication of this problem when finding that the patient has:
    1. Chills
    2. Cloudy urine
    3. Polyuria
    4. Bladder distention

45. Stress incontinence is associated with:
    1. Irritation of the bladder
    2. Neurological trauma
    3. Alcohol or caffeine ingestion
    4. Coughing or sneezing

46. For patients with diabetes mellitus, a nurse anticipates that the patients will experience:
    1. Dribbling
    2. Hesitancy
    3. Polyuria
    4. Hematuria

47. A nurse recognizes that one of the specific purposes of intermittent catheterization is for:
    1. Prevention of obstruction
    2. Assessment of residual urine
    3. Urinary drainage during surgical procedures
    4. Recording of output for comatose patients

48. A nurse notes that there is no urine in a drainage bag since it was emptied 1½ hours ago. The nurse should first:
    1. Remove the catheter
    2. Provide additional fluids
    3. Check for kinks or bends in the tubing
    4. Apply external pressure on the patient's bladder

49. The best way to remove urine from a patient's skin is for the nurse to use:
    1. Alcohol
    2. Mild soap
    3. An antibacterial agent
    4. A hydrogen peroxide mix

50. A nurse manager is observing a new nurse staff member provide care for a patient with a condom catheter. The manager determines that correction and additional instruction are required for the new employee if the staff nurse is observed:
    1. Draping the patient and exposing only the genitalia
    2. Attaching the urinary drainage bag to the lower bed frame
    3. Using adhesive tape to secure the catheter to the patient's penis
    4. Clipping the hair at the base of the penile shaft

51. A patient who is taking pyridium needs to be instructed that a specific side effect of this medication is that:
    1. The urine will turn orange
    2. There will be an increased frequency of urination
    3. Back pain will be moderately severe
    4. Occasional dizziness may be experienced

52. A nurse anticipates that a treatment option for a patient with functional incontinence will include:
    1. Catheterization
    2. Bladder training
    3. Electrical stimulation
    4. Hormone replacement

STUDY GROUP QUESTIONS

- What is the normal anatomy and physiology of the urinary system?
- What factors may influence urination?
- What are some common urinary elimination problems, their causes, and patient signs and symptoms?
- How do growth and development influence urinary function and patterns?
- How can urinary drainage be surgically altered, and why would an alteration be necessary?
- What measures may be implemented to prevent infection in the urinary tract?
- How does a nurse assess a patient's urinary function/elimination?
- What noninvasive and invasive procedures may be used to determine urinary function?
- What diagnostic tests are used to determine the characteristics of urine?
- What are the expected characteristics of urine?
- What nursing interventions are appropriate for promoting urination in the health care and home care settings?
- What information should be included in teaching patients/families about promotion of urination and prevention of infection?

Answers available through your instructor.

CHAPTER 33 • Urinary Elimination

Name _____ Date _____ Instructor's Name _____

Performance Checklist Skill 33-1: Inserting and Removing Straight or Indwelling Catheters

	S	U	NP	Comments

Assessment
1. Assess status of patient and allergy history. Assess for previous catheterization, including catheter size and patient's response.
2. Review patient's medical record, including prescriber's order and nurses' notes.
3. Perform hand hygiene, apply clean gloves, and assess for perineal anatomical landmarks, erythema, drainage, and odor. Remove gloves, and perform hand hygiene.
4. Assess bladder for fullness via palpation or bladder scanner.
5. Review medical record for any pathological condition that will impair passage of catheter (e.g., enlarged prostate gland in men).
6. Assess patient's knowledge of the purpose of catheterization and past experience.

Planning
1. Collect appropriate equipment. Explain procedure to patient.
2. Arrange for extra nursing personnel to assist as necessary.
3. Verify patient's identity by using at least two patient identifiers. Compare patient's name and one other identifier, such as hospital identification number, with medication administration record (MAR). Ask patient to state name as a third identifier.

Implementation
1. Perform hand hygiene.
2. Close curtain or door.
3. Raise bed to appropriate working height.
4. Facing patient, stand on left side of bed if right-handed (on right side if left-handed). If side rails in use, raise side rail on opposite side of bed and lower side rail on working side. Clear bedside table and arrange equipment.
5. Place waterproof pad under patient.
6. Position patient.
   A. **Female Patient**
      (1) Assist to dorsal recumbent position (supine with knees flexed). Ask patient to relax thighs so she is able to externally rotate the hip joints.
      (2) Optional position for female patient is side-lying (Sims') position with upper leg flexed at knee and hip if unable to be supine. Take extra precautions to cover rectal area with drape during procedure to reduce chance of cross-contamination.
   B. **Male Patient**
      (1) Assist to supine position. Ensure thighs are slightly abducted.
7. Drape patient.
   A. **Female Patient**
      (1) Drape with bath blanket. Place blanket diamond fashion over patient, with one corner at patient's neck, side corners over each arm and side, and last corner over perineum.
   B. **Male Patient**
      (1) Drape upper trunk with bath blanket. Cover lower extremities with bed sheet, exposing only genitalia.
8. Apply clean gloves, wash perineal area with soap and water as needed; dry and dispose of gloves.
9. Position lamp to illuminate perineal area. (When using flashlight, have assistant hold it.)

Copyright © 2011, 2007, 2003 by Mosby, Inc., an affiliate of Elsevier Inc. All rights reserved.

214 CHAPTER 33 • Urinary Elimination

	S	U	NP	Comments

10. Perform hand hygiene. When inserting an indwelling catheter open package containing drainage system; place drainage bag over edge of bottom bed frame and bring drainage tube up between side rail and mattress.
11. Open catheterization kit according to directions, keeping bottom of container sterile.
12. Place plastic bag that contains kit within reach of work area to use as waterproof bag to dispose of used supplies.
13. Apply sterile gloves.
14. Organize supplies on sterile field. Open inner sterile package containing catheter. Pour sterile antiseptic solution into correct compartment containing sterile cotton balls. Open lubricant packet. Remove specimen container (lid should be placed loosely on top) and prefilled syringe from collection compartment of tray and set them aside on sterile field if needed.
15. Lubricate catheter 2.5 to 5 cm (1 to 2 inches) for women and 12.5 to 17.5 cm (5 to 7 inches) for men. NOTE: Some catheter kits will have a plastic sheath over the catheter that must be removed before lubrication. (*Optional:* Physician may order use of lubricant containing local anesthetic.)
16. Apply sterile drape, keeping gloves sterile.
    A. **Female Patient**
       (1) Allow top edge of drape to form cuff over both hands. Place drape on bed between patient's thighs. Slip cuffed edge just under buttocks, taking care not to touch contaminated surface with gloves.
       (2) Pick up fenestrated sterile drape and allow it to unfold without touching an unsterile object. Apply drape over perineum, exposing labia and being sure not to touch contaminated surface.
    B. **Male Patient:** You will use one of two methods for draping, depending on preference.
       (1) First method: Apply drape over thighs and below penis without completely opening drape.
       (2) Second method: Apply drape over thighs just below penis. Pick up fenestrated sterile drape, allow it to unfold, and drape it over penis with fenestrated slit resting over penis.
17. Place sterile tray and contents on sterile drape between legs. Open specimen container. NOTE: Patient's size and positioning will dictate exact placement.
18. Cleanse urethral meatus.
    A. **Female Patient**
       (1) With nondominant hand, carefully retract labia to fully expose urethral meatus. **Maintain position of nondominant hand throughout procedure.**
       (2) Holding forceps in sterile dominant hand, pick up cotton ball saturated with antiseptic solution and clean perineal area, wiping front to back from clitoris toward anus. Using a new cotton ball for each area, wipe along the far labial fold, near labial fold, and directly over center of urethral meatus.
    B. **Male Patient**
       (1) If patient is not circumcised, retract foreskin with nondominant hand. Grasp penis at shaft just below glans. Retract urethral meatus between thumb and forefinger. **Maintain nondominant hand in this position throughout procedure.**

Copyright © 2011, 2007, 2003 by Mosby, Inc., an affiliate of Elsevier Inc. All rights reserved.

CHAPTER 33 • Urinary Elimination

	S	U	NP	Comments

    (2) With dominant hand, pick up antiseptic-soaked cotton ball with forceps and clean penis. Move cotton ball in circular motion from urethral meatus down to base of glans. Repeat cleansing three more times, using clean cotton ball each time.

19. Pick up catheter with gloved dominant hand 2.5 to 5 cm (1 to 2 inches) from catheter tip. Hold end of catheter loosely coiled in palm of dominant hand. (*Optional:* May grasp catheter with forceps.) Place distal end of catheter in urine tray receptacle if performing a straight catheterization.

20. Insert catheter.
    A. **Female Patient**
        (1) Ask patient to bear down gently as if to void and slowly insert catheter through urethral meatus.
        (2) Advance catheter a total of 5 to 7.5 cm (2 to 3 inches) in adult **or until urine flows out catheter's end.** When urine appears, advance the indwelling catheter another 2.5 to 5 cm (1 to 2 inches). Further insertion of a straight catheter is not necessary. Do not force against resistance.
        (3) Release labia, and hold catheter securely with nondominant hand.
    B. **Male Patient**
        (1) Lift penis to position perpendicular to patient's body, and apply light traction.
        (2) Ask patient to bear down as if to void and slowly insert catheter through urethral meatus.
        (3) In the adult, advance a straight catheter until urine flows out catheter's end. For an indwelling catheter, advance to the bifurcation of the drainage and balloon inflation port. If you meet resistance, do not attempt forceful catheter insertion.
        (4) Lower penis and hold catheter securely in nondominant hand. Reposition the foreskin if necessary.

21. Collect urine specimen as needed. Fill specimen cup to correct level (20 to 30 mL) by holding end of catheter in dominant hand over cup. A residual volume requires all urine to be drained.

22. Remove the straight catheter at this time. Withdraw slowly while gently palpating over patient's bladder. Check the amount of urine collected by placing in graduated cylinder.

23. Inflate balloon fully per manufacturer's recommendations, and then release catheter with nondominant hand and pull gently to feel resistance.

24. Attach end of catheter to collecting tube of drainage system, if necessary. Drainage bag must be below level of bladder; do not place bag on side rails of bed.

25. Anchor indwelling catheter.
    A. **Female Patient**
        (1) Secure catheter tubing to inner thigh with strip of nonallergenic tape (use paper tape if allergic) or use a commercial multipurpose tube holder with a Velcro strap if available. Allow for slack so movement of thigh does not create tension on catheter.
    B. **Male Patient**
        (1) Secure catheter tubing to top of thigh or lower abdomen (with penis directed toward chest). Allow slack in catheter so movement does not create tension on catheter. Clip drainage tubing to edge of mattress.

CHAPTER 33 • Urinary Elimination

	S	U	NP	Comments

(2) Be sure there are no obstructions in tubing. Coil excess tubing on bed, and fasten it to bottom sheet with clip from kit or with rubber band and safety pin.

26. Assist patient to comfortable position. Wash and dry perineal area as needed.
27. Remove gloves and dispose of equipment, drapes, and urine in proper receptacles.
28. Straight or intermittent catheterization
    A. Follow steps 1 to 16. Note the differences between an indwelling and straight catheter.

Removal of Indwelling Foley Catheter

29. Perform hand hygiene, put on clean gloves, and provide privacy.
30. Prepare the patient.
    A. Provide an explanation of procedure.
    B. Position the patient in the same position as during catheterization (see step 5).
    C. Remove the tape or Velcro strap securing the catheter tubing.
31. Place a towel between a female patient's thighs or over a male patient's thighs.
32. Insert the syringe tip into the balloon injection port. Slowly and completely withdraw all the solution to deflate the balloon completely.
33. Gently withdraw the catheter, and gather it in the towel. Discard supplies. Wash and dry perineal area, and position patient to comfort.
34. Empty urine collection bag into graduated container, and measure amount for I&O. Discard items into trash receptacle. Perform hand hygiene.

Evaluation

1. Ask about patient's comfort.
2. Observe character and amount of urine in drainage system.
3. Determine that there is no urine leaking from catheter or tubing connections.
4. Report and record type and size of catheter inserted, amount of fluid used to inflate balloon, characteristics of urine, amount of urine, reasons for catheterization, specimen collection if appropriate, and patient's response to procedure and teaching concepts.
5. Initiate I&O records.
6. If catheter is definitely in bladder and no urine is produced within an hour, absence of urine should be reported to physician immediately.
7. Ensure that times for catheter care are indicated in the care plan. Patients with indwelling catheters receive perineal and catheter care every 8 hours and after bowel movements.
8. Record in nurses' notes when catheter care was given and condition of urethral meatus.

Name _____ Date _____ Instructor's Name _____

Procedural Guidelines 33-1: Applying a Condom Catheter

	S	U	NP	Comments
1. Check health care provider's order.	___	___	___	_____
2. Perform hand hygiene.	___	___	___	_____
3. Assess urinary elimination patterns, patient's ability to voluntarily urinate, and continence.	___	___	___	_____
4. Assess mental status of patient and explain procedure.	___	___	___	_____
5. Provide for privacy by closing room door or bedside curtain. Raise bed to working height and lower side rail on working side.	___	___	___	_____
6. Prepare condom catheter and drainage bag (see manufacturer's directions).	___	___	___	_____
7. Assist patient to a supine or sitting position. Place bath blanket over upper torso, fold a sheet over lower torso so that only penis is exposed.	___	___	___	_____
8. Apply clean gloves; provide perineal care and dry thoroughly.	___	___	___	_____
9. If patient is uncircumcised, return foreskin to normal position.	___	___	___	_____
10. If needed, clip hair at base of penile shaft. Do not shave pubic area. An alternative to trimming pubic hair is placement of a hair guard (see manufacturer's directions) over the penis before applying the catheter.	___	___	___	_____
11. *Option:* Apply skin prep to penile shaft, and allow to dry.	___	___	___	_____
12. Secure condom catheter according to manufacturer's directions.	___	___	___	_____
13. Connect drainage tubing to end of condom catheter. Connect catheter to large-volume drainage bag or leg bag. Attach large-volume drainage bag to lower bed frame. Coil excess tubing on bed.	___	___	___	_____
14. Make patient comfortable and raise side rails as needed.	___	___	___	_____
15. Observe urinary drainage, drainage tube patency, condition of penis, and tape placement.	___	___	___	_____

34 Bowel Elimination

CASE STUDIES

1. You have arranged with your instructor and the home care agency to visit a 76-year-old woman. In completing your initial assessment, the patient tells you that she has been having difficulty over the past 2 years in "moving her bowels." She takes you to the bathroom, where she shows you a collection of over-the-counter laxatives and enemas. The patient also tells you that, since the death of her husband, she does not do a lot of cooking, relying on sandwiches and prepared foods.
   a. Based on this information, identify a nursing diagnosis, patient goal(s)/outcomes, and nursing interventions related to bowel elimination.
2. A patient is scheduled to have a colonoscopy performed.
   a. Identify the patient teaching that is provided before the procedure.

CHAPTER REVIEW

Match the description/definition in Column A with the correct term in Column B.

	Column A	Column B
_____	1. Propulsion of food through the gastrointestinal (GI) tract	a. Valsalva maneuver
_____	2. Agent used to empty the bowel	b. Stoma
_____	3. Artificial opening in the abdominal wall	c. Hemorrhoids
_____	4. Dilated rectal veins	d. Peristalsis
_____	5. Blood in the stool	e. Melena
_____	6. Contraction of abdominal muscles, while forcing expiration against a closed airway	f. Cathartic

Complete the following:

7. Constipation in the older adult is usually the result of:

8. What types of patients should be cautioned against straining during defecation and why?

9. As a result of persistent diarrhea, a patient is at risk for:

10. Provide an example of the effect that fecal incontinence can have on an individual:

11. Which of the following factors will interfere with bowel elimination and decrease peristalsis? Select all that apply.
    a. Slower esophageal emptying _____
    b. Eating raw vegetables _____
    c. Immobilization _____
    d. Consumption of lean meats _____
    e. Anxiety _____
    f. Emotional depression _____
    g. Abdominal surgery _____
    h. Use of antibiotics _____
    i. Food allergies _____
    j. Parkinson disease _____
    k. Use of narcotic analgesics _____
    l. Drinking fruit juices _____
    m. Tube feedings _____

12. Taking into account patients' cultural backgrounds, a nurse recognizes that individuals who are _____ try to avoid exposure of the lower torso.

13. Identify a risk factor for colon cancer.

14. Identify two nursing interventions for a patient who is experiencing:
    a. Constipation

    b. Diarrhea

Copyright © 2011, 2007, 2003 by Mosby, Inc., an affiliate of Elsevier Inc. All rights reserved.

CHAPTER 34 • Bowel Elimination

15. Provide an example of how each of the following factors influences bowel elimination.
    a. Positioning
    b. Pregnancy
    c. Diagnostic tests

16. How can a nurse promote comfort for a patient with hemorrhoids?

17. Identify one possible cause for an increase in both the total bilirubin and alkaline phosphatase levels.

18. What is the correct position for an adult patient to receive an enema?

19. An enema that is used to treat patients with hyperkalemia is:

20. a. A hypertonic enema works by:

    b. A commonly used over-the-counter hypertonic enema is:

21. A patient receiving tube feedings may experience diarrhea as a result of:

22. Identify what should be included in a focused assessment of a patient's bowel function.

23. What surgical procedures are anticipated for patients with:
    a. Colorectal cancer

    b. Diverticulitis

24. Which of the following are correct practices that should be included in the teaching plan for a patient with an ostomy? Select all that apply.
    a. Using creams around the peristomal skin _____
    b. Emptying the pouch when it is one-fourth to one-half full _____
    c. Washing the peristomal skin with a detergent soap _____
    d. Applying Kenalog spray for a yeast infection _____
    e. Anticipating a significant amount of bleeding _____
    f. Changing the entire pouching system daily _____
    g. Using the same manufacturer's flange and pouch _____
    h. Cutting the pouch opening $1/16$ to $1/8$ inch larger than the stoma _____
    i. Applying a skin barrier around the stoma _____

25. Which of the following fecal characteristics are expected findings? Select all that apply.
    a. Yellow infant's stool _____
    b. A defecation frequency greater than 3 times per day for an adult _____
    c. White-colored stool _____
    d. Tarry stool _____
    e. Soft, formed stool _____
    f. 150 mg/day average amount of stool _____

26. Before giving a patient a bedpan, the nurse should:

27. Select which of the following interventions may be delegated to assistive personnel.
    a. Digital removal of an impaction _____
    b. Enema administration _____
    c. Ostomy pouching _____

28. For an adult patient who will receive an enema, the nurse recognizes that the tube should be inserted _____ inches, and the height of the bag for a regular enema should be _____ inches above the anus.

29. a. *Clostridium difficile* is transmitted by:

    b. Transmission of *C. difficile* can be prevented or reduced by:

30. Identify a positive outcome for a patient who has a colostomy.

31. Normal defecation in the acute or long-term care environment may be promoted by:

32. Nasogastric tube irrigation is usually done with _____ mL of _____ (solution). Suction applied to the NG tube is usually _____.

33. Place the following steps for nasogastric tube insertion in the correct order:
    a. Have the patient drink water and swallow. _____
    b. Perform hand hygiene. _____
    c. Auscultate for bowel sounds. _____
    d. Insert the tube past the nasopharynx. _____
    e. Prepare the equipment. _____
    f. Measure the distance to insert the tube. _____
    g. Ask the patient to talk. _____

CHAPTER 34 • Bowel Elimination

34. What are the correct actions for pouching an ostomy? Select all that apply.
    a. Change the skin barrier daily. _____
    b. Cleanse the skin with warm tap water. _____
    c. Use sterile technique. _____
    d. Scrub the skin to remove excess skin adhesive. _____
    e. Cut the opening of the barrier $1/16$ inch to $1/8$ inch larger than the stoma. _____
    f. Place a hole in the pouch to release flatus. _____

Select the best answer for each of the following questions:

35. For a patient with a nasogastric tube who has a painful, distended abdomen, the first most appropriate action by the nurse is to:
    1. Remove the tube
    2. Irrigate the tube
    3. Pull the tube out farther
    4. Notify the supervisor

36. A patient expresses a feeling of mild cramping during the administration of a saline enema. The nurse should first:
    1. Discontinue the procedure
    2. Change the solution
    3. Lower the bag to slow the infusion
    4. Allow the solution to cool

37. A patient in a senior day care center is experiencing some constipation. A commonly prescribed medication is a wetting agent or stool softener, such as:
    1. Bisacodyl
    2. Phenolphthalein
    3. Magnesium hydroxide
    4. Docusate sodium

38. A nurse observes a nursing assistant carrying out bowel retraining with a patient in the extended care facility. The nurse identifies that the assistant implements an incorrect procedure when:
    1. Allowing the patient adequate time in the bathroom
    2. Taking the patient to the bathroom at regular times throughout the day
    3. Pulling the curtain around the patient while on the commode
    4. Restricting fluids with breakfast and lunch meals

39. For patients that have been prescribed extended bed rest, the prolonged immobility may result in reduced peristalsis and fecal impaction. A nurse is alert to one of the first signs of an impaction when the patient experiences:
    1. Headaches
    2. Abdominal distention
    3. Overflow diarrhea
    4. Abdominal pain with guarding

40. A patient has been admitted to an acute care unit with a diagnosis of biliary disease. When assessing the patient's feces, the nurse expects that they will be:
    1. Bloody
    2. Pus filled
    3. Black and tarry
    4. White or clay colored

41. Upon review of a patient's laboratory results, a nurse notes that the patient is experiencing hypocalcemia. The nurse will plan to implement measures to prevent:
    1. Gastric upset
    2. Malabsorption
    3. Constipation
    4. Fluid secretion

42. A nurse is preparing to administer an enema to a 7-year-old child. When assembling the equipment, the nurse will prepare an enema of:
    1. 150 to 250 mL of fluid
    2. 250 to 350 mL of fluid
    3. 400 to 500 mL of fluid
    4. 500 to 750 mL of fluid

43. A nurse recognizes that the greatest challenge for skin care will be for a patient with a(n):
    1. Ileostomy
    2. Sigmoid colostomy
    3. Descending ostomy
    4. Ileoanal pouch

44. A nurse evaluates that a patient has normal bowel sounds by auscultating all four quadrants and finding:
    1. 4 sounds per minute
    2. 15 sounds per minute
    3. 40 sounds per minute
    4. No bowel sounds after 1 minute

45. A nurse instructs a patient who is taking an iron supplement that his stool may be:
    1. Red and liquid
    2. Pale and frothy
    3. Mucus filled
    4. Black and tarry

46. A nurse is caring for a patient with a Salem sump tube for gastric decompression. Which of the following actions by the nurse requires correction?
    1. Clamping off the blue lumen or air vent
    2. Using clean technique to insert the tube
    3. Anchoring the tube to the patient's gown
    4. Keeping the nares lubricated

47. A nurse recognizes that the intake of mineral oil to promote bowel elimination interferes with the absorption of:
    1. Vitamin A
    2. Vitamin B_6
    3. Vitamin C
    4. Niacin

48. Further follow-up is required if a patient informs the nurse that he uses:
    1. Fleet enemas
    2. Tap water enemas
    3. Castile soap enemas
    4. Normal saline enemas

49. During a digital removal of a fecal impaction, a nurse notes that the patient has bradycardia. The nurse should:
    1. Provide oxygen
    2. Discontinue the procedure
    3. Turn the patient on the right side
    4. Instruct the patient to take rapid, deep breaths
50. In the teaching plan for a patient who will be having a fecal occult blood test, which of the following foods should be noted for producing a false positive result?
    1. Fish
    2. Pasta
    3. Vitamin B
    4. Whole grain bread

STUDY GROUP QUESTIONS

- What is the normal anatomy and physiology of the gastrointestinal system?
- How is bowel elimination influenced by the process of growth and development?
- What are some common bowel elimination problems?
- How are continent and incontinent bowel diversions/ostomies different?
- What is included in the nursing assessment of a patient to determine bowel elimination status?
- What diagnostic tests may be used to determine the presence of bowel elimination disorders?
- How are the critical thinking and nursing processes applied to situations in which patients are experiencing alterations in bowel elimination?
- What nursing interventions may be implemented to promote bowel elimination and comfort for patients in the health promotion, acute care, and restorative care settings?
- What information should be included in the teaching plan for patients/families with regard to promotion and/or restoration of bowel elimination?

STUDY CHART

Create concept maps with nursing diagnoses, related assessment data, and nursing interventions for the following: constipation, diarrhea, and incontinence.

Answers available through your instructor.

Name _____ Date _____ Instructor's Name _____

Performance Checklist Skill 34-1: Administering a Cleansing Enema

	S	U	NP	Comments

Assessment
1. Assess status of patient: last bowel movement, normal versus most recent bowel pattern, bowel sounds, hemorrhoids, mobility, external sphincter control, presence of abdominal pain.
2. Assess for presence of increased intracranial pressure, glaucoma, or recent abdominal, rectal, or prostate surgery.
3. Inspect abdomen for distention.
4. Determine patient's level of understanding of purpose of enema.
5. Review health care provider's order for type of enema and number to administer.

Planning
1. Collect appropriate equipment.
2. Verify patient's identity by using at least two patient identifiers. Compare patient's name and one other identifier, such as hospital identification number, with medication administration record (MAR). Ask patient to state name as a third identifier, and explain procedure.
3. Assemble enema bag with appropriate solution and rectal tube.

Implementation
1. Perform hand hygiene, and apply gloves.
2. Provide privacy by closing curtains around bed or closing door.
3. Raise bed to appropriate working height for nurse: stand on right side of bed, and raise side rail on opposite side.
4. Assist patient into left side-lying (Sims') position with right knee flexed. Children may be placed in dorsal recumbent position.
5. Place waterproof pad under hips and buttocks.
6. Cover patient with bath blanket, exposing only rectal area, clearly visualizing anus.
7. Separate buttocks and inspect perianal region for abnormalities including hemorrhoids, anal fissure, and rectal prolapse.
8. Place bedpan or commode in easily accessible position. If patient will be expelling contents in toilet, ensure that toilet is free. (If patient will be getting up to bathroom to expel enema, place patient's slippers and bathrobe in easily accessible position.)
9. Administer enema:
    A. Enema Bag
    (1) Add warmed solution to enema bag (warm tap water as it flows from faucet), place saline container in basin of hot water before adding saline to enema bag, and check temperature of solution by pouring small amount of solution over inner wrist. If soap suds enema is ordered, add castile soap.

	S	U	NP	Comments

    (2) Raise container, release clamp, and allow solution to flow long enough to fill tubing.

    (3) Reclamp tubing.

    (4) Lubricate 6 to 8 cm (2½ to 3 inches) of tip of rectal tube with lubricating jelly.

    (5) Gently separate buttocks and locate anus. Instruct patient to relax by breathing out slowly through mouth.

    (6) Insert tip of enema tube slowly by pointing tip in direction of patient's umbilicus. Length of insertion varies:
        Adult and adolescent: 7.5 to 10 cm (3 to 4 inches)
        Child: 5 to 7.5 cm (2 to 3 inches)
        Infant: 2.5 to 3.75 cm (1 to 1½ inches)

    (7) Hold tubing in rectum constantly until end of fluid instillation.

    (8) Open regulating clamp, and allow solution to enter slowly while holding container at patient's hip level.

    (9) Raise height of enema container slowly to appropriate level above anus: 30 to 45 cm (12 to 18 inches) for high enema, 30 cm (12 inches) for regular enema, 7.5 cm (3 inches) for low enema. Instillation time varies with volume of solution being administered.

    (10) Lower container or clamp tubing if patient complains of cramping or if fluid escapes around rectal tube.

    (11) Clamp tubing after all solution is instilled.

B. Prepackaged Disposable Container

    (1) Remove plastic cap from rectal tip. Tip is already lubricated, but more jelly can be applied as needed.

    (2) Gently separate buttocks and locate rectum. Instruct patient to relax by breathing out slowly through mouth. Expel any air from the enema container.

    (3) Insert tip of enema container gently into rectum toward the umbilicus.
        Adult: 7.5 to 10 cm (3 to 4 inches)
        Child: 5 to 7.5 cm (2 to 3 inches)
        Infant: 2.5 to 3.75 cm (1 to 1½ inches)

    (4) Squeeze enema container until all of solution has entered rectum and colon. Instruct patient to retain solution until the urge to defecate occurs, usually 2 to 5 minutes.

10. Place layers of toilet tissue around tube at anus and gently withdraw rectal tube.

11. Explain to patient that feeling of distention is normal, as well as some abdominal cramping. Ask patient to retain solution as long as possible while lying quietly in bed. (For infant or young child, gently hold buttocks together for a few minutes.)

12. Discard enema container and tubing in proper receptacle, or rinse out thoroughly with warm soap and water if container is to be reused.

	S	U	NP	Comments

13. Assist patient to bathroom or help position patient on bedpan.
14. Assist patient as needed in washing anal area with warm soap and water. If you administer perineal care, use gloves.
15. Remove and discard gloves, and perform hand hygiene.

Evaluation

1. Observe character of feces and solution evacuated (caution patient against flushing toilet before inspection). Inspect color, consistency, and amount of stool, odor and fluid passed.
2. Auscultate bowel sounds. Assess condition of abdomen; cramping, rigidity, or distention indicates a serious problem.
3. Record type and volume of enema given and characteristics of results.
4. Record and report patient's tolerance of and response to procedure.

CHAPTER 34 • Bowel Elimination

Name _____ Date _____ Instructor's Name _____

Performance Checklist Skill 34-2: Inserting and Maintaining a Nasogastric Tube for Gastric Decompression

	S	U	NP	Comments

Assessment
1. Perform hand hygiene. Inspect condition of patient's nasal and oral cavity.
2. Ask if patient has history of nasal surgery, and note if deviated nasal septum is present.
3. Auscultate for bowel sounds. Palpate patient's abdomen for distention, pain, and rigidity.
4. Assess patient's level of consciousness and ability to follow instructions.
5. Determine if patient has had a NG tube insertion in the past and which naris was used.
6. Check medical record for health care provider's order, type of NG tube to be placed, and whether tube is to be attached to suction.

Planning
1. Prepare equipment at the bedside. Have a 10-cm (4-inch) piece of tape ready with one end split in half to form a V or have NG fixation device available.
2. Identify patient by using at least two patient identifiers. Compare patient's name and one other identifier, such as hospital identification number, with medication administration record (MAR). Ask patient to state name as a third identifier, and explain procedure. Let patient know there will be a burning sensation in nasopharynx as tube is passed.
3. Position patient in high-Fowler's position with pillows behind head and shoulders. Raise bed to a horizontal level comfortable for the nurse.

Implementation
1. Perform hand hygiene. Apply clean gloves.
2. Place bath towel over patient's chest; give facial tissues to patient. Place emesis basin within reach.
3. Pull curtain around the bed or close room door. Wash bridge of nose with soap and water or alcohol swab.
4. Stand on patient's right side if right-handed, left side if left-handed.
5. Instruct patient to relax and breathe normally while occluding one naris. Then repeat this action for other naris. Select nostril with greater airflow.
6. Measure distance to insert tube:
    A. *Traditional method:* Measure distance from tip of nose to earlobe to xiphoid process.
    B. *Hanson method:* First mark 50-cm point on tube; then do traditional measurement. Tube insertion should be to midway point between 50 cm (20 inches) and traditional mark.
7. Mark length of tube to be inserted with small piece of tape loosely placed around tube so it can be easily removed.
8. Curve 10 to 15 cm (4 to 6 inches) of end of tube tightly around index finger; then release.
9. Lubricate 7.5 to 10 cm (3 to 4 inches) of end of tube with water-soluble lubricating gel.
10. Alert patient that procedure is to begin.

Copyright © 2011, 2007, 2003 by Mosby, Inc., an affiliate of Elsevier Inc. All rights reserved.

	S	U	NP	Comments

11. Initially instruct patient to extend neck back against pillow; insert tube slowly through naris with curved end pointing downward.
12. Continue to pass tube along floor of nasal passage, aiming down toward ear. When resistance is felt, apply gentle downward pressure to advance tube (do not force past resistance).
13. If resistance is met, try to rotate the tube and see if it advances. If still resistant, withdraw tube, allow patient to rest, relubricate tube, and insert into other naris.
14. Continue insertion of tube until just past nasopharynx by gently rotating tube toward opposite naris.
    A. Once past nasopharynx, stop tube advancement, allow patient to relax, and provide tissues.
    B. Explain to patient that next step requires that patient swallow. Give patient glass of water unless contraindicated.
15. With tube just above oropharynx, instruct patient to flex head forward, take a small sip of water, and swallow. Advance tube 2.5 to 5 cm (1 to 2 inches) with each swallow of water. If patient is not allowed fluids, instruct to dry swallow or suck air through straw. Advance tube with each swallow.
16. If patient begins to cough, gag, or choke, withdraw slightly and stop tube advancement. Instruct patient to breathe easily and take sips of water.
17. If patient continues to cough during insertion, pull tube back slightly.
18. If patient continues to gag and cough or complains that the tube feels as though it is coiling in the back of the throat, check back of oropharynx using flashlight and tongue blade. If tube is coiled, withdraw it until the tip is back in the oropharynx. Then reinsert with the patient swallowing.
19. After patient relaxes, continue to advance tube with swallowing until you reach the tape or mark on tube, which signifies the tube is at the desired distance. Temporarily anchor tube to patient's cheek with a piece of tape until tube placement is verified.
20. Verify tube placement: Check agency policy for preferred methods for checking tube placement.
    A. Ask patient to talk.
    B. Inspect posterior pharynx for presence of coiled tube.
    C. Attach Asepto or catheter tipped syringe to end of tube and aspirate gently back on syringe to obtain gastric contents. Observe color.
    D. Measure pH of aspirate with color-coded pH paper with range of whole numbers from 1 to 11.
    E. Have ordered x-ray film of chest/abdomen performed.
    F. If tube is not in stomach, advance another 2.5 to 5 cm (1 to 2 inches) and repeat step 20 A to D to check tube position.
21. Anchoring tube:
    A. After tube is properly inserted and positioned, either clamp end or connect it to suction machine.
    B. Tape tube to nose; avoid putting pressure on nares. Take prepared 4-inch strip of tape and split halfway.

CHAPTER 34 • Bowel Elimination   227

	S	U	NP	Comments

(1) Before taping tube to nose, apply small amount of tincture of benzoin to lower end of nose and allow to dry *(optional)*. Apply tape to nose, leaving the split end free. Be sure top end of tape over nose is secure. ___ ___ ___ _____

(2) Carefully wrap two split ends of tape around tube. ___ ___ ___ _____

(3) *Alternative:* Apply tube fixation device using shaped adhesive patch. ___ ___ ___ _____

C. Fasten end of NG tube to patient's gown by looping rubber band around tube in slipknot. Pin rubber band to gown (provides slack for movement). Do not attach pin to NG tube itself. ___ ___ ___ _____

D. Unless health care provider orders otherwise, head of bed should be elevated 30 degrees. When using a Salem sump tube, keep pigtail above level of stomach. ___ ___ ___ _____

E. Explain to patient that sensation of tube should decrease somewhat with time. ___ ___ ___ _____

F. Remove gloves, discard, and perform hand hygiene. ___ ___ ___ _____

22. Once placement is confirmed:
    A. Place a mark, either a red mark or tape, on the tube to indicate where the tube exits the nose. ___ ___ ___ _____
    B. *Option:* Measure the tube length from naris to connector as an alternative method. ___ ___ ___ _____
    C. Document the tube length in the patient record. ___ ___ ___ _____

23. Attach NG tube to suction as ordered. Usual setting is low intermittent. ___ ___ ___ _____

24. Tube irrigation:
    A. Perform hand hygiene, and apply clean gloves. ___ ___ ___ _____
    B. Check for tube placement in stomach (see step 20). Then temporarily clamp tube or reconnect to connecting syringe and remove syringe. ___ ___ ___ _____
    C. Draw 30 mL of normal saline into Asepto or catheter-tip syringe. ___ ___ ___ _____
    D. Clamp NG tube. Disconnect from connecting tubing, and lay end of connection tubing on towel. ___ ___ ___ _____
    E. Insert tip of irrigating syringe into end of NG tube. Remove clamp. Hold syringe with tip pointed at floor, and inject saline slowly and evenly. Do not force solution. ___ ___ ___ _____
    F. If resistance occurs, check for kinks in tubing. Turn patient onto left side. Report repeated resistance to health care provider. ___ ___ ___ _____
    G. After instilling saline, immediately aspirate or pull back slowly on syringe to withdraw fluid. If amount aspirated is greater than amount instilled, record the difference as output. If amount aspirated is less than amount instilled, record the difference as intake. ___ ___ ___ _____
    H. Reconnect NG tube to drainage or suction. (If solution does not return, repeat irrigation.) ___ ___ ___ _____
    I. Remove gloves and perform hand hygiene. ___ ___ ___ _____

25. Discontinuation of NG tube:
    A. Verify order to discontinue NG tube. ___ ___ ___ _____
    B. Explain procedure to patient, and reassure that removal is less distressing than insertion. ___ ___ ___ _____
    C. Perform hand hygiene, and apply clean gloves. ___ ___ ___ _____
    D. Turn off suction and disconnect NG tube from drainage bag or suction. Remove tape or fixation device from bridge of nose and unpin tube from gown. ___ ___ ___ _____

Copyright © 2011, 2007, 2003 by Mosby, Inc., an affiliate of Elsevier Inc. All rights reserved.

		S	U	NP	Comments

    E. Stand on patient's right side if right-handed, left side if left-handed.

    F. Hand the patient facial tissue; place clean towel across chest. Instruct patient to take and hold a deep breath.

    G. Clamp or kink tubing securely and then pull tube out steadily and smoothly into towel held in other hand while patient holds breath.

    H. Measure amount of drainage, and note character of content. Dispose of tube and drainage equipment into proper container.

    I. Clean nares and provide mouth care.

    J. Position patient comfortably and explain procedure for drinking fluids, if not contraindicated.

26. Clean equipment and return to proper place. Place soiled linen in utility room or proper receptacle.
27. Remove gloves, and perform hand hygiene.

Evaluation

1. Observe amount and character of contents draining from NG tube. Ask if patient feels nauseated.
2. Auscultate for the presence of bowel sounds. Turn off suction while auscultating. Then, palpate patient's abdomen periodically, noting any distention, pain, and rigidity.
3. Inspect condition of nares and nose.
4. Observe position of tubing.
5. Ask if patient feels sore throat or irritation in pharynx.
6. Record length, size, and type of gastric tube inserted and naris used, patient's tolerance to procedure, confirmation of tube placement, character of gastric contents, pH value, whether the tube is clamped or connected to drainage or to suction, and the amount of suction supplied.
7. Record difference between amount of normal saline instilled and amount of gastric aspirate removed on intake and output (I&O) sheet. Record in nurses' notes or flow sheet amount and character of contents draining from NG tube every shift. Record removal of tube as "intact."
8. Report any unexpected outcomes.

Name _____ Date _____ Instructor's Name _____

Performance Checklist Skill 34-3: Pouching an Ostomy

	S	U	NP	Comments

Assessment

1. Perform hand hygiene, and apply clean gloves. Auscultate for bowel sounds.
2. Observe existing skin barrier and pouch for leakage and length of time in place. Depending on type of pouching system used (such as opaque pouch), remove the pouch to fully observe the stoma.
3. Observe stoma for color, swelling, trauma, and healing; make sure stoma is moist and reddish pink. Assess type of stoma.
4. Observe abdominal contour and abdominal incision (if present).
5. Observe effluent from stoma, and keep a record of intake and output. Ask patient about skin tenderness.
6. Assess condition of peristomal skin, check that pouching system is not leaking.
7. To minimize skin irritation, avoid unnecessary changing of pouching system.
8. Assess abdomen for best type of pouching system to use.
9. Assess the patient's self-care ability to determine the best type of pouching system to use. Assess the patient's vision, dexterity or mobility, and cognitive function.
10. Remove existing pouch by gently pushing skin away from adhesive barrier; properly dispose of soiled pouch (save clamp if attached to pouch). After skin barrier and pouch removal, assess skin around stoma, noting scars, folds, skin breakdown, and peristomal suture line if present.
11. Remove gloves, and perform hand hygiene.
12. Determine patient's emotional response, knowledge and understanding of an ostomy and its care.

Planning

1. Identify patient by using at least two patient identifiers. Compare patient's name and one other identifier, such as hospital identification number, with medical record. Ask patient to state name as a third identifier.
2. Explain procedure to patient; encourage patient's interaction and questions.
3. Assemble equipment, and close room curtains or door.

Implementation

1. Position patient either standing or supine and drape, leaving area around stoma exposed. If seated, position patient either on or in front of toilet.
2. Perform hand hygiene, and apply clean gloves.
3. Place towel or disposable waterproof barrier under patient.
4. Cleanse peristomal skin gently with warm tap water using gauze pads or clean washcloth; do not scrub skin. Dry completely by patting skin with gauze or towel. If portions of the skin barrier remain, use an adhesive remover to gently remove them.
5. Measure stoma for correct size of pouching system needed using the manufacturer's measuring guide.

	S	U	NP	Comments

6. Select appropriate pouch for patient based on patient assessment. With a custom cut-to-fit pouch, use an ostomy guide to cut opening on the pouch 1/16 to 1/8 inch larger than stoma before removing backing. Prepare pouch by removing backing from barrier and adhesive. With ileostomy, apply thin circle of barrier paste around opening in pouch; allow to dry.
7. Apply skin barrier and pouch. If creases next to stoma occur, use barrier paste to fill in; let dry 1 to 2 minutes.
   A. **For One-Piece Pouching System**
      (1) Use skin sealant wipes on skin directly under adhesive skin barrier or pouch; allow to dry. Press adhesive backing of pouch and/or skin barrier smoothly against skin, starting from the bottom and working up and around sides.
      (2) Hold pouch by barrier, center over stoma, and press down gently on barrier; bottom of pouch should point toward patient's knees.
      (3) Maintain gentle finger pressure around barrier for 1 to 2 minutes.
   B. **For Two-Piece Pouching System**
      (1) Apply barrier-paste flange (barrier with adhesive) as in steps above for one-piece system. Snap on pouch and maintain finger pressure.
   C. **For Both Pouching Systems**
      (1) Gently tug on pouch in a downward direction.
8. Gently press on pectin or karaya flange to facilitate adhesion.
9. Although many ostomy pouches are odor-proof, explain to patient not to use "home remedies," which will harm the stoma, to control ostomy odor. Do not make a hole in pouch to release flatus.
10. Fold bottom of drainable open-ended pouches up once, and close using a closure device such as a clamp (or follow manufacturer's instructions for closure).
11. Properly dispose of old pouch and soiled equipment. Some patients will also request you to spray the room with air freshener.
12. Remove gloves, and perform hand hygiene.
13. Change one- or two-piece pouch every 3 to 7 days unless leaking. Pouch remains in place for tub bath or shower. After bath, pat adhesive dry.

Evaluation
1. Ask if patient feels discomfort around stoma.
2. Note appearance of stoma, peristomal skin, and existing incision (if present) while removing pouch and cleansing skin. Inspect condition of skin barrier and adhesive. Inspect edges of pouch for "tracking" of effluent under edges. This indicates a potential leak due to skin fold or wrinkles.
3. Auscultate bowel sounds, and observe characteristics of stool.
4. Observe patient's nonverbal behaviors as pouch is applied. Ask if patient has any questions about pouching.
5. Document type of pouch and skin barrier applied.
6. Record amount and appearance of stool, texture, condition of peristomal skin, and sutures.
7. Record and report any of the following to nurse in charge and/or health care provider:

	S	U	NP	Comments

A. Abnormal appearance of stoma, suture line, peristomal skin, character of output, abdominal tenderness or distention, and absence of bowel sounds.

B. No flatus in 24 to 36 hours and no stool by third day.

8. Record patient's level of participation and need for teaching.

Name _____ Date _____ Instructor's Name _____

Procedural Guidelines 34-1: Measuring Fecal Occult Blood

	S	U	NP	Comments

1. Explain purpose of test and ways patient will assist. Some patients collect own specimen, if possible.
2. Perform hand hygiene.
3. Apply clean, disposable gloves.
4. Use tip of wooden applicator to obtain a small portion of uncontaminated stool specimen. Be sure specimen is free of toilet paper.
5. Perform Hemoccult slide test:
   A. Open flap of slide and, using a wooden applicator, thinly smear stool in first box of the guaiac paper. Apply a second fecal specimen from a different portion of the stool to slide's second box.
   B. Close slide cover and turn the packet over to reverse side. After waiting 3 to 5 minutes, open cardboard flap and apply two drops of developing solution on each box of guaiac paper. A blue color indicates a positive guaiac, or presence of fecal occult blood. Interpret the color of the guaiac paper after 30 to 60 seconds.
   C. After determining if the patient's specimen is positive or negative, apply one drop of developer to the quality control section and interpret within 10 seconds.
   D. Dispose of test slide in proper receptacle.
6. Wrap wooden applicator in paper towel, remove gloves, and discard in proper receptacle.
7. Perform hand hygiene.
8. Record results of test; note any unusual fecal characteristics.

Name _____ Date _____ Instructor's Name _____

Procedural Guidelines 34-2: Assisting Patient On and Off a Bedpan

	S	U	NP	Comments

1. Assess the patient's level of mobility, strength, ability to help, and presence of any condition (e.g., orthopedic) that interferes with the use of a bedpan.
2. Explain to the patient the technique you will use for turning and positioning.
3. Offer the bedpan at a time that coincides with the peristaltic reflex.
4. Perform hand hygiene, and apply clean gloves.
5. Close the room curtain for privacy.
6. Raise the bed to a comfortable working height. Position the patient high in bed with head elevated 30 degrees (unless contraindicated). Raise the side rail opposite the side where you are standing.
7. Fold back top linen to patient's knees.
8. Assist with positioning an independent patient: Instruct patient to bend knees and place weight on heels. Place your hand, palm up, under patient's sacrum, resting elbow on mattress. Then have patient lift hips while you slip bedpan into place with other hand.
9. Dependent patient: Lower head of bed flat and have patient roll onto side opposite nurse. Apply powder lightly to lower back and buttocks (optional). Place bedpan firmly against buttocks and push down into mattress with open rim toward patient's feet. Keeping one hand against bedpan, place other hand around patient's forehip. Ask patient to roll onto pan, flat on bed. With patient positioned comfortably, raise head of bed 30 degrees.
10. Place rolled towel under lumbar curve of patient's back.
11. Place call light and toilet tissue within patient's reach, and keep side rails up as needed. Give patient time to defecate.
12. Remove bedpan as patient lifts hips up or as patient carefully rolls off pan and to side. Hold pan firmly as patient moves.
13. Assist in cleansing anal area. Wipe from pubic area toward anus. Replace top covers.
14. If you collect a specimen for intake and output, do not dispose of tissue in bedpan.
15. Have patient wash and dry hands.
16. Empty pan's contents, dispose of gloves, and perform hand hygiene.
17. Inspect stool for color, amount, consistency, odor, or presence of abnormal substances. Document findings.

Name _____ Date _____ Instructor's Name _____

Procedural Guidelines 34-3: Digital Removal of Stool

	S	U	NP	Comments
1. Perform hand hygiene, pull curtains around bed, obtain patient's baseline vital signs and assess level of comfort, auscultate for bowel sounds, and palpate for abdominal distention before the procedure.	___	___	___	_____
2. Explain the procedure, and help the patient to lie on the left side in Sims' position with knees flexed and back toward you.	___	___	___	_____
3. Drape the trunk and lower extremities with a bath blanket, and place a waterproof pad under the buttocks. Keep a bedpan next to the patient.	___	___	___	_____
4. Apply clean gloves, and lubricate the index finger of dominant hand with water soluble lubricant.	___	___	___	_____
5. Instruct the patient to take slow, deep breaths. Gradually and gently insert the index finger into the rectum and advance the finger slowly along the rectal wall toward the umbilicus.	___	___	___	_____
6. Gently loosen the fecal mass by massaging around it. Work the finger into the hardened mass.	___	___	___	_____
7. Work the feces downward toward the end of the rectum. Remove small pieces at a time and discard into bedpan.	___	___	___	_____
8. Periodically reassess the patient's heart rate and look for signs of fatigue. Stop the procedure if the heart rate drops significantly (check agency policy) or the rhythm changes.	___	___	___	_____
9. Continue to clear rectum of feces, and allow the patient to rest at intervals.	___	___	___	_____
10. After completion, wash and dry the buttocks and anal area.	___	___	___	_____
11. Remove bedpan; inspect feces for color and consistency. Dispose of feces. Remove gloves by turning them inside out; then discard.	___	___	___	_____
12. Assist patient to toilet or clean bedpan if urge to defecate develops.	___	___	___	_____
13. Perform hand hygiene. Record results of procedure by describing fecal characteristics and amount.	___	___	___	_____
14. Follow procedure with enemas or cathartics as ordered by health care provider.	___	___	___	_____
15. Reassess patient's vital signs and level of comfort, auscultate bowel sounds, and observe status of abdominal distention.	___	___	___	_____

Immobility

35

CASE STUDIES

1. A patient has just gone to the rehabilitation facility. She has been immobilized with a spinal cord injury from an automobile accident. You are aware of the physical hazards of immobility, but her withdrawn behavior is your concern now.
   a. What can you do to prevent the possible psychological and emotional effects of the patient's period of immobility?
2. A patient will be getting out of bed for the first time after having surgery and receiving general anesthesia.
   a. What actions should be taken by the nurse to promote the patient's safety?

CHAPTER REVIEW

Match the descriptions/definitions in Column A with the correct term in Column B.

Column A
_____ 1. Characterized by bone resorption
_____ 2. Temporary decrease in blood supply to an organ or tissue
_____ 3. Capacity to maneuver around freely
_____ 4. Permanent plantar flexion
_____ 5. Lung inflammation from stasis or pooling of secretions
_____ 6. Increased urine excretion
_____ 7. Collapse of alveoli
_____ 8. Bathing, dressing, eating
_____ 9. Calcium stones in the kidney
_____ 10. Accumulation of platelets, fibrin, clotting factors, and cellular elements attached to the interior wall of an artery or vein

Column B
a. Renal calculi
b. Diuresis
c. Hypostatic pneumonia
d. Mobility
e. Ischemia
f. Atelectasis
g. Thrombus
h. Activities of daily living
i. Disuse osteoporosis
j. Footdrop

Complete the following:

11. The objectives or advantages of bed rest are:

12. Which of the following pathophysiological changes occur with immobility? Select all that apply.
    a. Increased basal metabolic rate _____
    b. Decreased gastrointestinal motility _____
    c. Orthostatic hypotension _____
    d. Increased appetite _____
    e. Increased oxygen availability _____
    f. Hypercalcemia _____
    g. Increased lung expansion _____
    h. Decreased cardiac output _____
    i. Increased dependent edema _____
    j. Decreased stressors _____
    k. Increased urinary stasis _____
    l. Decreased passive behaviors _____
    m. Increased sensory overload _____

13. An example of a fluid and electrolyte imbalance that may occur with prolonged immobility is:

14. An example of a common behavioral change that may be observed in an immobilized patient is:

15. A nurse anticipates that a patient on prolonged bed rest will have a heart rate that is faster by _____ beats per minute.

16. Virchow triad is related to _____, and the three associated problems are:

17. With an immobilized child, the nurse's focus is on:

Copyright © 2011, 2007, 2003 by Mosby, Inc., an affiliate of Elsevier Inc. All rights reserved.

236 CHAPTER 35 • Immobility

18. An important concept when working with patients who are immobilized is to maintain the patient's autonomy. The nurse can accomplish this by:

19. Identify at least one major change that may occur in the cardiovascular system as a result of immobility, and a nursing intervention to prevent or treat the change.

20. Identify at least one potential respiratory complication of immobility, and the nursing intervention to prevent or treat the complication.

21. What areas are included in a focused assessment of patient mobility?

22. Identify for each of the following illustrations what range-of-joint-motion (ROJM) exercise is being performed:

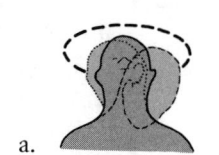

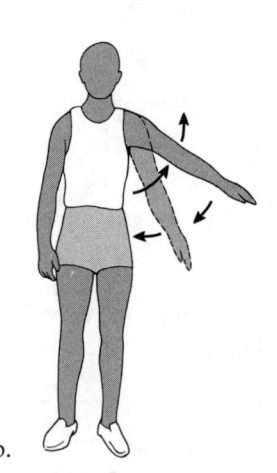

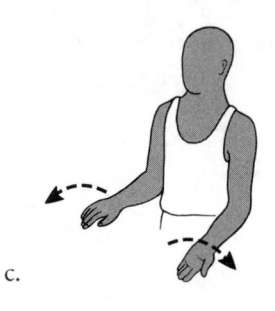

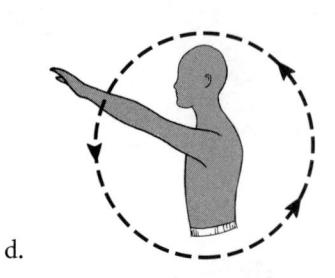

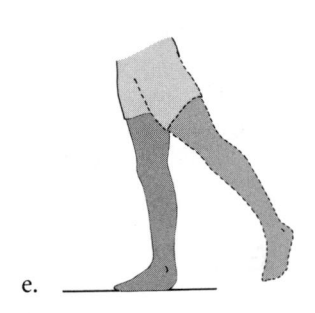

    a.

    b.

    c.

    d.

    e.

23. To evaluate muscle atrophy, a nurse should:

24. Where should a nurse check for edema in an immobilized patient?

25. For an immobilized patient, identify the usual frequency of assessment for the following:
    a. Respiratory status

    b. Anorexia

    c. Urinary elimination

    d. Intake and output

26. Specific ROJM exercises to prevent thrombophlebitis include:

27. For a patient who will have antiembolic stockings:
    a. The contraindications for their use are:

    b. How often are they are removed?

    c. A nurse makes sure that the stockings are NOT:

    d. Application of the stockings may be delegated to an unlicensed nursing assistant.
       True _____ False _____

28. Which of the following actions are correct for the use of a sequential compression device? Select all that apply.
    a. The back of the patient's ankle and knee are aligned with markings on the sleeve. _____
    b. A hand width is left between the sleeve and the patient's skin. _____

Copyright © 2011, 2007, 2003 by Mosby, Inc., an affiliate of Elsevier Inc. All rights reserved.

c. The sleeve and device are removed once daily. _____
d. The unit is observed through one complete cycle after application. _____

29. a. A medication that is used to reduce the risk of thrombophlebitis is:

    b. It is usually given every _____ hours by the _____ route.

30. An immobilized patient is experiencing shortness of breath and chest pain. The nurse suspects a pulmonary emboli. Which of the following independent or nurse-initiated actions should be taken immediately? Select all that apply.
    a. Administering heparin _____
    b. Placing the patient in an upright position _____
    c. Drawing arterial blood gases _____
    d. Administering fluids _____
    e. Checking the patient's oxygen saturation _____

31. Identify at least one change that may occur in the following systems as a result of immobility, a related nursing diagnosis, and a nursing intervention to prevent or treat the problem.
    a. Integumentary

    b. Gastrointestinal

    c. Urinary

    d. Musculoskeletal

32. For a patient who had a cerebrovascular accident (CVA, or stroke) with right-sided hemiplegia, identify how the patient can be involved in joint exercise.

33. The best way to prevent decubitus ulcers is to:

Select the best answer for each of the following questions:

34. After a CVA (stroke) a patient is prescribed prolonged bed rest. During assessment, the nurse is especially alert to the presence of:
    1. An increased JROM
    2. Warmth to the calf area
    3. Increased muscle mass
    4. An increased hemoglobin level

35. An older adult patient had a fractured hip repaired 2 days ago. The patient is having more difficulty than expected in moving around, and the nurse is concerned about possible respiratory complications. In assessing the patient for possible atelectasis, the nurse expects to find:
    1. A decreased respiratory rate
    2. Wheezing on inspiration
    3. Asymmetrical breath sounds
    4. Rubbing sounds during inspiration and expiration

36. For a patient who has been placed in a spica (full body) cast, the nurse remains alert to possible changes in the cardiovascular system as a result of immobility. The nurse may find that the patient has:
    1. Hypertension
    2. Tachycardia
    3. Hypervolemia
    4. An increased cardiac output

37. A possible complication for a patient who has been prescribed prolonged bed rest is thrombus formation. For the nurse to assess the presence of this serious problem, the nurse should:
    1. Attempt to elicit Chvostek sign
    2. Palpate the temperature of the feet
    3. Measure the patient's calf and thigh diameters
    4. Observe for hair loss and skin turgor in the lower legs

38. A patient was prescribed extended bed rest after abdominal surgery. The patient now has an order to be out of bed. The nurse should first:
    1. Assess respiratory function
    2. Obtain the patient's blood pressure measurement
    3. Ask if the patient feels light-headed
    4. Assist the patient to the edge of the bed

39. A patient has been placed in skeletal traction and will be immobilized for an extended period of time. The nurse recognizes that there is a need to prevent respiratory complications and intervenes by:
    1. Suctioning the airway every hour
    2. Changing the patient's position every 4 to 8 hours
    3. Using oxygen and nebulizer treatments regularly
    4. Encouraging deep breathing and coughing every hour

40. Patients who are immobilized in health care facilities require that their psychosocial needs be met along with their physiological needs. A nurse recognizes a patient's psychosocial needs when telling the patient the following:
    1. "The staff will limit your visitors so that you will not be bothered."
    2. "We will help you get dressed so you look more like yourself."
    3. "We can discuss the routine to see if there are any changes that we can make with you."
    4. "A roommate can sometimes be a real bother and very distracting. We can move you to a private room."

41. A patient is transferred to a rehabilitation facility from the medical center after a CVA (stroke). The CVA resulted in severe right-sided paralysis, and the patient is very limited in mobility. To prevent the complication of external hip rotation for this patient, the nurse uses a:
    1. Footboard
    2. Bed board
    3. Trapeze bar
    4. Trochanter roll

CHAPTER 35 • Immobility

42. A patient who has deep vein thrombosis is at risk for:
    1. Atelectasis
    2. Pulmonary emboli
    3. Orthostatic hypotension
    4. Hypostatic pneumonia
43. The equipment that is used on a bed to assist a patient to raise the torso is a:
    1. Sandbag
    2. Bed board
    3. Trapeze bar
    4. Wedge pillow
44. For exercise, which of the following is appropriate for an immobilized older adult?
    1. Gradual, extended warm-ups
    2. Rapid transitions and movements
    3. Sustained isometric exercises of at least a minute
    4. Slowing of exercise rate in the presence of angina or breathlessness
45. If all of the following are prescribed, the best nursing strategy for the prevention of renal calculi is:
    1. Administration of diuretics
    2. Provision of a high-fiber diet
    3. Insertion of a urinary catheter.
    4. Offering of 2 liters of fluid per day
46. A nurse is instructing a patient on joint range of motion and performance of shoulder abduction. The nurse correctly instructs the patient to:
    1. Raise the arm straight forward
    2. Move the arm in a full circle
    3. Move the arm until the thumb is turned inward and toward the back
    4. Raise the arm to the side to a position above the head
47. To prevent plantar flexion, a nurse will obtain:
    1. Trochanter rolls
    2. Foot boots
    3. Sandbags
    4. Hand splints
48. A nurse is instructing a patient on ROJM and performance of forearm supination. The nurse correctly instructs the patient to:
    1. Move the palm toward the inner aspect of the forearm
    2. Turn the lower arm and hand so the palm is up
    3. Straighten the elbow by lowering the hand
    4. Touch the thumb to each finger of the hand
49. A patient has weakness to the upper and lower extremities and has been on bed rest for several days. Which of the following actions performed by the new staff nurse requires correction?
    1. Performing passive ROJM exercises
    2. Having the patient do as much of the bath as possible
    3. Massaging the lower extremities
    4. Assisting the patient to different positions every 1½ hours
50. A patient is being instructed to perform dorsiflexion of the foot. The nurse observes the patient's ability to:
    1. Turn the foot and leg toward the other leg
    2. Move the foot so the toes point upward
    3. Turn the sole of the foot medially
    4. Straighten and spread the toes of the foot

STUDY GROUP QUESTIONS

- What are the basic concepts of mobility?
- What is immobility?
- How is bed rest used therapeutically?
- What physiological changes may occur throughout the body as a result of immobility?
- What psychosocial and developmental changes may occur as a result of immobility?
- What assessments should be made by a nurse to determine the effect of immobility on the patient?
- What nursing interventions should be implemented to prevent or treat the effects of immobility?

Answers available through your instructor.

Name _____ Date _____ Instructor's Name _____

Procedural Guidelines 35-1: Applying Antiembolic Elastic Stockings

		S	U	NP	Comments
1.	Assess patient for risk factors in Virchow triad.	___	___	___	_____
2.	Observe for signs, symptoms, and conditions that might contraindicate use of elastic stockings.	___	___	___	_____
3.	Assess and document the condition of patient's skin and circulation to the legs.	___	___	___	_____
4.	Obtain health care provider's order.	___	___	___	_____
5.	Assess patient's or caregiver's understanding of application of antiembolic elastic stockings.	___	___	___	_____
6.	Assess the condition of the patient's skin and circulation to the leg and foot.	___	___	___	_____
7.	Use tape measure to measure patient's legs to determine proper stocking size.	___	___	___	_____
8.	Explain procedure and reasons for applying stockings.	___	___	___	_____
9.	Perform hand hygiene. Provide hygiene to patient's lower extremities as needed.	___	___	___	_____
10.	Position patient in supine position.	___	___	___	_____
11.	Apply elastic stockings:				
	A. Turn elastic stocking inside out up to the heel. Place one hand into stocking, holding heel. Pull top of stocking with other hand inside out over foot of stocking.	___	___	___	_____
	B. Place patient's toes into foot of elastic stocking, making sure that stocking is smooth.	___	___	___	_____
	C. Slide remaining portion of stocking over patient's foot, being sure that the toes are covered. Make sure the foot fits into the toe and heel position of the stocking.	___	___	___	_____
	D. Slide top of stocking up over patient's calf until stocking is completely extended. Be sure stocking is smooth and no ridges or wrinkles are present, particularly behind the knee.	___	___	___	_____
	E. Instruct patient not to roll stockings partially down.	___	___	___	_____
12.	Reposition patient for comfort, and perform hand hygiene.	___	___	___	_____
13.	Remove stockings at least once per shift.	___	___	___	_____
14.	Inspect stockings for wrinkles or constriction.	___	___	___	_____
15.	Inspect elastic stockings to determine that there are no wrinkles, rolls, or binding.	___	___	___	_____
16.	Observe circulatory status of lower extremities. Observe color, temperature, and condition of skin. Palpate pedal pulses.	___	___	___	_____
17.	Observe the patient's response to wearing the antiembolic elastic stockings.	___	___	___	_____
18.	Observe patient or caregiver apply stockings.	___	___	___	_____

Name _____ Date _____ Instructor's Name _____

Procedural Guideline 35-2: Applying Sequential Compression Devices

		S	U	NP	Comments
1.	Assess patient's need for sequential compression stockings.	___	___	___	_____
2.	Obtain baseline assessment data about the status of circulation, pulses, and skin integrity on patient's lower extremities before initiating sequential compression stockings.	___	___	___	_____
3.	Verify patient's identity by using at least two patient identifiers. Compare patient's name and one other identifier, such as hospital identification number, with medication administration record (MAR). Ask patient to state name as a third identifier.	___	___	___	_____
4.	Perform hand hygiene. Provide hygiene to lower extremities, as needed.	___	___	___	_____
5.	Assemble and prepare equipment.				
6.	Arrange SCD sleeve under the patient's leg according to the leg position indicated on the inner lining of the sleeve.	___	___	___	_____
	A. Back of patient's ankle should align with the ankle marking on inner lining of the sleeve.	___	___	___	_____
	B. Position back of knee with the popliteal opening.	___	___	___	_____
7.	Wrap SCD sleeve securely around patient's leg.	___	___	___	_____
8.	Verify fit of SCD sleeves by placing two fingers between patient's leg and sleeve.	___	___	___	_____
9.	Attach SCD sleeve's connector to plug on mechanical unit. Arrows on compressor line up with arrows on plug from mechanical unit.	___	___	___	_____
10.	Turn mechanical unit on. Green light indicates unit is functioning.	___	___	___	_____
11.	Observe functioning of unit for one complete cycle.	___	___	___	_____
12.	Reposition patient for comfort and perform hand hygiene.	___	___	___	_____
13.	Remove compression stockings at least once per shift.	___	___	___	_____
14.	Monitor skin integrity and circulation to patient's lower extremities as ordered or as recommended by SCD manufacturer.	___	___	___	_____

Skin Integrity and Wound Care 36

CASE STUDY

1. You are a student nurse assigned to provide care to a patient in an extended care facility. While assisting the patient from the bed to the shower chair, you notice reddened areas on her sacral region, and on both elbows and heels. The skin on these areas is intact, but the redness does not go away.
    a. Identify a nursing diagnosis, patient goal/outcomes, and nursing interventions related to this patient's assessment data.

CHAPTER REVIEW

Match the description/definition in Column A with the correct term in Column B.

	Column A		Column B
_____	1. Localized collection of blood under the tissues	a.	Cachexia
_____	2. Separation of wound layers with protrusion of visceral organs	b.	Approximate
_____	3. Wound edges come together	c.	Abrasion
_____	4. Superficial loss of dermis	d.	Laceration
_____	5. Pressure exerted against the skin when the patient is moved	e.	Dehiscence
_____	6. General poor health and malnutrition with weakness and emaciation	f.	Fistula
_____	7. Removal of devitalized tissue	g.	Hematoma
_____	8. Torn, jagged damage to dermis and epidermis	h.	Evisceration
_____	9. Separation of skin and tissue layers	i.	Debridement
_____	10. Abnormal passage between two body organs or between an organ and the outside of the body	j.	Shearing force

Complete the following:

11. Mark the areas on the body that are common sites for pressure ulcer development.

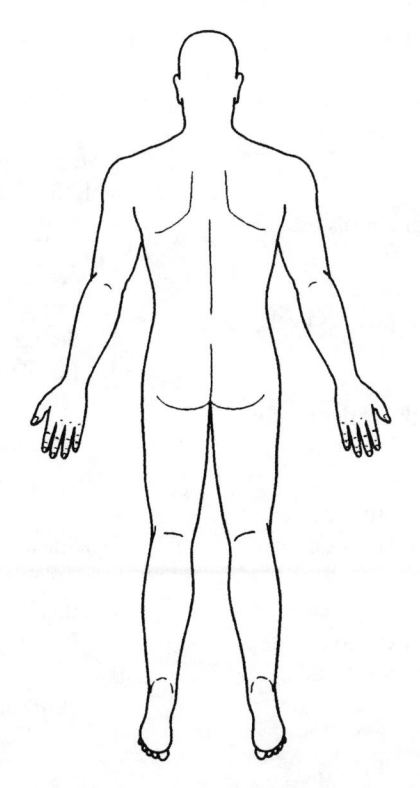

CHAPTER 36 • Skin Integrity and Wound Care

12. Identify the following stages of pressure ulcer development:
    a.

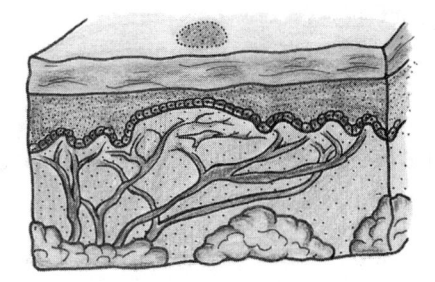

    b.

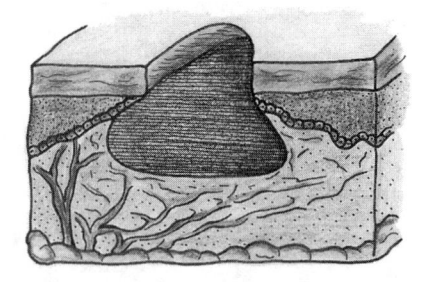

13. Provide an example of a contributing factor for pressure ulcer formation.

14. Patients in what age-groups are at the highest risk for sensitivity to heat and cold applications?

15. The major change in an older adult's skin that contributes to pressure ulcer development is:

16. Identify the following related to wound healing.
    a. A clean surgical wound with little tissue loss heals by:

    b. A severe laceration or chronic wound heals by:

17. Identify if the following statements are true or false.
    a. Wounds that are kept moist for several days heal faster than those that are kept dry.
       True _____ False _____
    b. Reddened areas that are noted on the patient's skin should be massaged.
       True _____ False _____
    c. Use of a foam ring or "donut" is effective for pressure reduction for the patient sitting out of bed.
       True _____ False _____
    d. Specimens for aerobic wound cultures should be taken from wound areas with clean, healthy skin.
       True _____ False _____

18. Identify a complication of wound healing that is assessed by the nurse in the following examples.
    a. Separation of the layers of the skin with serosanguineous drainage noted

    b. Bluish swelling or mass at the site

    c. Fever, general malaise, and increased white blood cell (WBC) count

    d. Green, odorous local drainage

    e. Decreased blood pressure, increased pulse rate, increased respirations

    f. Visceral organs protruding through abdominal wall

    g. Wound edges swollen, painful, with redness extending from the edges outward

19. Identify the methods or indicators that are used for assessing darkly pigmented skin.
    a. Lighting source

    b. Unexpected consistency

    c. Unexpected change in color

20. Identify an example of how each of the following factors influences wound healing.
    a. Age

    b. Obesity

    c. Diabetes

    d. Immunosuppression

21. Match each of the following types of wound drainage with their correct description.

    Drainage
    a. Serous
    b. Sanguineous
    c. Serosanguineous
    d. Purulent

    Description
    1. Pale, more watery, with plasma and red blood cells
    2. Thick, yellow, green, or brown with organisms and white blood cells
    3. Clear, watery plasma
    4. Fresh bleeding

22. Provide at least one nursing intervention that should be implemented to prevent pressure ulcer formation specifically related to:
    a. Pressure reduction

    b. Skin care

23. Arrange the steps for obtaining an aerobic wound culture in correct order.
    a. Return the swab to the culture tube _____
    b. Apply pressure to express fluid from wound onto swab _____
    c. Moisten swab with normal saline _____
    d. Swab wound in a 1 × 1 cm area _____
    e. Cleanse the wound and allow to dry _____
24. A nurse investigates whether a patient had a tetanus toxoid injection within the past year if the patient has a(n):

25. Identify how the nurse determines whether a wound is healing.

26. A patient who is sitting out of bed in a chair and requires assistance to move around should be limited to _____ hours sitting and should be repositioned every _____ hour(s).
27. A nurse can reduce friction or shear by:

28. Nursing care of an abrasion or laceration includes:

29. For use of a negative pressure wound therapy system:
    a. The purpose of the therapy is to:

    b. The tube is attached to:

    c. The dressing that is used for this system is:

    d. The transparent dressing should:

30. For wound irrigation, identify the following that are considered as safe guidelines.
    a. Syringe size

    b. Needle gauge

    c. psi

    d. The syringe should be held how far above the wound?

e. During an irrigation, the nurse notes sanguineous return. The nurse should:

f. It is noted that there is retained debris in the wound. The nurse should:

31. Identify what is pictured in the following illustrations:
    a.

    b.

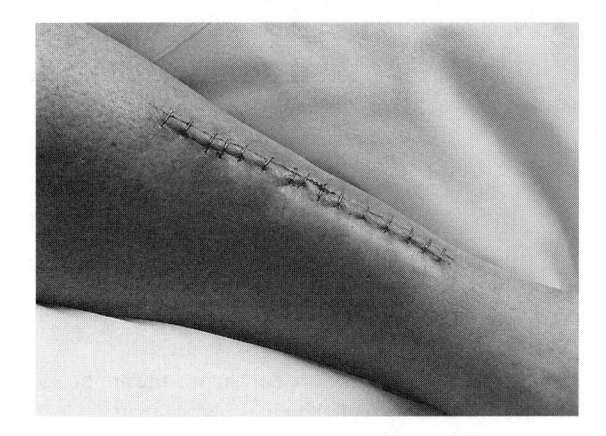

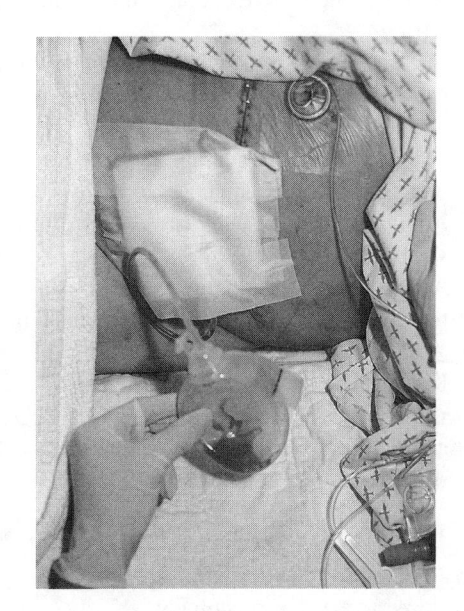

32. Which of the following are correct nursing interventions for elastic bandages? Select all that apply.
    a. Placing the body part to be bandaged in anatomical position _____
    b. Applying a bandage to an extremity from proximal to distal _____
    c. Positioning pins or knots toward the wound _____

CHAPTER 36 • Skin Integrity and Wound Care

d. Overlapping turns by one-half to two-thirds the width of the bandage _____
e. Assessing circulation once daily _____

33. Identify the steps in caring for a traumatic wound.

34. Specify whether the following effects are a result of heat (H) or cold (C) therapy.
    a. Vasoconstriction _____
    b. Decreased blood viscosity _____
    c. Increased tissue metabolism _____
    d. Decreased muscle tension _____
    e. Increased capillary permeability _____

35. a. Provide an instance in which the application of heat is contraindicated.

    b. Provide an instance in which the application of cold is contraindicated.

36. The usual duration of time for the application of heat or cold is:

37. Which of the following are correct for the application of heat or cold? Select all that apply.
    a. Providing a timer or clock so the patient may help time the application _____
    b. Allowing the patient to adjust the temperature setting _____
    c. Not placing the patient in a position that prevents movement away from the temperature source _____
    d. Maintaining the temperature as hot or cold as the patient is able to tolerate _____
    e. Applying a heating pad or cold pack directly to the skin _____
    f. Adding hotter solution to a soak to maintain temperature while the patient remains immersed _____
    g. Keeping the rest of the patient draped or covered while receiving treatment _____

38. Using the Braden Scale, what is this patient's risk for pressure ulcer development?

		Score
Sensory	Very Limited	_____
Moisture	Occasionally	_____
Activity	Chairfast	_____
Mobility	Very Limited	_____
Nutrition	Probably Inadequate	_____
Friction/Shear	Potential Problem	_____
	Total Score	_____
	Patient Risk	_____

39. Which of the following are correct for application of a moist dressing? Select all that apply.
    a. Wringing out excess moisture from the dressing _____
    b. Pouring the solution directly onto the dressing in the wound _____
    c. Loosely packing sinus tracks or dead spaces in the wound _____
    d. Avoiding the use of secondary dressings _____
    e. Using Montgomery ties or straps perpendicular to the wound _____

40. a. Nonblanchable hyperemia is:

    b. This assessment signifies:

    c. When nonblanchable hyperemia is assessed, the stage is reversible if pressure is relieved.
       True _____ False _____

41. Which of the following are correct actions for a postoperative dressing? Select all that apply.
    a. Routinely changing the dressing after the procedure _____
    b. Reinforcing saturated dressings _____
    c. Providing the patient with an analgesic 30 minutes before the dressing change _____
    d. Expecting inflammation of the wound edges for at least a week after the surgery _____
    e. Noting the amount, color, consistency, and odor of wound drainage _____
    f. Expecting that a primary intention wound with no drainage will have the dressing discontinued _____

42. A patient will need to continue to perform dressing changes when he is discharged to his home. Identify the necessary nursing assessments/evaluations before the patient's discharge.

Select the best answer for each of the following questions:

43. To avoid pressure ulcer development for an immobilized patient at home, a nurse recommends a surface to use on the bed. A surface type that is low-cost and easy to use in the home is a(n):
    1. Foam overlay surface
    2. Air overlay surface
    3. Air fluidized surface
    4. Low air loss surface

44. For a patient in the extended care facility who has a nursing diagnosis of *Impaired physical mobility*, a nurse will implement:
    1. Massage of reddened skin areas
    2. Movement of the patient in the chair every 3 hours
    3. Maintenance of a position while in bed at 30 degrees or lower
    4. Placement of plastic absorptive pads directly beneath the patient

45. A patient has experienced a traumatic injury that will require applications of heat. The nurse implements the treatment based on the principle that:
    1. Long exposures help the patient develop tolerance to the procedure

CHAPTER 36 • Skin Integrity and Wound Care

2. The foot and the palm of the hand are the most sensitive to temperature
3. Patient response is best to minor temperature adjustments
4. Patients are more tolerant to temperature changes over a large body surface area

46. A severely overweight patient has returned to the unit after having major abdominal surgery. When the nurse enters the room, it is evident that the patient has moved or coughed and the wound has eviscerated. The nurse should immediately:
    1. Assess vital signs
    2. Contact the physician
    3. Apply light pressure on the exposed organs
    4. Place sterile towels soaked in saline over the area

47. A patient with a knife protruding from his upper leg is taken into the emergency department. A nurse is waiting for the physician to arrive when a newly hired nurse comes to assist. The nurse delegates the new staff member to do all of the following as soon as possible except:
    1. Assess vital signs
    2. Remove the knife to cleanse the wound
    3. Wrap a bandage around the knife and injured site
    4. Apply pressure to the surrounding area to stop bleeding

48. A nurse is assessing a patient's wound and notices that it has very minimal tissue loss and drainage. There are a number of dressings that may be used according to the protocol on the unit. The nurse selects:
    1. Gauze
    2. Alginate
    3. Negative pressure wound therapy
    4. Transparent film

49. A nurse is completing an assessment of the patient's skin integrity and identifies that an area is a full-thickness wound with damage to the subcutaneous tissue. The nurse identifies this stage of ulcer formation as:
    1. Stage I
    2. Stage II
    3. Stage III
    4. Stage IV

50. A patient has a large wound to the sacral area that requires irrigation. The nurse explains to the patient that irrigation will be performed to:
    1. Decrease scar formation
    2. Decrease wound drainage
    3. Remove debris from the wound
    4. Improve circulation in the wound

51. A nurse is working with an older adult patient in an extended care facility. While turning the patient, the nurse notices that there is a reddened area on the patient's coccyx. The nurse implements skin care that includes:
    1. Soaking the area with normal saline
    2. Cleaning the area with mild soap, drying, and applying a protective moisturizer
    3. Washing the area with an astringent and painting it with povidone-iodine solution
    4. Applying a dilute solution of hydrogen peroxide and water and using a heat lamp to dry the area

52. A patient has a wound to the left lower extremity that has minimal exudates and collagen formation. The nurse identifies the healing phase of this wound as:
    1. Primary intention
    2. Proliferative phase
    3. Secondary intention
    4. Inflammatory phase

53. After neurosurgery, a nurse assesses the patient's bandage and finds that there is fresh bleeding coming from the operative site. The nurse describes this drainage to the surgeon as:
    1. Serous
    2. Purulent
    3. Sanguineous
    4. Serosanguineous

54. A patient has a surgical wound on the right upper aspect of the chest that requires cleansing. The nurse implements appropriate aseptic technique by:
    1. Opening the cleansing solution with sterile gloves
    2. Moving from the outer region of the wound toward the center
    3. Cleaning the wound twice and discarding the swab
    4. Starting at the drainage site and moving outward with circular motions

55. A nurse is working in a physician's office and is asked by one of the patients when heat or cold should be applied. In providing an example, the nurse identifies that cold therapy should be applied for the patient with:
    1. A newly fractured ankle
    2. Menstrual cramping
    3. An infected wound
    4. Degenerative joint disease

56. A patient will require the application of a binder to provide support to the abdomen. When applying the binder, the nurse uses the principle that:
    1. The binder should be kept loose for patient comfort
    2. The patient should be sitting or standing when it is applied
    3. The patient must maintain adequate ventilatory capacity
    4. The binder replaces the need for underlying bandages or dressings

57. A nurse is aware that malnutrition places a patient at a greater risk for tissue damage. The patient with the greatest risk is the individual who:
    1. Experienced a 7% weight loss in 4 months
    2. Is between 45 and 60 years of age
    3. Has an albumin level of 3 mg/dL
    4. Has a transferrin level of 120 mg/dL

58. The agent that is most effective and safest for cleaning a granular wound is:
    1. Acetic acid
    2. Normal saline
    3. Povidone-iodine
    4. Hydrogen peroxide
59. A nurse is working with a patient who has a stage III, clean ulcer with significant exudate. The nurse anticipates that which of the following dressings will be used?
    1. Composite film dressing
    2. Transparent dressing
    3. Calcium alginate dressing
    4. Hydrogel dressing
60. For a patient's optimal nutritional intake that will promote formation of new blood vessels and collagen synthesis, the nurse plans to teach the patient to include a sufficient intake of:
    1. Fats
    2. Proteins
    3. Carbohydrates
    4. Fat-soluble vitamins

STUDY GROUP QUESTIONS

- What are pressure ulcers and what contributes to their development?
- Where are pressure ulcers most likely to develop?
- What are the stages of pressure ulcer development?
- What are the classifications of wounds?
- How do wounds heal?
- What are the possible complications of wound healing?
- How do pressure ulcers affect health care costs?
- What tools may be used to predict patients' risks for pressure ulcer development?
- What should be included in the nursing assessment of patients to determine their risk for pressure ulcer development?
- How are wounds managed in both emergency and nonemergency health care settings?
- What types of drainage may be seen in wounds?
- How are wound cultures obtained?
- How can the nurse prevent pressure ulcer development?
- What nursing interventions may be implemented to treat pressure ulcers and wounds?
- What are the procedures for dressing changes and wound care?
- What criteria are used in the selection of dressings and sutures or staples?
- What are the principles involved in heat and cold therapy, including patient safety?
- What information should be included in patient/family teaching for prevention and treatment of pressure ulcers, wound care, and use of heat and cold therapy?

Answers available through your instructor.

CHAPTER 36 • Skin Integrity and Wound Care 247

Name _____ Date _____ Instructor's Name _____

Performance Checklist Skill 36-1: Assessment of Patient for Pressure Ulcer: Risk and Skin Assessment

	S	U	NP	Comments

Assessment
1. Perform hand hygiene. Close room door or bedside curtains.
2. Identify patient's risk for pressure ulcer formation using the Braden Scale; assign a score for each of the subscales.
3. Obtain the risk score and evaluate based upon patient's overall condition.
4. Conduct a systematic skin assessment of bony prominences. Apply clean gloves when applying pressure to reddened areas.
5. Assess the following potential areas of skin breakdown: back of head, shoulders, ribs, hips, sacral region, ischium, inner and outer knees, inner and outer ankles, heels, feet, ears, nares, lips, tube sites, and sites of orthopedic and positioning devices
6. Assess all skin surfaces for absence of superficial skin layers, blisters, and loss of epidermis and dermis.
7. Determine the patient's ability to respond meaningfully to pressure-related discomfort (sensory perception).
8. Assess the degree to which the patient's skin is exposed to moisture.
9. Evaluate the patient's activity level.

Implementation
1. If any of the risk factors receive low scores on the risk assessment tool, consider one or more interventions.
2. Assist patient when changing positions during the assessment.
3. When you note a reddened area, inspect for skin discoloration, blanchable erythema, nonblanchable erythema, pallor, or mottling.
4. Remove gloves, perform hand hygiene, and reposition patient.

Evaluation
1. Evaluate patient's skin daily, especially those areas at high risk for breakdown (check agency policy).
2. Compare current risk score with previous scores.
3. Record risk score and frequency of risk assessment.
4. Record appearance of skin, especially pressure points.
5. Describe positioning and turning schedule.
6. Describe preventative skin interventions.
7. Report changes in skin care protocol.
8. Document consultation from skin or wound care specialists.

CHAPTER 36 • Skin Integrity and Wound Care

Name _____ Date _____ Instructor's Name _____

Performance Checklist Skill 36-2: Treating Pressure Ulcers

	S	U	NP	Comments

Assessment

1. Assess the patient's comfort level and need for pain medication. Administer analgesic if needed.
2. Determine if patient has allergies to latex or topical agents.
3. Review the order for topical agent or dressing.
4. Assess each of the patient's pressure ulcers and surrounding skin to determine ulcer characteristics, including the stage.
5. Assess the type of tissue in the wound bed. Chart the approximate amount of each tissue found in the wound bed.
6. Assess need for revisions to therapy during each dressing change.
   A. Note color, temperature, edema, moisture, and condition of skin around the ulcer. Modify the assessment technique based on the patient's individual skin color.
   B. Measure the wound's length and width per agency policy.
   C. Measure the depth of the pressure ulcer using a sterile cotton-tipped applicator or other device that will allow measurement of wound depth. Place the applicator gently into the pressure ulcer until it touches the bottom. Mark the place on the applicator where it reaches the top of the wound, and then remove the applicator from the ulcer. Measure the distance from the tip of the applicator to the mark using a measuring tape or ruler to determine the depth of the pressure ulcer.
   D. Measure depth of undermining tissue. Use a cotton-tipped applicator, and gently probe under skin edges.
7. Remove gloves, discard appropriately, and perform hand hygiene.

Planning

1. Explain procedure to patient and family. Individualize the teaching plan for older adult patients, taking into account the normal aging changes that affect learning.
2. Prepare the following necessary equipment and supplies:
   A. Washbasin, warm water, soap, washcloth, and bath towel
   B. Normal saline or other wound-cleansing agent in sterile solution container
   C. Prescribed topical agent
   D. Appropriate dressing and tape

	S	U	NP	Comments

Implementation
1. Close room door or bedside curtains. Perform hand hygiene and apply clean gloves. Open sterile packages and topical solution containers. (Apply goggles and moisture-proof cover gown if indicated.)   ___   ___   ___   _____
2. Remove bed linen and patient's gown to expose ulcer and surrounding skin. Keep remaining body parts draped.   ___   ___   ___   _____
3. Gently wash skin surrounding ulcer with warm water and soap.   ___   ___   ___   _____
4. Rinse area thoroughly with water.   ___   ___   ___   _____
5. Gently dry skin thoroughly by patting lightly with towel.   ___   ___   ___   _____
6. Perform hand hygiene and change gloves.   ___   ___   ___   _____
7. Cleanse ulcer thoroughly with normal saline or prescribed wound-cleansing agent.   ___   ___   ___   _____
8. Use whirlpool treatments if needed to assist with wound debridement. Keep the wound away from the water jets.   ___   ___   ___   _____
9. Apply topical agents, if prescribed.   ___   ___   ___   _____
   A. **Enzymes:**
      (1) Using a wooden tongue blade, apply a small amount of enzyme debridement ointment directly to the necrotic areas on the base of pressure ulcer. Avoid getting the enzyme on the surrounding skin. Do not apply enzyme to surrounding skin.   ___   ___   ___   _____
      (2) Place gauze dressing directly over ulcer, and tape it in place. Follow specific manufacturer's recommendation for type of dressing material to use to cover a pressure ulcer when using enzymatic agent.   ___   ___   ___   _____
      (3) If using an antibiotic solution, apply per order and cover with gauze pad. Generally, solution is applied every 12 hours.   ___   ___   ___   _____
   B. **Hydrogel agents:**
      (1) Cover surface of ulcer with hydrogel using applicator or gloved hand.   ___   ___   ___   _____
      (2) Apply a secondary dressing, such as dry gauze, hydrocolloid, or transparent dressing, over gel to completely cover ulcer.   ___   ___   ___   _____
   C. **Calcium alginates:**
      (1) Pack wound with alginate using applicator or gloved hand.   ___   ___   ___   _____
      (2) Apply a secondary dressing, such as dry gauze, foam, or hydrocolloid, over alginate.   ___   ___   ___   _____
10. Reposition patient comfortably off pressure ulcer.   ___   ___   ___   _____
11. Remove gloves, and dispose of soiled supplies. Perform hand hygiene.

	S	U	NP	Comments

Evaluation
1. Observe skin surrounding ulcer for inflammation, edema, and tenderness. ____ ____ ____ _____
2. Inspect dressings and exposed ulcers, observing for drainage, foul odor, and tissue necrosis. Monitor patient for signs and symptoms of infection, including fever and elevated WBC count. ____ ____ ____ _____
3. Compare subsequent ulcer measurements. ____ ____ ____ _____
4. Use one of the scales designed to measure wound healing such as the PUSH Scale (Nix, 2007a) or the PSST (Bates-Jensen, 1990). ____ ____ ____ _____
5. Record appearance of ulcer in patient's record. ____ ____ ____ _____
6. Describe the type of topical agent used, dressing applied, and patient's response. ____ ____ ____ _____
7. Report any deterioration in ulcer appearance. ____ ____ ____ _____

Name _____ Date _____ Instructor's Name _____

Performance Checklist Skill 36-3: Negative Pressure Wound Therapy

	S	U	NP	Comments

Assessment
1. Assess location, appearance, and size of wound to be dressed.
2. Review health care provider's orders for frequency of dressing change, type of foam to use, and amount of negative pressure to be used.
3. Assess patient's level of comfort using a scale of 0 to 10.
4. Assess patient's and family member's knowledge of purpose of dressing.

Planning
1. Collect appropriate equipment and arrange at bedside.
2. Explain procedure to patient.
3. Position patient to allow access to wound site.
4. Plan dressing change to occur 30 minutes after any analgesic is administered.

Implementation
1. Close room door or cubicle curtains.
2. Position patient, expose wound site, and cover patient.
3. Cuff top of disposable waterproof bag, and place within reach of work area.
4. Perform hand hygiene, and put on clean gloves. If risk for spray exists, apply protective gown, goggles, and mask.
5. Push therapy on/off button on the negative pressure wound therapy system.
6. Raise the tubing connectors above the level of the negative pressure wound therapy unit. Engage clamp on the canister tubing.
7. Gently stretch transparent film horizontally, and slowly pull up from the skin.
8. Remove the foam dressing. Observe the appearance of drainage on dressing. Use caution to remove dressing around drains. Dispose of soiled dressings in waterproof bag. Remove gloves by pulling them inside out, and dispose of them in waterproof bag. Avoid having patient see old dressing. Perform hand hygiene.
9. Apply sterile or clean gloves. Irrigate the wound with normal saline or other solution ordered by the health care provider. Gently blot to dry.
10. Measure wound as ordered: at baseline, first dressing change, weekly, and discharge from therapy. Remove and discard gloves. Perform hand hygiene.
11. Depending on the type of wound, apply new sterile or clean gloves.
12. Prepare wound edges with a skin preparation product to enhance dressing seal and to protect the periwound skin.

Copyright © 2011, 2007, 2003 by Mosby, Inc., an affiliate of Elsevier Inc. All rights reserved.

		S	U	NP	Comments

13. Select appropriate foam dressing depending on wound type and stage of healing. Use sterile scissors to cut foam to exact wound size, making sure to fit the size and shape of the wound, including tunnels and undermined areas.
14. Gently place foam in wound, making sure that the foam is in contact with entire wound (base, margins, and tunneled and undermined areas). Multiple pieces of foam can be used to adequately fill the wound providing the pieces of foam are in direct contact with each other.
15. Size and trim the transparent dressing to cover wound, and overlap onto intact healthy surrounding skin.
16. Secure tubing to the unit to transparent film, aligning drainage hole to ensure an occlusive seal. Do not apply tension to drape and tubing.
17. Secure tubing several centimeters away from the dressing.
18. After the wound is completely covered, connect the tubing from the dressing to the tubing from the negative pressure wound therapy canister.
    A. Remove new canister from sterile packaging and push into the negative therapy pressure wound therapy unit until a click is heard. **An alarm will sound if the canister is not properly engaged.**
    B. Connect the dressing tubing to the canister tubing. Make sure both clamps are open.
    C. Place negative pressure wound therapy unit on a level surface or hang from the foot of the bed. **The unit will alarm and deactivate therapy if the unit is tilted beyond 45 degrees.**
    D. Power on the system using the green-lit power button, and set negative pressure as ordered.
19. Discard soiled dressing change materials properly. Remove gloves. Perform hand hygiene.
20. Inspect the negative pressure wound therapy unit to verify that negative pressure is achieved.
    A. Verify that display screen reads "THERAPY ON."
    B. Be sure clamps are open and tubing is patent.
    C. Identify air leaks by listening with stethoscope or by moving hand around edges of wound while applying light pressure.
    D. If a leak is present, use strips of transparent film to patch areas around the edges of the wound.
21. Assist patient to a comfortable position.

	S	U	NP	Comments

Evaluation
1. Inspect condition of wound on ongoing basis; note drainage and odor.
2. Ask patient to rate pain using a scale of 0 to 10.
3. Verify airtight dressing seal and correct negative pressure setting.
4. Measure wound drainage output in canister on a regular basis.
5. Observe patient's or family member's ability to perform dressing change.
6. Record wound appearance, color and characteristics of any drainage, presence of wound healing, and patient tolerance to procedure. Record date and time of new dressing on the dressing as per agency policy.
7. Report any brisk, bright red bleeding; evidence of poor wound healing; evisceration or dehiscence; and possible wound infection.

Name _____ Date _____ Instructor's Name _____

Performance Checklist Skill 36-4: Applying Dressings: Dry or Moist-to-Dry and Transparent

	S	U	NP	Comments

Assessment

1. Assess size of wound to be dressed.
2. Assess location of wound.
3. Ask patient to rate pain using a scale of 0 to 10.
4. Assess patient's knowledge of purpose of dressing change.
5. Assess need and readiness for patient or family member to participate in dressing wound.
6. Review medical orders for dressing change procedure.
7. Identify patients with risk factors for wound-healing problems.

Planning

1. Explain procedure to patient.
2. Position patient to allow access to area to be dressed.
3. Plan dressing change to occur 30 to 60 minutes after administration of analgesic.

Implementation

1. Close room or cubicle curtains. Perform hand hygiene. Apply gown, goggles, and mask if risk for spray exists.
2. Position patient comfortably and drape to expose only wound site. Instruct patient not to touch wound or sterile supplies.
3. Place disposable bag within reach of work area. Fold top of bag to make cuff. Put on clean gloves.
4. Remove tape: Pull parallel to skin, toward dressing, and hold down uninjured skin. If over hairy areas, remove in the direction of hair growth. Remove remaining adhesive from skin.
5. With clean-gloved hand or forceps, remove dressings. Carefully remove outer secondary dressing first, and then remove inner primary dressing that is in contact with the wound bed. If drains are present, slowly and carefully remove dressing one layer at a time. Keep soiled undersurface from patient's sight.
6. Inspect wound for color, edema, drains, exudate, and integrity. Observe appearance of drainage on dressing. Assess for odor. Gently palpate the wound edges for drainage, bogginess, or patient report of increased pain. Measure wound size.
7. Describe the appearance of the wound and any indicators of wound healing to the patient.

	S	U	NP	Comments

8. Dispose of soiled dressings in disposable bag. Remove gloves by pulling them inside out. Dispose of gloves in bag. Perform hand hygiene.
9. Open sterile dressing tray or individually wrapped sterile supplies. Place on bedside table.
10. Open prescribed cleansing solution and pour over sterile gauze.
11. Put on gloves, clean or sterile depending on institution policy.
12. Cleanse wound:
    A. Use separate swab for each cleansing stroke or spray wound surface.
    B. Clean from least contaminated area to most contaminated.
    C. Cleanse around the drain (if present), using circular stroke starting near drain and moving outward and away from the insertion site.
13. Use dry gauze to blot in same manner as in step 12 to dry wound. Dry thoroughly.
14. Apply antiseptic ointment if ordered, using same technique as for cleansing.
15. Apply dressings to incision or wound site:
    A. **Dry Dressing**
       (1) Apply loose woven gauze as contact layer.
       (2) Cut 4 × 4 gauze flat to fit around drain if present or use precut split gauze.
       (3) Apply additional layers of gauze as needed.
       (4) Apply thicker woven pad (e.g., Surgipad abdominal dressing).
    B. **Moist Dressing**
       (1) Moisten dressing with prescribed solution.
       (2) Wring out excess fluid and apply moist fluffed gauze or packing strip directly onto wound surface without allowing the gauze touch the surrounding skin.
       (3) Make sure any dead space from sinus tracts, undermining, or tunneling is loosely packed with gauze.
       (4) Apply dry sterile gauze over wet gauze.
       (5) Cover the packed wound with a secondary dressing such as an ABD pad, Surgipad, or gauze.
    C. **Transparent Dressing**
       (1) Apply dressing according to manufacturer's directions. Do not stretch film during application. Avoid wrinkles in film.

	S	U	NP	Comments
16. Secure dressing with roll gauze, tape, Montgomery ties or straps, or binder.	___	___	___	_____
17. Remove gloves, gown if worn, and dispose of them in bag. Dispose of all supplies. Remove goggles if worn.	___	___	___	_____
18. Assist patient to comfortable position.	___	___	___	_____
19. Perform hand hygiene.	___	___	___	_____

Evaluation

	S	U	NP	Comments
1. Inspect condition of wound and presence of any drainage.	___	___	___	_____
2. Ask if patient had pain during procedure.	___	___	___	_____
3. Inspect condition of dressing at least every shift.	___	___	___	_____
4. Ask patient to describe steps and techniques of dressing change.	___	___	___	_____
5. Record appearance of wound; color, presence, and characteristics of exudate; change in wound characteristics (especially drainage amount); type and amount of dressings applied; and tolerance of patient to dressing change.	___	___	___	_____
6. Report unexpected appearance of wound drainage or accidental removal of drain, bright red bleeding, or evidence of wound dehiscence or evisceration.	___	___	___	_____
7. Write your initials, date, and time of dressing change on a piece of tape in ink (not marker) and place on dressing.	___	___	___	_____

CHAPTER 36 • Skin Integrity and Wound Care

Name _____ Date _____ Instructor's Name _____

Performance Checklist Skill 36-5: Performing Wound Irrigation

	S	U	NP	Comments

Assessment

1. Review health care provider's order for irrigation of open wound and type of solution to be used. ___ ___ ___ _____
2. Assess recent recording of signs and symptoms assessments related to patient's open wound:
   A. Extent of impairment of skin integrity, including size of wound: Measure wound in centimeters and in the following order: Length, width, and depth. ___ ___ ___ _____
   B. Drainage from wound (amount, color, and consistency): Amount can be measured by part of dressing saturated or in terms of quantity. ___ ___ ___ _____
   C. Odor ___ ___ ___ _____
   D. Wound color ___ ___ ___ _____
   E. Consistency of drainage ___ ___ ___ _____
   F. Culture report ___ ___ ___ _____
   G. Dressing: dry and clean, evidence of bleeding, profuse drainage ___ ___ ___ _____
3. Assess comfort level or pain on a scale of 0 to 10, and identify symptoms of anxiety. ___ ___ ___ _____
4. Assess patient for history of allergies to antiseptics, tapes, or dressing material. ___ ___ ___ _____

Planning

1. Explain procedure of wound irrigation and cleansing. ___ ___ ___ _____
2. Administer prescribed anesthetic 30 to 60 minutes before starting wound irrigation procedure. ___ ___ ___ _____
3. Position patient.
   A. Position patient comfortably to permit gravitational flow of irrigating solution through wound and into collection receptacle. ___ ___ ___ _____
   B. Position patient so that wound is vertical to collection basin. Place container of irrigant/cleaning solution in basin of hot water to warm solution to body temperature. ___ ___ ___ _____
   C. Place padding or extra towels on the bed. ___ ___ ___ _____
   D. Expose wound only. ___ ___ ___ _____

Implementation

1. Perform hand hygiene. ___ ___ ___ _____
2. Form cuff on waterproof biohazard bag, and place it near bed. ___ ___ ___ _____
3. Close room door or bed curtains. ___ ___ ___ _____
4. Apply gown and goggles and mask. ___ ___ ___ _____
5. Apply clean gloves, remove soiled dressing, and discard in waterproof bag. Discard gloves. ___ ___ ___ _____
6. Prepare equipment; open sterile supplies. ___ ___ ___ _____
7. Apply sterile gloves. ___ ___ ___ _____

Copyright © 2011, 2007, 2003 by Mosby, Inc., an affiliate of Elsevier Inc. All rights reserved.

		S	U	NP	Comments

8. To irrigate wound with wide opening:
   A. Fill 35-mL syringe with irrigation solution.
   B. Attach 19-gauge angiocatheter.
   C. Hold syringe tip 2.5 cm (1 inch) above upper end of wound and over area being cleansed.
   D. Using continuous pressure, flush wound; repeat steps 8 A through C until solution draining into basin is clear.
9. To irrigate deep wound with small opening:
   A. Attach angiocatheter to filled irrigating syringe.
   B. Lubricate tip of catheter with irrigating solution and gently insert tip of catheter and pull out about 1 cm (½ inch).
   C. Using slow, continuous pressure, flush wound.
   D. Remove and refill syringe. Reconnect to catheter and repeat until solution draining into basin is clear.
10. When indicated, obtain cultures after cleansing with nonbacteriostatic saline.
11. Dry wound edges with gauze; dry patient if shower or whirlpool is used.
12. Apply appropriate dressing.
13. Remove gloves, mask, goggles, and gown.
14. Assist patient to comfortable position.
15. Dispose of equipment and soiled supplies, and perform hand hygiene.

Evaluation

1. Assess type of tissue in wound bed.
2. Inspect dressing periodically.
3. Evaluate skin integrity.
4. Observe patient for signs of discomfort.
5. Observe for presence of retained irrigant.
6. Record wound irrigation and patient response on progress notes.
7. Immediately report to health care provider any evidence of fresh bleeding, sharp increase in pain, retention of irrigant, or signs of shock.

CHAPTER 36 • Skin Integrity and Wound Care

Name _____ Date _____ Instructor's Name _____

Procedural Guidelines 36-1: Applying Abdominal or Breast Binders

	S	U	NP	Comments
1. Observe patient with need for support of thorax or abdomen. Observe ability to breathe deeply and cough effectively.	___	___	___	_____
2. Review medical record if medical prescription for particular binder is necessary and evaluate reasons for application.	___	___	___	_____
3. Inspect skin for actual or potential alterations in integrity. Observe for irritation, abrasion, skin surfaces that rub against each other, or allergic response to adhesive tape used to secure dressing.	___	___	___	_____
4. Inspect any surgical dressing.	___	___	___	_____
5. Assess patient's comfort level using analog scale of 0 to 10 and noting any objective signs and symptoms.	___	___	___	_____
6. Gather necessary data regarding size of patient and appropriate binder.	___	___	___	_____
7. Explain procedure to patient.	___	___	___	_____
8. Perform hand hygiene, and apply gloves (if likely to contact wound drainage).	___	___	___	_____
9. Close curtains or room door.	___	___	___	_____
10. Apply binder.				
A. Abdominal binder:				
(1) Position patient in supine position with head slightly elevated and knees slightly flexed.	___	___	___	_____
(2) Fanfold far side of binder toward midline of binder.	___	___	___	_____
(3) Instruct and assist patient in rolling away from you toward raised side rail while firmly supporting abdominal incision and dressing with hands.	___	___	___	_____
(4) Place fanfolded ends of binder under patient.	___	___	___	_____
(5) Instruct or assist patient in rolling over folded ends toward you.	___	___	___	_____
(6) Unfold and stretch ends out smoothly on far side of bed.	___	___	___	_____
(7) Instruct patient to roll back into supine position.	___	___	___	_____
(8) Adjust binder so that supine patient is centered over binder using symphysis pubis and costal margins as lower and upper landmarks, respectively.	___	___	___	_____
(9) Close binder. Pull one end of binder over center of patient's abdomen. While maintaining tension on that end of binder, pull opposite end of binder over center and secure with Velcro closure tabs, metal fasteners, or horizontally placed safety pins.	___	___	___	_____

Copyright © 2011, 2007, 2003 by Mosby, Inc., an affiliate of Elsevier Inc. All rights reserved.

	S	U	NP	Comments
(10) Assess patient's comfort level.	___	___	___	_____
(11) Adjust binder as necessary.	___	___	___	_____

B. **Breast binder:**
   (1) Assist patient in placing arms through binder's armholes. ___ ___ ___ _____
   (2) Assist patient to supine position in bed. ___ ___ ___ _____
   (3) Pad area under breasts if necessary. ___ ___ ___ _____
   (4) Using Velcro closure tabs or horizontally placed safety pins, secure binder at nipple level first. Continue closure process above and then below nipple line until entire binder is closed. ___ ___ ___ _____
   (5) Make appropriate adjustments, including individualizing fit of shoulder straps and pinning waistline darts to reduce binder size. ___ ___ ___ _____
   (6) Instruct and observe skill development in self-care related to reapplying breast binder. ___ ___ ___ _____

11. Remove gloves, and perform hand hygiene. ___ ___ ___ _____
12. Observe site for skin integrity, circulation, and characteristics of the wound. ___ ___ ___ _____
13. Assess comfort level of patient using analog scale of 0 to 10 and noting any objective signs and symptoms. ___ ___ ___ _____
14. Evaluate patient's ability to ventilate properly, including deep breathing and coughing. ___ ___ ___ _____

Name _____ Date _____ Instructor's Name _____

Procedural Guidelines 36-2: Applying Elastic Bandages

	S	U	NP	Comments

1. Review patient's medical record and order for application of elastic bandage.
2. Inspect areas to be dressed for the following:
   A. Intact skin
   B. Abrasions
   C. Draining wounds
   D. Skin discoloration
3. Note circulation to the area requiring an elastic dressing.
   A. Palpate skin, noting temperature, color.
   B. Palpate pulse, noting pulse quality.
   C. Observe extremity for edema or dehydration.
4. Determine level of function of affected extremity.
5. Assess level of pain severity to area (0 to 10 scale).
6. Explain procedure to patient.
7. Perform hand hygiene, and apply gloves, if indicated.
8. Close curtains or room door.
9. Hold roll of elastic dressing in dominant hand, and use other hand to tightly hold the beginning of dressing at distal body part.
10. Apply dressing from distal point toward proximal boundary, stretching the bandage slightly, using a variety of dressing turns to cover various body shapes. Prevent uneven dressing tension or circulatory impairment by overlapping turns by one-half to two-thirds width of dressing roll. NOTE: Be sure dressing is smooth (without creases).
11. Secure each roll with clip or tape before applying additional roll(s).
12. When finished with application, secure last elastic roll with clip, adhesive tape, or mesh to prevent wrap from becoming dislodged and thus decreasing extremity support.
13. Remove gloves, and perform hand hygiene.
14. Evaluate circulation to dressing area every 4 hours.
    A. Palpate distal pulse.
    B. Palpate skin, noting temperature every 4 hours.
    C. Observe skin color.
15. Determine patient's level of comfort, using analog scale of 0 to 10 and noting any objective signs and symptoms.
16. Observe for changes from baseline assessment in level of extremity function.

37 Sensory Alterations

CASE STUDIES

1. You are making a home visit to a patient with diabetes mellitus who is losing his eyesight (diabetic retinopathy).
   a. What interventions may be implemented with the patient to assist in maintaining adequate sensory stimulation and personal safety?
2. You have been assigned to care for a patient in the intensive care unit (ICU).
   a. What sensory alterations may this patient experience, and how can you prevent their occurrence or reduce their impact?

CHAPTER REVIEW

Complete the following:

1. Identify other terms for the following.
   a. Sight:
   b. Hearing:
   c. Taste:
   d. Smell:
   e. Touch:
   f. Position sense:

2. Identify one of the major diseases that can lead to visual impairment.

3. Identify at least one factor that can lead to each of the following *Disturbed sensory perception* diagnoses, and possible signs and symptoms.
   a. Sensory deprivation
   b. Sensory overload

4. Provide the correct term for the following.
   a. A buildup of ear wax in the external auditory canal
   b. Hearing loss associated with aging
   c. Opacity of the lens resulting in blurred vision
   d. Decreased salivary production or dry mouth
   e. Intermittent hearing loss, vertigo, tinnitus, and pressure in the ears

5. Identify how the following factors may influence sensory function.
   a. Age: older adulthood
   b. Medications
   c. Smoking
   d. Environment

6. Identify a way that a nurse can evaluate a patient's vision and hearing during routine interactions or care.

7. a. A common cause of blindness in children is:
   b. Identify an area that should be included when teaching parents about eyesight safety.

8. A common cause of hearing impairment in children is:

9. Identify a way that a nurse can modify sensory stimulation in the health care environment.

10. A nurse may communicate with a hearing-impaired patient by:

11. Provide an example of a drug that may cause ototoxicity in patients.

CHAPTER 37 • Sensory Alterations 263

12. Identify how a nurse may assist patients with the following deficits to adapt their home environments for safety.
    a. Hearing deficit
    b. Diminished sense of smell
    c. Diminished sense of touch

13. Identify a nursing diagnosis that may be formulated for a patient with a sensory deficit.

14. Provide an example of a general screening that is conducted to determine visual and/or auditory deficits.

15. Which of the following are appropriate in promoting sensory stimulation in the home environment? Select all that apply.
    a. Reducing glare by using sheer curtains on windows _____
    b. Using pale colors on surfaces _____
    c. Serving bland foods with similar textures _____
    d. Using a pocket magnifier _____
    e. Introducing fragrant flowers _____
    f. Playing recorded music with high-frequency sound _____

16. A patient has gone to the local walk-in emergency center with flu-like symptoms. After seeing the physician, the patient shows the nurse the prescriptions the physician has written. The patient should be informed that ototoxicity may occur with the administration of which of the following medications? Select all that apply.
    a. Furosemide _____
    b. Vitamin C _____
    c. Acetaminophen _____
    d. Erythromycin _____
    e. Cough suppressant with codeine _____
    f. Aspirin _____

17. Identify at least one rationale for why a patient may not use his or her hearing aid.

18. A patient with a diminished tactile sense may be assisted with hygiene and grooming by:

Select the best answer for each of the following questions:

19. An expected outcome for a patient with an auditory deficit should include:
    1. Minimizing use of affected sense(s)
    2. Preventing additional sensory losses
    3. Promoting the patient's acceptance of dependency
    4. Controlling the environment to reduce sensory stimuli

20. A nurse is working with patients at the senior day care center and recognizes that changes in sensory status may influence the older adult's eating patterns. For patients who are experiencing changes in their dietary intake, the nurse will assess for:
    1. Presbycusis
    2. Xerostomia
    3. Vestibular ataxia
    4. Peripheral neuropathy

21. Parents arrive at the pediatric clinic with their 1½-year-old child. The parents ask the nurse if there are signs that may indicate that the child is not able to hear well. The nurse explains to the parents that they should be alert to the child:
    1. Awakening to loud noises
    2. Responding reflexively to sounds
    3. Having delayed speech development
    4. Remaining calm when unfamiliar people approach

22. A nurse is assessing a patient for a potential gustatory impairment. This may be indicated if the patient has a(n):
    1. Weight loss
    2. Blank look or stare
    3. Increased sensitivity to odors
    4. Period of excessive clumsiness or dizziness

23. Which of the following is a priority safety measure in the acute care environment for a patient with a sensory deficit?
    1. Encouraging the family to visit the patient
    2. Refering the patient to a support group
    3. Determining the patient's medical history
    4. Orienting the patient to the surroundings

24. A responsive patient had eye surgery, and patches have been temporarily placed on both eyes for protection. The evening meal has arrived, and the nurse will be assisting the patient. In this circumstance, the nurse should:
    1. Feed the patient the entire meal
    2. Encourage family members to feed the patient
    3. Allow the patient to be totally independent and feed himself
    4. Orient the patient to the locations of the foods on the plate and provide the utensils

25. After a cerebrovascular accident (CVA, or stroke), a patient is found to have receptive aphasia. The nurse may assist this patient with communication by:
    1. Obtaining a referral for a speech therapist
    2. Using a system of simple gestures and repeated behaviors
    3. Providing the patient with a letter chart to use to answer questions
    4. Offering the patient a notepad and pen to write down questions and concerns

26. A patient has been diagnosed with glaucoma. The nurse anticipates that the patient will report a history of:
    1. Severe redness and itching of the eyes
    2. Cloudy and blurred vision

3. Painless loss of peripheral and central vision
4. Dark spaces blocking forward vision and distortion of lines

27. A mother is taking her newborn for his first physical examination. She expresses concern because during her pregnancy she may have been exposed to an infectious disease, and the baby's hearing could be affected. The nurse inquires if the patient was exposed to:
   1. Rubella
   2. Pneumonia
   3. Excessive oxygen
   4. A urinary tract infection

28. For a patient with a hearing deficit, the best way for the nurse to communicate is to:
   1. Approach the patient from the side
   2. Use visible facial expressions
   3. Shout or speak very loudly to the patient
   4. Repeat the entire conversation if it is not totally understood

STUDY GROUP QUESTIONS

- What are the human senses and their functions?
- What factors influence sensory function?
- What are some common sensory alterations?
- What types of patients are at risk for developing sensory alterations?
- How should a nurse assess a patient's sensory function?
- What behaviors or changes in lifestyle patterns or socialization may indicate a sensory alteration?
- How can a nurse promote sensory function and prevent injury and isolation in the health promotion and acute and restorative care settings?
- What screening processes are used to determine the presence of sensory alterations?
- How may the family/significant others be involved in the care of a patient with a sensory alteration?
- What information should be included in patient/family teaching for promotion of sensory function and prevention of injury?

Answers available through your instructor.

Surgical Patient 38

CASE STUDIES

1. Your patient is scheduled to have extensive abdominal surgery with a large, midline incision.
   a. How can you assist this patient to promote respiratory function postoperatively?
2. A patient is having outpatient surgery.
   a. How may preoperative teaching be conducted and what information should be included?
3. While completing the preoperative checklist, a nurse discovers that a patient's temperature is 101° F.
   a. What should the nurse do?
4. A patient insists that his good luck medallion must go with him everywhere, even to surgery.
   a. What should you do?
5. A patient had laparoscopic surgery on his right knee and is going to be discharged to his home. His wife and young children have visited often during his hospital stay.
   a. What general information do you need in order to prepare the patient and the family for the discharge?

CHAPTER REVIEW

Match the description/definition in Column A with the correct term in Column B.

	Column A		Column B
___	1. Performed on the basis of the patient's choice; not essential for health	a.	Palliative surgery
___	2. Involves extensive reconstruction or alteration in body parts; poses risks to well-being	b.	Transplant surgery
___	3. Relieves or reduces intensity of disease symptoms; will not produce cure	c.	Major surgery
___	4. Must be done immediately to save life or preserve function of body part	d.	Ablative surgery
___	5. Surgical exploration that allows physician to confirm medical status; may involve removal of body tissue for analysis	e.	Cosmetic surgery
___	6. Performed to improve personal appearance	f.	Emergency surgery
___	7. Amputation or removal of diseased body part	g.	Elective surgery
___	8. Performed to replace malfunctioning organs or structures	h.	Diagnostic surgery

Complete the following:

9. a. In relation to the operative experience, A patient who smokes cigarettes is at a greater risk for:

   b. Postoperative care for this patient will require more aggressive:

10. a. Identify a medical condition that may increase a patient's surgical risk.

    b. Malignant hyperthermia is associated with:

11. Identify an example of how changes in each of the following body systems place the older adult patient at risk during surgery.
    a. Cardiovascular
    b. Pulmonary
    c. Renal
    d. Neurological

12. Obesity places a patient at greater risk for surgery as a result of:

CHAPTER 38 • Surgical Patient

13. Identify a consideration for surgical patients who are taking the following medications.
    a. Insulin
    b. Antibiotics
    c. NSAIDs

14. Provide two examples of information that is usually included in preoperative teaching.

15. Identify a routine screening test that may be ordered for a patient preoperatively.

16. Identify the commonly used types of preoperative medications.

17. Identify two nursing diagnoses that may be formulated for a patient who will be having his or her first surgery.

18. The patient is going to receive general anesthesia for the surgical procedure. Specify the general NPO criteria for the following.
    a. No food or fluids _____ hours before surgery
    b. No meat or fried foods _____ hours before surgery

19. Identify the adverse effects associated with the following types of anesthesia.
    a. General anesthesia
    b. Regional anesthesia
    c. Local anesthesia
    d. Conscious sedation

20. Which of the following preoperative interventions are appropriate? Select all that apply.
    a. Completing bowel preparation before GI surgery _____
    b. Shaving the surgical site with a razor _____
    c. Providing antimicrobial soap for bathing _____
    d. Removing the patient's wig _____
    e. Leaving artificial fingernails intact _____
    f. Removing a hearing aid when the patient gets to the operating room (OR) _____

21. In the presurgical care unit (PSCU) and OR, verification is done to determine:

22. Identify whether of the following tasks are responsibilities of the circulating nurse (C) or scrub nurse (S).
    a. Completion of preoperative assessments/verification _____
    b. Application of sterile drapes _____
    c. Establishment of the intraoperative plan of care _____
    d. Calculation of blood loss and urinary output _____
    e. Provision of sterile equipment for the surgeon _____
    f. Documentation of the procedure _____
    g. Maintenance of the sterile field _____

23. For the following, identify a nursing intervention for intraoperative patient care.
    a. Prevention of injury
    b. Maintenance of patient's body temperature
    c. Prevention of infection

24. Identify a specific nursing intervention to prevent the following postoperative complications.
    a. Pulmonary stasis
    b. Venous stasis
    c. Wound infection
    d. Gastrointestinal stasis

25. Which of the following assessment findings for a patient in the postanesthesia care unit (PACU) signify that the patient is qualified to be discharged from the unit? Select all that apply.
    a. Oxygen saturation 96% _____
    b. Rales on auscultation _____
    c. Pulse rate 110 beats per minute _____
    d. Bilateral peripheral pulses _____
    e. Abdominal distention _____
    f. Response to verbal stimuli _____
    g. Sluggish hand grasp and pupillary response _____
    h. Quarter-size sanguineous spot maintained on incisional dressing _____
    i. 30 mL per hour urinary output _____

26. A nurse is aware that a patient should void within _____ hours after surgery. For the patient who has not voided, what should the nurse do?

27. After general anesthesia, postoperative oral intake usually begins with an order for _____ (diet).

28. With regard to postoperative wound healing and care, which of the following statements are correct? Select all that apply.
    a. The surgical dressing is changed after the patient leaves the PACU. _____
    b. Any visible drainage on the surgical dressing should be marked. _____
    c. The patient who has an order for an oral analgesic should be medicated 20 minutes before an uncomfortable dressing change. _____

d. Redness, warmth, and edema should be expected at the incision site. _____
e. Wound drainage should be measured once a day. _____
f. The patient should be draped during a dressing change to minimize exposure. _____

29. a. The patient in the illustration is demonstrating the use of a(n):

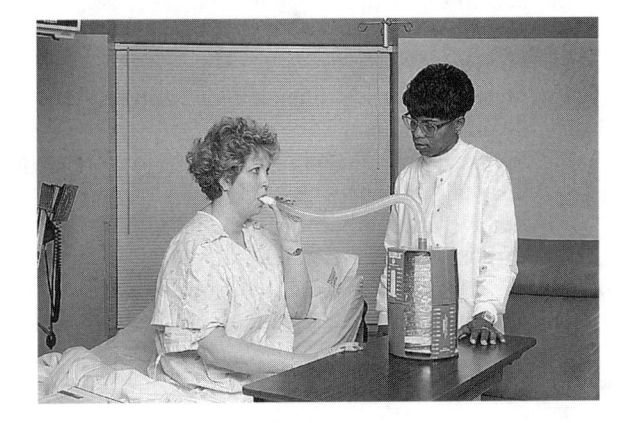

b. This device is used to prevent:

30. For a patient who will be alert during a surgical procedure, what support should be provided by the nurse?

31. Identify at least three examples of routine postoperative patient assessments.

Select the best answer for each of the following questions:

32. A nurse is starting the preparations for a patient who is having surgery tomorrow morning. The nurse prepares to have the consent form completed. The nurse recognizes that informed consent:
    1. Is valid if the patient is disoriented
    2. Is signed by the patient after the administration of preoperative medications
    3. Indicates that the patient is aware of the procedure and its possible complications
    4. Requires that the nurse provide information about the surgery before the consent can by signed

33. A patient is taken to PACU after surgery. A nurse is assessing the patient and is alert to the indication of a postoperative hemorrhage if the patient exhibits:
    1. Restlessness
    2. Warm, dry skin
    3. A slow, steady pulse rate
    4. A decreased respiratory rate

34. A nurse is checking the vital signs of a patient who had major surgery yesterday. The nurse discovers that the patient's temperature is slightly elevated. This finding is usually indicative of:
    1. A postoperative wound infection
    2. An allergic response to latex
    3. A response to the anesthesia
    4. Extensive neural damage

35. A nurse is completing the preoperative checklist for a woman who will be having surgery. The nurse determines that the surgeon and anesthesiologist should be informed of which of the patient's laboratory results?
    1. Hemoglobin level: 10 g/dL
    2. Potassium level: 4.2 mEq/L
    3. Platelet count: 210,000/mm^3
    4. Prothrombin time: 11 seconds

36. A patient has received a spinal anesthetic during the surgical procedure. The nurse is alert to possible complications of the anesthetic and is assessing the patient for a:
    1. Rash
    2. Headache
    3. Nephrotoxic response
    4. Hyperthermic response

37. A patient is being evaluated for transfer from the PACU to the patient's unit. The nurse determines that the patient will be approved for transfer if the patient exhibits:
    1. Increased wound drainage
    2. Pulse oximetry of 95%
    3. Respirations of 30 breaths per minute
    4. Nonpalpable peripheral pulses

38. A patient is scheduled to have abdominal surgery later in the morning. At 9:00 AM, while completing the preoperative checklist, the nurse recognizes the need to contact the surgeon immediately. The nurse has identified that the patient:
    1. Received an enema at 6:00 AM
    2. Admitted to recent substance abuse
    3. Ate a hamburger last evening at 6:00 PM
    4. Has bowel sounds in all four quadrants of the abdomen

39. A patient is being positioned in the PACU after surgery. Unless contraindicated, the nurse should place the patient:
    1. Prone
    2. In high-Fowler's
    3. Supine with arms across the chest
    4. On the side with the face turned downward

40. When a patient first arrives at PACU, the nurse will:
    1. Provide oral fluids
    2. Allow the patient to sleep
    3. Provide a warm blanket
    4. Remove the urinary catheter

41. A nurse is visiting a patient who had surgery 9 hours ago. The nurse asks if the patient has voided, and the patient responds negatively. At this time, the nurse:
    1. Provides more oral fluids
    2. Inserts an IV and administers fluids
    3. Obtains an order for urinary catheterization
    4. Recognizes that this is a normal outcome

CHAPTER 38 • Surgical Patient

42. During a patient assessment in the PACU, a nurse finds that the patient's operative site is swollen and appears tight. The nurse suspects:
    1. Infection
    2. Hemorrhage
    3. Lymphedema
    4. Subcutaneous emphysema
43. An immediate postoperative priority in providing nursing care for a patient is:
    1. Airway patency
    2. Relief of pain
    3. Sufficient circulation to the extremities
    4. Prevention of wound infection
44. A 54-year-old patient is scheduled to have a gastric resection. The nurse informs the surgeon preoperatively of the patient's history of:
    1. A tonsillectomy at age 10
    2. Employment as a telephone repair person
    3. Smoking two packs of cigarettes per day
    4. Taking acetaminophen for minor body aches
45. A patient has been taking warfarin at home. The patient is going to be admitted for a surgical procedure, and the nurse anticipates that this prescribed medication will be:
    1. Administered as usual
    2. Increased in dose immediately before the procedure
    3. Reduced in dose by half immediately before the procedure
    4. Discontinued at least 2 days before the procedure
46. During the intraoperative phase, a nurse's responsibility is reflected in the statement:
    1. "I think that the patient requires more information about the procedure and its consequences."
    2. "There seems to be a missing sponge, so a recount must be done to see that all of the sponges were removed."
    3. "The patient has signed the request. I will prepare the medications and then get the record completed."
    4. "The patient appears reactive and stable. Dressing to wound is dry and intact. Analgesic administered per order."
47. A nurse is assisting a patient with postoperative exercises. The patient tells the nurse, "Blowing into this thing (incentive spirometer) is a waste of time." The nurse explains to the patient that the specific purpose of this therapy is to:
    1. Stimulate the cough reflex
    2. Promote lung expansion
    3. Increase pulmonary circulation
    4. Directly remove excess secretions from the respiratory tract
48. A patient is scheduled for surgery, and a nurse is completing the final areas of the preoperative checklist. After administering the preoperative medications, the nurse should:
    1. Assist the patient to void
    2. Obtain the informed consent
    3. Prepare the skin at the surgical site
    4. Place the side rails up on the bed or stretcher
49. At the ambulatory surgery center, a patient is having surgery using general anesthesia. The nurse will expect this patient to:
    1. Ambulate immediately after being admitted to the recovery area
    2. Meet all of the identified criteria in order to be discharged home
    3. Remain in the phase I recovery area longer than a hospitalized patient
    4. Receive large amounts of oral fluids immediately entering the recovery area
50. A nurse is preparing a patient for surgery and recognizes that the greatest risk of bleeding is for the patient with:
    1. Diabetes mellitus
    2. Emphysema
    3. Thrombocytopenia
    4. Immunodeficiency syndrome
51. A patient has a nasogastric tube in place after surgery and complains to the nurse of nausea. The nurse should first:
    1. Remove the NG tube
    2. Provide oral fluids
    3. Move the patient side to side
    4. Irrigate the tube with normal saline
52. Which of the following individuals is most at risk for postoperative wound infection?
    1. A pregnant patient
    2. A patient who smokes cigarettes
    3. A patient with poorly controlled diabetes
    4. A patient experiencing periods of sleep apnea
53. A patient's surgeon has previously discussed the procedure with the patient, but she has a few more questions. The best way for the nurse to approach this is to first:
    1. Refer the patient back to the surgeon
    2. Determine what the patient has been told already
    3. Provide details of what the procedure will be like
    4. Get the consent form for the patient to read

STUDY GROUP QUESTIONS

- How are surgeries classified?
- What are some surgical risk factors, and why do they increase the patient's risk?
- How does the incision site influence a patient's recovery?
- How may previous surgical experiences influence the patient's expectations of surgery?
- What general information should be included in preoperative teaching?

- What is the purpose of the preoperative exercises that are explained and demonstrated to patients?
- What preoperative assessments should be made by a nurse?
- What are some common preoperative diagnostic tests that may be ordered for a patient?
- What nursing interventions are implemented in the preoperative care of patients?
- How does a nurse prepare and assist a patient in the acute care setting on the day of surgery?
- What are the roles of nurses in the operating room and in the recovery setting?
- What interventions are implemented to maintain patient safety and well-being in the operating room and postanesthesia care area?
- What nursing care is critical in the immediate postoperative stage?
- What are the similarities and differences between preanesthesia and postanesthesia care for patients in the acute care and ambulatory surgery settings?
- What general information should be included in postoperative teaching for patients/families in the acute care and ambulatory surgery settings?
- How may the family/significant other be involved in the patient's perioperative experience?

STUDY CHART

Create a study chart on Surgical Risk Factors that identifies how age, nutritional status, obesity, immunocompetence, fluid/electrolyte balance, and pregnancy may affect the patient's perioperative experience.

Answers available through your instructor.

CHAPTER 38 • Surgical Patient

Name _____ Date _____ Instructor's Name _____

Performance Checklist Skill 38-1: Teaching Postoperative Exercises

	S	U	NP	Comments

Assessment
1. Assess patient's risk for postoperative respiratory complications: review medical history to identify presence of chronic pulmonary condition (e.g., emphysema, asthma), any condition that affects chest wall movement, history of smoking, and presence of reduced hemoglobin (low red blood cell [RBC] count).
2. Auscultate lungs.
3. Assess patient's ability to cough and deep breathe by having patient take a deep breath and observing movement of shoulders, chest wall, and abdomen. Measure chest excursion during a deep breath. Ask patient to cough after taking a deep breath.
4. Assess patient's risk for postoperative thrombus formation (e.g., older patients, those with active cancer, immobilized patients, those with personal or family history of clots, women older than 35 years who smoke and are taking oral contraceptives). Observe the calves for redness, warmth, and tenderness, swollen calf or thigh, calf swelling more than 3 cm compared with asymptomatic leg, pitting edema in symptomatic leg, and collateral superficial veins. Compare legs for bilateral equality.
5. Assess patient's ability to move independently while in bed.
6. Assess patient's willingness and capability to learn exercises; note attention span, anxiety, level of consciousness, and language level.
7. Assess family members' or significant others' willingness to learn and to support patient postoperatively.
8. Assess patient's medical orders preoperatively and postoperatively.

Planning
1. Prepare equipment as needed.
2. Plan teaching sessions to occur when patient is not in pain.
3. Explain the postoperative exercises to patient, including importance to recovery and physiological benefits.
4. Prepare room for teaching.

Implementation
1. Demonstrate exercises.
   A. Diaphragmatic Breathing
   (1) Assist patient to a comfortable semi-Fowler's position in bed or in a sitting position on side of bed or in a chair.
   (2) Stand or sit facing patient.
   (3) Instruct patient to place palms of hands across from each other, down, and along lower borders of anterior rib cage; place fingers lightly together on upper abdomen. Demonstrate for patient.
   (4) Instruct patient to take slow, deep breaths, inhaling through nose and pushing abdomen against hands. Tell patient to feel middle fingers separate during inhalation. Explain that patient will feel normal downward movement of diaphragm during inhaling and that abdominal organs descend and chest wall expands. Demonstrate for patient.
   (5) Instruct patient to avoid using chest and shoulders while inhaling.
   (6) Have patient hold a slow, deep breath; hold for count of three; and then slowly exhale through mouth as if blowing out a candle (through pursed lips). Demonstrate for patient. Tell patient middle fingertips will touch as chest wall contracts during exhalation.

	S	U	NP	Comments

(7) Repeat breathing exercise 3 to 5 times.
(8) Have patient practice exercise. Instruct patient to take 10 slow, deep breaths every hour while awake during postoperative period.

B. Incentive Spirometry (IS)
(1) Perform hand hygiene.
(2) Instruct patient to assume semi-Fowler's or high-Fowler's position. For a patient who is obese, consider the reverse Trendelenburg position.
(3) Indicate to patient on the IS device the volume level to be obtained with each inhalation. Use the manufacturer's guidelines to set the volume for the patient.
(4) Demonstrate and then have patient place mouthpiece of incentive spirometer so that lips completely cover mouthpiece.
(5) Instruct patient to inhale slowly and maintain constant flow through unit, while attempting to reach goal volume. When patient reaches maximal inspiration, have patient hold his or her breath for 3 to 5 seconds and then exhale slowly. Make sure number of breaths does not exceed 10 to 12 per minute.
(6) Instruct patient to breathe normally for short period between the 10 breaths on spirometer.
(7) Have patient repeat maneuver until goals are achieved.
(8) Perform hand hygiene.

C. Positive Expiratory Pressure Therapy and "Huff" Coughing
(1) Perform hand hygiene.
(2) Set positive expiratory pressure (PEP) device for setting ordered.
(3) Instruct patient to assume semi-Fowler's or high-Fowler's position, and place nose clip on patient's nose.
(4) Have patient place lips around mouthpiece or demonstrate placement. Instruct patient to take a full breath and then exhale 2 or 3 times longer than inhalation. Repeat pattern for 10 to 20 breaths.
(5) Remove device from mouth, and have patient take a slow, deep breath and hold for 3 seconds.
(6) Then have patient exhale in quick, short, forced "huffs."

D. Controlled Coughing
(1) Explain importance of maintaining an upright position.
(2) If surgical incision is to be either abdominal or thoracic, teach patient to place pillow or bath blanket over incisional area and place hands over pillow to splint incision. During breathing and coughing exercises, press gently against incisional area for splinting or support.
(3) Demonstrate coughing. Take 2 slow, deep breaths, inhaling through nose and exhaling through mouth.
(4) Inhale deeply a third time, and hold breath to count of three. Cough fully for 2 or 3 consecutive coughs without inhaling between coughs. (Tell patient to push all air out of lungs.)
(5) Caution patient against just clearing throat instead of coughing. Explain that coughing will not cause injury to incision.
(6) Have patient continue to practice coughing exercises, splinting imaginary incision. Instruct the patient to cough 2 or 3 times every 2 hours while awake.
(7) Instruct patient to examine sputum for consistency, odor, amount, and color changes.

	S	U	NP	Comments

E. Turning
(1) Instruct patient to assume supine position and move toward left side of bed by bending knees and pressing heels against the mattress to raise and move buttocks.
(2) Instruct patient to place the right hand over incisional area to splint it.
(3) Instruct patient to keep right leg straight and flex left knee up.
(4) Have patient grab right side rail with left hand, pull toward right, and roll onto right side.
(5) Instruct patient to turn every 2 hours while awake.

F. Leg Exercises
(1) Have patient assume supine position in bed. Demonstrate leg exercises by performing passive range-of-motion exercises and simultaneously explaining exercise.
(2) Rotate each ankle in complete circle. Instruct patient to draw imaginary circles with big toe. Repeat 5 times.
(3) Alternate dorsiflexion and plantar flexion of both feet. Direct patient to feel calf muscles contract and relax alternately.
(4) Perform quadriceps stretching by tightening thigh and bringing knee down toward mattress, then relaxing. Repeat 5 times.
(5) Have patient alternately raise each leg up from bed surface, keeping legs straight, and then have patient bend leg at hip and knee. Repeat 5 times.

2. Have patient continue to practice exercises at least every 2 hours while awake. Instruct patient to coordinate turning and leg exercises with diaphragmatic breathing, incentive spirometry, and coughing exercises.

Evaluation
1. Observe patient performing exercises independently.
2. Observe family members' or significant other's ability to coach patient.
3. Palpate calves for redness, warmth, and tenderness. Assess pedal pulses.
4. Observe patient's chest expansion.
5. Auscultate patient's lungs.
6. Record which exercises have been demonstrated to patient and whether patient can perform exercises independently or needs continued assistance.
7. Record physical assessment findings.
8. Report any problems patient has in practicing exercises to nurse assigned to patient on next shift for follow-up.